# Rotaviruses and Rotavirus Vaccines: Current Topics in Microbiology and Immunology

# Rotaviruses and Rotavirus Vaccines: Current Topics in Microbiology and Immunology

Editor: Connor Riley

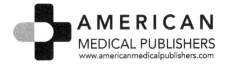

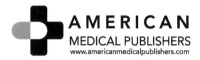

Cataloging-in-Publication Data

Rotaviruses and rotavirus vaccines : current topics in microbiology and immunology / edited by Connor Riley.
   p. cm.
Includes bibliographical references and index.
ISBN 979-8-88740-444-8
1. Rotaviruses. 2. Rotavirus infections--Vaccination. 3. Viral vaccines. 4. Rotavirus infections--Microbiology.
5. Rotavirus infections--Immunological aspects. I. Riley, Connor.
QR201.R67 R68 2023
616.019 4--dc23

© American Medical Publishers, 2023

American Medical Publishers,
41 Flatbush Avenue,
1st Floor, New York,
NY 11217, USA

ISBN 979-8-88740-444-8 (Hardback)

This book contains information obtained from authentic and highly regarded sources. Copyright for all individual chapters remain with the respective authors as indicated. All chapters are published with permission under the Creative Commons Attribution License or equivalent. A wide variety of references are listed. Permission and sources are indicated; for detailed attributions, please refer to the permissions page and list of contributors. Reasonable efforts have been made to publish reliable data and information, but the authors, editors and publisher cannot assume any responsibility for the validity of all materials or the consequences of their use.

**Trademark Notice:** Registered trademark of products or corporate names are used only for explanation and identification without intent to infringe.

# Contents

Preface ..................................................................................................................................................... VII

Chapter 1  **Rotavirus Infection and Vaccination: Knowledge, Beliefs and Behaviors among Parents in Italy** ........................................................................................................................ 1
Francesco Napolitano, Abdoulkader Ali Adou, Alessandra Vastola and Italo Francesco Angelillo

Chapter 2  **First Detection of Rotavirus Group C in Asymptomatic Pigs of Smallholder Farms in East Africa** ................................................................................................................. 12
Joshua Oluoch Amimo, Eunice Magoma Machuka and Edward Okoth

Chapter 3  **Differences of Rotavirus Vaccine Effectiveness by Country: Likely Causes and Contributing Factors** ........................................................................................................... 17
Ulrich Desselberger

Chapter 4  **Genome Characterization of a Pathogenic Porcine Rotavirus B Strain Identified in Buryat Republic, Russia in 2015** ......................................................................................... 30
Konstantin P. Alekseev, Aleksey A. Penin, Alexey N. Mukhin, Kizkhalum M. Khametova, Tatyana V. Grebennikova, Anton G. Yuzhakov, Anna S. Moskvina, Maria I. Musienko, Sergey A. Raev, Alexandr M. Mishin, Alexandr P. Kotelnikov, Oleg A. Verkhovsky, Taras I. Aliper, Eugeny A. Nepoklonov, Diana M. Herrera-Ibata, Frances K. Shepherd and Douglas G. Marthaler

Chapter 5  **Rotavirus Burden, Genetic Diversity and Impact of Vaccine in Children under Five in Tanzania** ..................................................................................................................... 41
Joseph J. Malakalinga, Gerald Misinzo, George M. Msalya and Rudovick R. Kazwala

Chapter 6  **Histo-Blood Group Antigens in Children with Symptomatic Rotavirus Infection** ........... 56
Raúl Pérez-Ortín, Susana Vila-Vicent, Noelia Carmona-Vicente, Cristina Santiso-Bellón, Jesús Rodríguez-Díaz and Javier Buesa

Chapter 7  **Epidemiological Trends of Five Common Diarrhea-Associated Enteric Viruses Pre- and Post-Rotavirus Vaccine Introduction in Coastal Kenya** ....................................... 66
Arnold W. Lambisia, Sylvia Onchaga, Nickson Murunga, Clement S. Lewa, Steven Ger Nyanjom and Charles N. Agoti

Chapter 8  **Phylogenetic Analyses of Rotavirus A from Cattle in Uruguay Reveal the Circulation of Common and Uncommon Genotypes and Suggest Interspecies Transmission** ........................................................................................................................ 80
Matías Castells, Rubén Darío Caffarena, María Laura Casaux, Carlos Schild, Samuel Miño, Felipe Castells, Daniel Castells, Matías Victoria, Franklin Riet-Correa, Federico Giannitti, Viviana Parreño and Rodney Colina

Chapter 9 **Molecular Epidemiology of Rotavirus A Strains Pre- and Post-Vaccine (Rotarix®) Introduction in Mozambique, 2012–2019: Emergence of Genotypes G3P[4] and G3P[8]** .................................................................................................................. 97
Eva D. João, Benilde Munlela, Assucênio Chissaque, Jorfélia Chilaúle, Jerónimo Langa, Orvalho Augusto, Simone S. Boene, Elda Anapakala, Júlia Sambo, Esperança Guimarães, Diocreciano Bero, Marta Cassocera, Idalécia Cossa-Moiane, Jason M. Mwenda, Isabel Maurício, Hester G. O'Neill and Nilsa de Deus

Chapter 10 **Rotavirus A in Brazil: Molecular Epidemiology and Surveillance during 2018–2019** .................... 112
Meylin Bautista Gutierrez, Alexandre Madi Fialho, Adriana Gonçalves Maranhão, Fábio Correia Malta, Juliana da Silva Ribeiro de Andrade, Rosane Maria Santos de Assis, Sérgio da Silva e Mouta, Marize Pereira Miagostovich, José Paulo Gagliardi Leite and Tulio Machado Fumian

Chapter 11 **Uncovering the First Atypical DS-1-like G1P[8] Rotavirus Strains That Circulated during Pre-Rotavirus Vaccine Introduction Era in South Africa** .................... 126
Peter N. Mwangi, Milton T. Mogotsi, Sebotsana P. Rasebotsa, Mapaseka L. Seheri, M. Jeffrey Mphahlele, Valantine N. Ndze, Francis E. Dennis, Khuzwayo C. Jere and Martin M. Nyaga

Chapter 12 **Whole Genome Characterization and Evolutionary Analysis of G1P[8] Rotavirus A Strains during the Pre- and Post-Vaccine Periods in Mozambique (2012–2017)** ..................... 143
Benilde Munlela, Eva D. João, Celeste M. Donato, Amy Strydom, Simone S. Boene, Assucênio Chissaque, Adilson F. L. Bauhofer, Jerónimo Langa, Marta Cassocera, Idalécia Cossa-Moiane, Jorfélia J. Chilaúle, Hester G. O'Neill and Nilsa de Deus

Chapter 13 **Retrospective Case-Control Study of 2017 G2P[4] Rotavirus Epidemic in Rural and Remote Australia** ........................................................................................ 161
Bianca F. Middleton, Margie Danchin, Helen Quinn, Anna P. Ralph, Nevada Pingault, Mark Jones, Marie Estcourt and Tom Snelling

Chapter 14 **Group A Rotavirus Detection and Genotype Distribution before and after Introduction of a National Immunisation Programme in Ireland: 2015–2019** ..................... 173
Zoe Yandle, Suzie Coughlan, Jonathan Dean, Gráinne Tuite, Anne Conroy and Cillian F. De Gascun

Chapter 15 **Molecular Characterisation of a Rare Reassortant Porcine-Like G5P[6] Rotavirus Strain Detected in an Unvaccinated Child in Kasama, Zambia** ........................ 188
Wairimu M. Maringa, Peter N. Mwangi, Julia Simwaka, Evans M. Mpabalwani, Jason M. Mwenda, Ina Peenze, Mathew D. Esona, M. Jeffrey Mphahlele, Mapaseka L. Seheri and Martin M. Nyaga

Chapter 16 **Multiple Introductions and Predominance of Rotavirus Group A Genotype G3P[8] in Kilifi, Coastal Kenya, 4 Years after Nationwide Vaccine Introduction** ............... 209
Mike J. Mwanga, Jennifer R. Verani, Richard Omore, Jacqueline E. Tate, Umesh D. Parashar, Nickson Murunga, Elijah Gicheru, Robert F. Breiman, D. James Nokes and Charles N. Agoti

**Permissions**

**List of Contributors**

**Index**

# Preface

The main aim of this book is to educate learners and enhance their research focus by presenting diverse topics covering this vast field. This is an advanced book which compiles significant studies by distinguished experts in the area of analysis. This book addresses successive solutions to the challenges arising in the area of application, along with it; the book provides scope for future developments.

Rotavirus is a genus of double-stranded RNA viruses in the family Reoviridae. It is the most common cause of diarrhea and other intestinal symptoms. It is contagious and most commonly affects infants and young children across the world. Some common symptoms of rotavirus are fever, vomiting, and abdominal pain followed by diarrhea. It causes inflammation in the stomach and intestines. There is no treatment for a rotavirus infection. Rotavirus vaccine is the most efficient method of preventing the rotavirus disease. It is highly recommended that the parents get their children vaccinated against rotavirus, as it will make the symptoms less severe in case the child is infected with this virus. This book outlines the role of rotavirus vaccine in the management of rotavirus infection. Researchers and students associated with the study of this virus and its management will find this book full of crucial and unexplored topics.

It was a great honour to edit this book, though there were challenges, as it involved a lot of communication and networking between me and the editorial team. However, the end result was this all-inclusive book covering diverse themes in the field.

Finally, it is important to acknowledge the efforts of the contributors for their excellent chapters, through which a wide variety of issues have been addressed. I would also like to thank my colleagues for their valuable feedback during the making of this book.

Editor

# Rotavirus Infection and Vaccination: Knowledge, Beliefs and Behaviors among Parents in Italy

Francesco Napolitano, Abdoulkader Ali Adou, Alessandra Vastola and Italo Francesco Angelillo *

Department of Experimental Medicine, University of Campania "Luigi Vanvitelli", Via L. Armanni, 5 80138 Naples, Italy; francesco.napolitano2@unicampania.it (F.N.); kadermed88@hotmail.it (A.A.A.); alexia291@hotmail.it (A.V.)
* Correspondence: italof.angelillo@unicampania.it;

**Abstract:** This study was designed to investigate the knowledge, beliefs, and behaviors about rotavirus infection and its vaccination in a sample of parents in Naples, Italy. The survey was conducted between June and December 2018 among parents of children aged 3 months to 3 years. A total of 40.7% of the study subjects declared that they had heard about rotavirus infection and 60.8% and 59.2% were aware about the vaccination and of its availability in Italy. Parents with a child aged <1 year and those who reported the physicians as source of information were more likely to have heard about rotavirus infection and to know that the vaccination is available in Italy. More than half (56.4%) were worried that their children could have a rotavirus gastroenteritis and this was most likely to occur in those who have heard about rotavirus infection. Only 15.3% declared that they had immunized their children against rotavirus infection. Parents who considered it dangerous for their children to contract the rotavirus gastroenteritis, those who considered the rotavirus vaccine useful, and those who had received information by physicians were more likely to have vaccinated their children against the infection. More than half of the parents who did not immunize their children expressed their willingness to vaccinate them. Developing and implementing additional public education programs are needed for better knowledge toward rotavirus infection and vaccination and a high coverage among parents.

**Keywords:** behaviors; knowledge; parents; rotavirus vaccination; survey

## 1. Introduction

Rotavirus is one of the leading causes of gastroenteritis among children younger than 5 years of age and data worldwide estimated that it globally caused approximately 37% of all diarrhea-associated hospitalizations and 215,000 deaths [1], whereas in Italy the estimated incidence is 5 cases per 100 [2].

The World Health Organization has recommended the introduction of the vaccine against rotavirus in all national immunization programs since 2009 [3,4]. In Italy, childhood vaccinations are provided by public centers and in Campania region rotavirus vaccination is recommended and free of charge since 2018 [5,6]. The schedule included two doses administered at 6 and 10 weeks of age with hexavalent vaccine (diphtheria-tetanus-pertussis, polio, hepatitis B, *H. influenzae*) and pneumococcal conjugate vaccine [5]. However, despite the vaccination's implementation having resulted as a safe and effective public health strategy with a sustained reduction in rotavirus disease burden and deaths [7,8], coverage rates remain low in many countries [9]. In Italy, the vaccination uptake in 2018 was 16.5% for the 2015 birth cohort [10]. Primary care for children ≤6 years old is provided free of charge by primary care pediatricians and for those aged >6 years either by pediatricians or general practitioners.

The low coverage rates are still public health challenges and various factors have been cited for why parents and informal caregivers' declined childhood vaccinations, such as vaccine hesitancy [11,12], lack of appropriate information [13,14], and perception of vaccine safety and benefits [15–17]. Therefore, an understanding of the parents' knowledge, beliefs, and behaviors regarding vaccination against rotavirus could provide useful information on the factors that influence the uptake and to design and to develop interventions to increase the coverage. To date, there have been few attempts worldwide on what parents know, beliefs, and experiences on this topic [18–20], while there is a knowledge gap in this geographic area of Italy with the attention on different groups mainly focused on Human Papillomavirus (HPV) [21–25] and on vulnerable populations [17,26,27]. Therefore, the present cross-sectional study was designed to investigate the knowledge, beliefs, and behaviors about rotavirus infection and the relative childhood vaccination and to investigate their determinants in a sample of parents in Italy.

## 2. Materials and Methods

### 2.1. Settings and Participants

Data collection occurred between June and December 2018 in the geographic area of Naples, Italy. The population of interest was parents of children aged from 3 months to 3 years of age. A one-stage cluster sample has been used. From the list of all public nurseries, eight of them were selected using a computer-generated list of random numbers, and all children attendees were recruited. In Italy, children can attend nurseries from three months of age. The sample size calculation was based on the expected positive attitude of parents towards the willingness to vaccinate their children with rotavirus vaccine of 80% [19,20], a confidence interval of 95%, and an error of 5%. Assuming a response rate of 80%, the final sample size was calculated to be of 307 individuals.

### 2.2. Procedure

Before starting the study, the research team contacted by letter the heads of the selected nurseries and asked the approval to conduct the survey. The heads received information about the study's purposes and procedure. After getting the permission, two researchers contacted the teachers of each class, who delivered to all parents a sealed envelope that contained a letter with information regarding the purposes of the study, an informed consent form, a questionnaire, and an envelope to return the completed questionnaire along with the signed consent form. In the letter it was also made clear that completing the questionnaire was voluntary and that all of information collected would be processed anonymously and confidentially. Those who agreed to participate completed the questionnaire at home. Only one parent of each child filled out the questionnaire. After three weeks, the researchers contacted the teachers to collect the questionnaires. No monetary compensation or gift has been given to the surveyed parents.

### 2.3. Questionnaire

The structured self-administered questionnaire developed by the Authors comprised 26 items grouped into the following five sections: (a) socio-demographic characteristics (gender, age, nationality, marital status, education, employment status, husband/wife/partner education and employment status, number and ages of children); (b) knowledge regarding the rotavirus infection and the relative vaccination (having heard about the infection, clinical symptoms, modes of transmission, preventive measures, availability of the vaccination against rotavirus in Italy); (c) attitudes about rotavirus gastroenteritis and related vaccination (preoccupation that their children may acquire the infection, concern about the dangerousness of the infection, agree that the vaccine is important to protect their children, concern about the dangerousness of the vaccination, willingness or unwillingness to vaccinate their children); (d) behaviors regarding vaccination (whether or not they had vaccinated their children); and (e) trusted rotavirus infection and vaccination information sources. The questions regarding the knowledge had the response yes, no, or do not know. A ten-point Likert scale was used for questions regarding beliefs, with possible responses ranging from "1" to "10" with higher values corresponding to a stronger attitude. The remaining questions had multiple-choice alternatives.

The developed questionnaire was assessed in a pilot involving 20 mothers of children of vaccination age prior to administering it to the study population, in order to ensure that the questions were understood as intended, and to omit questions that were misinterpreted.

The study was approved by the Ethics Committee of the Teaching Hospital of the University of Campania "Luigi Vanvitelli" (approval number 484).

*2.4. Statistical Analysis*

Data were analyzed using STATA version 15, StataCorp LLC: College Station, TX, USA [28]. The first level of analysis comprised a descriptive analysis of the responses. The second level of analysis involved univariate tests of association. Chi-square for categorical variables and Student's *t*-test for continuous variables were used to check whether there was an association between the outcomes of interest and the independent variables. Those determinants that showed an association with a *p*-value less or equal than 0.25 with the outcomes of interest in the univariate analyses were entered simultaneously in the multivariate model to assess their unique contribution to the explanation of the outcomes. The third level of analysis included multivariate stepwise logistic regression performed to identify the association of independent characteristics with the following outcomes of interest: Having heard about the rotavirus infection and having the knowledge that the vaccination against rotavirus is available in Italy (Model 1), parents who were very worried that their children could have a rotavirus gastroenteritis (Model 2), and having immunized their children against the rotavirus infection (Model 3). The following variables were included in all Models: Age (<40 years = 0; ≥40 years = 1), gender (male = 0; female = 1), educational level (none or primary/middle/high schools = 0; college degree or higher = 1), at least one parent who is a healthcare worker (no = 0; yes = 1), having a child aged <1 year (no = 0; yes = 1), having more than one child (no = 0; yes = 1), having received information on rotavirus infection and relative vaccination from physicians (no = 0; yes = 1), need to receive additional information about rotavirus infection and relative vaccination (no = 0; yes = 1). Moreover, the following variables were included in Models 2 and 3: Having heard about rotavirus infection (no = 0; yes = 1) and having the knowledge that the vaccination against rotavirus is available in Italy (no = 0; yes = 1). Finally, the following variables were included in Model 3: Being very worried that their children could have a rotavirus gastroenteritis (no = 0; yes = 1), considering dangerous for their children to contract the rotavirus gastroenteritis (continuous), considering useful the rotavirus vaccine (continuous), and considering dangerous for their children the rotavirus vaccine (continuous).

The significance level for variables entering in the stepwise logistic regression models was set at 0.2 and for removing at 0.4. Odds ratios (ORs) were calculated along with their associated 95% confidence intervals (CIs) in the multivariate logistic regression analysis. All tests were two-tailed and the results were evaluated at a significance level of 0.05 or less.

## 3. Results

*3.1. Participants*

In total, 500 individuals were approached to participate and 307 consented and were enrolled in the survey for a response rate of 61.4%. Selected characteristics of the parents who participated in the study are presented in Table 1. Only 4.3% had ≤25 years, the majority (52.9%) were aged between 26 and 34, 42.8% had ≥35 years with an overall mean and median age of 33.5 and 34, respectively. The respondents were predominately female, more than two thirds were married, 55.9% have more than one child, one third had a college degree or above, and two thirds were employed.

**Table 1.** Main characteristics of the study respondents.

| | Total (n = 307) | |
|---|---|---|
| | n | % |
| Gender | | |
| Female | 257 | 84.5 |
| Male | 47 | 15.5 |
| Age (years) | 33.5 ± 4.9 (18–47) * | |
| Marital status | | |
| Married | 250 | 82.3 |
| Other | 54 | 17.7 |
| Educational level (years) | | |
| None/Primary school (<9) | 4 | 1.4 |
| Middle school (9–11) | 54 | 17.9 |
| High school (12–16) | 158 | 52.5 |
| College degree or higher (>16) | 85 | 28.2 |
| Employment status | | |
| Employed | 211 | 69.9 |
| Unemployed | 91 | 30.1 |
| At least one parent who is a healthcare professional | | |
| No | 280 | 96.2 |
| Yes | 11 | 3.8 |
| Number of children | | |
| 1 | 135 | 44.1 |
| ≥2 | 171 | 55.9 |

Number for each item may not add up to total number of study population due to missing value; * Mean ± Standard deviation (Range).

### 3.2. Knowledge

The results regarding the knowledge about rotavirus infection of the study population are presented in Table 2. Less than half declared that they had heard about rotavirus infection (40.7%), and similar values had been observed among those who had a child aged <1 year (40.9%) and with more than one child (40.3%). More than half of those who had heard about rotavirus infection were aware that it can be transmitted by contaminated water (60.8%) and foods (56%), and more than one third by contact with contaminated surfaces (38.4%) and through person-to-person (36%). Regarding the vaccination, 60.8% and 59.2% were aware about it and of the availability in Italy, 44.1% of them knew that there are two vaccines (two or three doses schedule) for children, but none indicated correctly the schedule. Univariate analysis showed that participants with a college degree or above ($p = 0.001$) and those who have received information about rotavirus infection and vaccination by physicians ($p < 0.001$) have heard about rotavirus infection and know that the vaccination is available in Italy. Table 3 showed the multivariate stepwise logistic regression analysis results on the potential factors affecting the different outcomes of interest. The results demonstrated that only two determinants were significantly associated with the knowledge. Indeed, parents with a child aged <1 year and those who reported the physicians as source of information were almost 3 (95% CI 1.42–7.36) and 21 times (95% CI 9.84–46.17) respectively more likely to have heard about rotavirus infection and to know that the vaccination is available in Italy (Model 1).

Table 2. Knowledge about rotavirus infection of the study respondents.

|  | n | % |
|---|---|---|
| Have heard about the rotavirus infection [a] | 125 ÷ 307 | 40.7 |
| Knowledge that the vaccination against rotavirus is a preventive measure [b] | 76 ÷ 125 | 60.8 |
| Knowledge that the rotavirus vaccine is available in Italy [b] | 74 ÷ 125 | 59.2 |
|  | Correct response | |
| Modes of transmission of rotavirus [b] | n | % |
| Contaminated water (true) | 76 ÷ 125 | 60.8 |
| Contaminated food (true) | 70 ÷ 125 | 56 |
| Contaminated surfaces (true) | 48 ÷ 125 | 38.4 |
| Person-to-person (true) | 45 ÷ 125 | 36 |

[a] All sample (n = 307); [b] Only for those who reported that they have heard about rotavirus infection.

Table 3. Multivariate analysis results.

| Variable | OR | SE | 95% CI | p |
|---|---|---|---|---|
| **Model 1. Having heard about rotavirus infection and having the knowledge that the vaccination against rotavirus is available in Italy** | | | | |
| Log-likelihood = −109.22, $\chi^2$ = 86.37, p value < 0.0001 | | | | |
| Parents who received information on rotavirus infection and relative vaccination from physicians | 21.31 | 8.4 | 9.84–46.17 | <0.001 |
| Having a child aged <1 year | 3.23 | 1.35 | 1.42–7.36 | 0.005 |
| Having more than one child | 0.55 | 0.2 | 0.26–1.13 | 0.106 |
| Age ≥40 years | 2.2 | 1.12 | 0.82–5.95 | 0.119 |
| At least one parent who is a healthcare worker | 3.49 | 2.94 | 0.67–18.19 | 0.137 |
| Female | Backward elimination | | | |
| Having college degree or higher level of education | Backward elimination | | | |
| Need to receive additional information | Backward elimination | | | |
| **Model 2. Parents who were very worried that their children could have a rotavirus gastroenteritis** | | | | |
| Log-likelihood = −91.44, $\chi^2$ = 19.2, p value = 0.003 | | | | |
| Having heard about rotavirus infection | 6.47 | 3.07 | 2.56–16.41 | <0.001 |
| Having more than one child | 0.57 | 0.23 | 0.26–1.27 | 0.172 |
| Having the knowledge that the vaccination against rotavirus is available in Italy | 0.51 | 0.27 | 0.18–1.45 | 0.211 |
| Parents who received information on rotavirus infection and relative vaccination from physicians | 0.57 | 0.32 | 0.19–1.71 | 0.320 |
| Having a child aged <1 year | 1.58 | 0.73 | 0.64–3.93 | 0.322 |
| Age <40 years | 0.49 | 0.39 | 0.11–2.29 | 0.369 |
| Female | Backward elimination | | | |
| Need to receive additional information | Backward elimination | | | |
| **Model 3. Having immunized their children against the rotavirus infection** | | | | |
| Log-likelihood = −45.82, $\chi^2$ = 150.18, p value < 0.0001 | | | | |
| Parents who received information on rotavirus infection and relative vaccination from physicians | 25.09 | 17.25 | 6.52–96.61 | <0.001 |
| Parents who considered dangerous for their children to contract the rotavirus gastroenteritis | 1.91 | 0.41 | 1.25–2.91 | 0.003 |
| Parents who considered useful the rotavirus vaccine | 1.45 | 0.26 | 1.02–2.07 | 0.037 |
| Parents who were very worried that their children could have a rotavirus gastroenteritis | 0.81 | 0.12 | 0.65–1.12 | 0.15 |
| Age ≥40 years | 4.56 | 4.45 | 0.67–30.83 | 0.119 |
| Having heard about rotavirus vaccine | 2.34 | 1.68 | 0.57–9.66 | 0.239 |
| Parents who considered dangerous for their children the rotavirus vaccine | 0.86 | 0.12 | 0.65–1.13 | 0.271 |
| Having a child aged <1 year | 2.31 | 1.87 | 0.49–11.21 | 0.286 |
| Having more than one child | 0.54 | 0.33 | 0.16–1.81 | 0.319 |
| Need to receive additional information | 0.57 | 0.33 | 0.18–1.81 | 0.341 |
| Having heard about rotavirus infection | 2.41 | 2.39 | 0.34–16.95 | 0.378 |
| Having college degree or higher level of education | Backward elimination | | | |

## 3.3. Beliefs

The results regarding parents' beliefs about rotavirus infection are presented in Table 4. More than half (56.4%) were worried that their children could have a rotavirus gastroenteritis and two thirds (63.7%) considered dangerous for their children to contract it with a mean value respectively of 6 and 6.4, out of a maximum score of 10. Almost two thirds (60.8%) considered that the rotavirus vaccine was important for their child with an average value of 6.5 and the vast majority (89%) believed that it was not harmful. In the bivariate analysis, having heard about rotavirus infection ($p < 0.001$) and having received information from physicians ($p < 0.001$) were significantly associated with the parents' worrying that their children could have a rotavirus gastroenteritis. The multivariate stepwise logistic regression analysis confirmed that parents who have heard about rotavirus infection (OR = 6.47; 95% CI 2.56–16.41) were more likely to be very worried that their children could have a rotavirus gastroenteritis compared with those who did not have this knowledge (Model 2 in Table 3).

Table 4. Beliefs about rotavirus vaccination of the study respondents.

|  | n | % |
| --- | --- | --- |
| Parents who believed that the vaccine was not harmful for their children | 259 ÷ 291 | 89 |
| Parents who considered dangerous for their children to contract the rotavirus gastroenteritis | 191 ÷ 300 | 63.7 |
| Parents who considered useful the rotavirus vaccine | 178 ÷ 293 | 60.8 |
| Parents who were worried that their children could have a rotavirus gastroenteritis | 172 ÷ 305 | 56.4 |

Number for each item may not add up to total number of study population due to missing value.

## 3.4. Behaviors

The results regarding the parents' behaviors about rotavirus infection are reported in Table 5. Only 15.3% of the total sample and 15% of those who had more than one child declared that they had immunized their children against rotavirus infection. The bivariate analysis revealed that ten variables were significantly associated with this behavior: Lower age ($p = 0.015$), having a college degree or above ($p < 0.001$), having heard about rotavirus infection ($p < 0.001$), having heard about rotavirus vaccination ($p < 0.001$), worry that their children could have a rotavirus gastroenteritis ($p < 0.001$), considering dangerous for their children to contract a rotavirus gastroenteritis ($p < 0.001$), considering useful the rotavirus vaccine ($p < 0.001$), believing that the vaccine was not harmful for their children ($p < 0.001$), having received information about rotavirus infection and relative vaccination by physicians ($p < 0.001$), and needing more information ($p < 0.001$). After adjustment for the potential confounding variables, logistic regression analysis showed that the variables that were significantly associated with a higher likelihood of having their children vaccinated against rotavirus infection were considering it dangerous for their children to contract a rotavirus gastroenteritis (OR = 1.91; 95% CI 1.25–2.91), having positive perception toward the effectiveness of the vaccine (OR = 1.45; 95% CI 1.02–2.07), and having received information about rotavirus infection and relative vaccination by physicians (OR = 25.09; 95% CI 6.52–96.61) (Model 3 in Table 3). Reasons for having immunized their children were: Wanted to reduce the chance of getting the disease (76.7%), had been told to do so by the pediatricians (75%), and fear that the infection could cause severe health problems (63.8%). The most frequent reasons for those who did not immunize their children were: Lack of knowledge about vaccination (77.9%), the vaccination had not been recommended by the pediatrician (31.6%), and concerns about the side effects of the vaccine (15.8%). Among those who did not immunize their children, more than half of the total sample (51.3%) and of those who had more than one child (52.7%) expressed their willingness to vaccinate their children. The most frequently selected reasons for this positive attitude were that the rotavirus vaccination is useful (55.7%), the infection could cause severe health problems (44.7%), and a recommendation by the pediatrician (20.5%). Reasons for being unwilling to immunize included lack of knowledge about vaccination (53.6%), concerns about the side effects of the vaccine (30.4%), and lack of recommendation by the pediatrician (30.1%).

Table 5. Behaviors about rotavirus vaccination of the study respondents.

| | n | % |
|---|---|---|
| Having immunized their children against the rotavirus infection | 47 ÷ 307 | 15.3 |
| Reasons for having immunized their children | | |
| Wanted to reduce the chance of getting the disease | 36 ÷ 47 | 76.7 |
| Had been told to do so by the pediatricians | 35 ÷ 47 | 75 |
| Fear that the infection could cause severe health problems | 30 ÷ 47 | 63.8 |
| Reasons for not having immunized their children | | |
| Lack of knowledge about the vaccination | 202 ÷ 259 | 77.9 |
| Vaccination had not been recommended by the pediatrician | 93 ÷ 258 | 36.1 |
| Concerns about the side effects of the vaccine | 41 ÷ 260 | 15.8 |

Number for each item may not add up to total number of study population due to missing value.

*3.5. Information Sources*

The most common sources of rotavirus infection and vaccination-related information were physicians (68%) and internet (63.9%), followed by media/advertisement (25.5%), and family (15.5%). Finally, two-thirds of the respondents (63.5%) wished to receive more information about vaccines.

## 4. Discussion

This study, conducted within the season when rotaviruses do not peak in temperate countries, is the first to specifically analyze the knowledge, beliefs, and behaviors towards rotavirus infection and relative vaccination for their children and of their influencing predictors in the population of parents in Italy. The results have several implications considering the Italian Immunization Prevention Plan 2017–2019, the recent legislation on mandatory and recommended vaccinations, and the low coverage for rotavirus vaccination in children that has been reported in Italy.

First, a striking observation in the present results was the low levels of knowledge regarding rotavirus infection, how it can be transmitted, and also about the vaccination currently available. Indeed, less than half had heard of the infection and only 59.2% of them knew that the vaccine was available in Italy. This lack of knowledge indicates that comprehensive information about rotavirus infection and relative vaccination is not being widely disseminated and this is a very worrying result because it is well known that rotavirus gastroenteritis could have serious health complications for children. Therefore, it is urgent to improve the level of knowledge of the population through effective pediatricians recommendation of vaccine and educational interventions using all occasions in which it is possible to meet the population interested in vaccination such as, for example, prenatal-classes or parents' utilization of the vaccinations service for their children. Moreover, parents could benefit from targeted communication strategies and promotion of vaccination education programs because effective physician-patient communication may increase the vaccines' knowledge, clarifies the concerns, and motivates the population to vaccinations acceptability [29–31].

Second, more than half were worried that their children could have a rotavirus gastroenteritis, two thirds considered it dangerous for their children to contract it, and the majority had positive attitudes towards rotavirus vaccination since almost two thirds considered that it is important for their child. Although the majority of participants (89%) agreed with the statement that the vaccine was not harmful, among those who did not immunize their children a large proportion reported that they will not be willing to obtain vaccination mainly because a lack of knowledge or concerns of side effects. This underlines the importance of health education towards targeting population, especially those with common misconceptions regarding vaccinations, to eliminate their worries about safety. Moreover, an association has been observed between knowledge and attitudes, since respondents who very worried that their children could have rotavirus gastroenteritis were those who have heard about rotavirus infection. This finding is in keeping with findings of previous studies that showed that vaccination might be accepted in those more knowledgeable [26,32,33]. These findings indicate that providing specific vaccine-related knowledge may help to change their attitudes.

Third, a concerning result from this study was, not surprisingly, the insufficient vaccination rate with only 15.3% of the participants reported having immunized their children against rotavirus infection. This result, in line with the rate in Italy [10], highlights the need for greater efforts by policymakers and pediatricians to recommend vaccination more effectively in order to improve the coverage. Moreover, the results showed that parents had high intention to get their children vaccinated in spite of the low uptake rate. As expected, those considering it dangerous for their children to contract rotavirus gastroenteritis and having positive perception toward the effectiveness of the vaccine were more likely to have immunized their children. These findings are consistent with several studies worldwide evaluating factors positively associated with vaccination [15,17,20,33–35]. These observations underlined the importance of not only adequately providing information about rotavirus infection to parents, but also explaining the utility of the vaccination in order to increase the coverage.

Fourth, the results of the multivariable regression analysis indicated other several interesting associations. The exposure to sources of information had a significant effect on rotavirus infection and vaccination-related knowledge and uptake. However, not all sources were equally effective. Pediatrician was the strongest predictor for the reported knowledge and child vaccination status: Parents who reported this source of information were 21 times more likely to have heard about rotavirus infection and to know that the vaccination is available in Italy and 25 times to have a child vaccinated against rotavirus. These findings corroborate previous research on the key role that they play in promoting vaccinations. Notably, having received information from healthcare professionals had a significantly stronger association with the level of knowledge and the vaccination rates [17,22,27,36–38]. This is a clear indication of the need to develop and to disseminate interventions to improve the interaction between pediatrician and all eligible patients, although more than two-thirds of participants identified pediatricians as a primary source of information. Similar results were also seen in previous studies [39–42]. Moreover, the majority of the participants indicated an interest in receiving additional information regarding vaccines, implying that this gap may not necessarily due to parent disinterest. The interventions should also address parents' barriers. For example, insufficient knowledge about vaccination, concerns regarding the side effects, and the lack of recommendation by the pediatrician were the most frequently cited barriers for not having immunized their children. The lack of recommendation by pediatricians underline the need that they should be aware of their role in providing adequate, clear, and accessible information and communications to parents regarding rotavirus infection, vaccine safety, and adverse effects, since this may be one way to reduce concerns and misconceptions. Moreover, almost two-thirds of the sample cited Internet as source of information and this may be of concern due the spread of anti-vaccine arguments online and this may be translated into lower vaccine coverage. Monitoring social media for anti-vaccine beliefs is essential and effective health communication must combat the anti-vaccination campaigns. Websites that address public health issues should provide clear and evidence-based information easily accessible to users.

This study has some methodological limitations that warrant discussion and the results must be interpreted and used with caution. Firstly, the survey was conducted in one geographical area and thus, the generalizability of the findings to the rest of Italy needs to be established. However, we are confident that the characteristics of the sample are similar to those of other areas of the country and the observed vaccination coverage is in line with the value throughout the whole country [10]. Secondly, the recruitment has been performed through public nurseries, and, therefore, parents of children who do not attend any pre-schools or private nurseries were excluded. It is well known that those attending public schools may belong to lower social groups and, therefore, they may not be representative of the parents' population. However, we believe that this would not have an impact on the conclusions of the study, although we cannot be certain, because attending pediatricians and preventive healthcare services is provided free of charge. Thirdly, caution should be taken when interpreting the findings owing to the cross-sectional study that allowed for identification of associations and prevent from making any statements regarding causality. Fourthly, the survey data, including child vaccination status, were collected based on self-reporting and were not verified by a certification and, therefore, the information is susceptible to forgetting and recall bias that may have resulted in an underestimation of vaccination. Moreover, the possible association of rotavirus vaccine with another multivalent vaccine may lead to some parents not realizing that their children have received it. The inclusion of parents of very young children may have reduced the bias. Fifthly, the possibility of the parents responding in a socially expected way and this would mean that the reported intentions would not correspond to the real situation or their future behaviors. However, the fact that the questionnaires were self-administered and completed anonymously should result in reducing this bias.

## 5. Conclusions

The current survey indicated low levels of knowledge and coverage on rotavirus vaccination and highlight the need for developing and implementing additional public education programs so that parents are informed, which should result in a better knowledge toward rotavirus infection and vaccination and in a high coverage.

**Author Contributions:** Conceptualization, F.N., A.A.A., A.V. and I.F.A.; methodology, F.N., A.A.A., A.V. and I.F.A.; validation, F.N., A.A.A., A.V. and I.F.A.; formal analysis, F.N., A.A.A. and I.F.A.; investigation, F.N., A.A.A., A.V.; data curation, F.N. and I.F.A.; writing—original draft preparation, I.F.A.; writing—review and editing, I.F.A.; visualization, F.N. and I.F.A.; supervision, F.N. and I.F.A.; project administration, I.F.A.

**Acknowledgments:** The authors wish to thank the heads of the participating nurseries for giving their permission to conduct the survey and the teachers for their assistance during data collection. We would also like to thank the participating parents for taking time to complete the questionnaire.

## References

1. Tate, J.E.; Burton, A.H.; Boschi-Pinto, C.; Parashar, U.D.; World Health Organization–Coordinated Global Rotavirus Surveillance Network. Global, regional, and national estimates of rotavirus mortality in children <5 years of age, 2000–2013. *Clin. Infect. Dis.* **2016**, *62*, S96–S105.
2. Van Damme, P.; Giaquinto, C.; Huet, F.; Gothefors, L.; Maxwell, M.; Van der Wielen, M. Multicenter prospective study of the burden of rotavirus acute gastroenteritis in Europe, 2004–2005: The REVEAL Study. *J. Infect. Dis.* **2007**, *195*, 4–16. [CrossRef]
3. World Health Organization. Rotavirus vaccines: An update. *Wkly. Epidemiol. Rec.* **2009**, *84*, 533–540.
4. World Health Organization. Rotavirus vaccines. WHO position paper. *Wkly. Epidemiol. Rec.* **2013**, *88*, 49–64.
5. Ministero Della Salute. Piano Nazionale Prevenzione Vaccinale 2017–2019. Available online: http://www.salute.gov.it/imgs/C_17_pubblicazioni_2571_allegato.pdf (accessed on 10 April 2019).
6. Ministero Della Salute. Legge di Conversione 31 Luglio 2017, n. 119. Available online: http://www.salute.gov.it/portale/vaccinazioni/dettaglioContenutiVaccinazioni.jsp?lingua=italiano&id=4824&area=vaccinazioni&menu=vuoto (accessed on 8 May 2019).
7. Troeger, C.; Khalil, I.A.; Rao, P.C.; Cao, S.; Blacker, B.F.; Ahmed, T.; Armah, G.; Bines, J.E.; Brewer, T.G.; Colombara, D.V.; et al. Rotavirus vaccination and the global burden of rotavirus diarrhea among children younger than 5 years. *JAMA Pediatr.* **2018**, *172*, 958–965. [CrossRef] [PubMed]
8. Shah, M.P.; Tate, J.E.; Mwenda, J.M.; Steele, A.D.; Parashar, U.D. Estimated reductions in hospitalizations and deaths from childhood diarrhea following implementation of rotavirus vaccination in Africa. *Expert Rev. Vaccines* **2017**, *16*, 987–995. [CrossRef]
9. Lo Vecchio, A.; Liguoro, I.; Dias, J.A.; Berkley, J.A.; Boey, C.; Cohen, M.B.; Cruchet, S.; Salazar-Lindo, E.; Podder, S.; Sandhu, B.; et al. Rotavirus immunization: Global coverage and local barriers for implementation. *Vaccine* **2017**, *35*, 1637–1644. [CrossRef]
10. Ministero della Salute. Vaccinazioni dell'età pediatrica e dell'adolescente–Coperture Vaccinali. Available online: http://www.salute.gov.it/portale/documentazione/p6_2_8_3_1.jsp?lingua=italiano&id=20 (accessed on 10 April 2019).

11. Napolitano, F.; D'Alessandro, A.; Angelillo, I.F. Investigating Italian parents' vaccine hesitancy: A cross-sectional survey. *Hum. Vaccin. Immunother.* **2018**, *14*, 1558–1565. [CrossRef]
12. Dubé, E.; Laberge, C.; Guay, M.; Bramadat, P.; Roy, R.; Bettinger, J.A. Vaccine hesitancy: An overview. *Hum. Vaccin. Immunother.* **2013**, *9*, 1763–1773. [CrossRef]
13. Bianco, A.; Mascaro, V.; Zucco, R.; Pavia, M. Parent perspectives on childhood vaccination: How to deal with vaccine hesitancy and refusal? *Vaccine* **2019**, *37*, 984–990. [CrossRef]
14. Smith, A.; Yarwood, J.; Salisbury, D.M. Tracking mothers' attitudes to MMR immunisation 1996–2006. *Vaccine* **2007**, *25*, 3996–4002. [CrossRef]
15. Yuen, W.W.Y.; Lee, A.; Chan, P.K.S.; Tran, L.; Sayko, E. Uptake of human papillomavirus (HPV) vaccination in Hong Kong: Facilitators and barriers among adolescent girls and their parents. *PLoS ONE* **2018**, *13*, e0194159. [CrossRef] [PubMed]
16. Gilbert, N.L.; Gilmour, H.; Dubé, È.; Wilson, S.E.; Laroche, J. Estimates and determinants of HPV non-vaccination and vaccine refusal in girls 12 to 14 y of age in Canada: Results from the Childhood National Immunization Coverage Survey, 2013. *Hum. Vaccin. Immunother.* **2016**, *12*, 1484–1490. [CrossRef]
17. D'Alessandro, A.; Napolitano, F.; D'Ambrosio, A.; Angelillo, I.F. Vaccination knowledge and acceptability among pregnant women in Italy. *Hum. Vaccin. Immunother.* **2018**, *14*, 1573–1579. [CrossRef]
18. MacDougall, D.M.; Halperin, B.A.; Langley, J.M.; MacKinnon-Cameron, D.; Li, L.; Halperin, S.A. Knowledge, attitudes, beliefs, and behaviors of parents and healthcare providers before and after implementation of a universal rotavirus vaccination program. *Vaccine* **2016**, *34*, 687–695. [CrossRef]
19. Veldwijk, J.; Lambooij, M.S.; Bruijning-Verhagen, P.C.; Smit, H.A.; de Wit, G.A. Parental preferences for rotavirus vaccination in young children: A discrete choice experiment. *Vaccine* **2014**, *32*, 6277–6283. [CrossRef] [PubMed]
20. Morin, A.; Lemaître, T.; Farrands, A.; Carrier, N.; Gagneur, A. Maternal knowledge, attitudes and beliefs regarding gastroenteritis and rotavirus vaccine before implementing vaccination program: Which key messages in light of a new immunization program? *Vaccine* **2012**, *30*, 5921–5927. [CrossRef] [PubMed]
21. Napolitano, F.; Navaro, M.; Vezzosi, L.; Santagati, G.; Angelillo, I.F. Primary care pediatricians' attitudes and practice towards HPV vaccination: A nationwide survey in Italy. *PLoS ONE* **2018**, *13*, e0194920. [CrossRef] [PubMed]
22. Napolitano, F.; Napolitano, P.; Liguori, G.; Angelillo, I.F. Human papillomavirus infection and vaccination: Knowledge and attitudes among young males in Italy. *Hum. Vaccin. Immunother.* **2016**, *12*, 1504–1510. [CrossRef] [PubMed]
23. Bianco, A.; Pileggi, C.; Iozzo, F.; Nobile, C.G.; Pavia, M. Vaccination against human papilloma virus infection in male adolescents: Knowledge, attitudes, and acceptability among parents in Italy. *Hum. Vaccin. Immunother.* **2014**, *10*, 2536–2542. [CrossRef] [PubMed]
24. Pelullo, C.P.; Di Giuseppe, G.; Angelillo, I.F. Human papillomavirus infection: Knowledge, attitudes, and behaviors among lesbian, gay men, and bisexual in Italy. *PLoS ONE* **2012**, *7*, e42856. [CrossRef] [PubMed]
25. Di Giuseppe, G.; Abbate, R.; Liguori, G.; Albano, L.; Angelillo, I.F. Human papillomavirus and vaccination: Knowledge, attitudes, and behavioural intention in adolescents and young women in Italy. *Br. J. Cancer* **2008**, *99*, 225–229. [CrossRef]
26. Napolitano, F.; Gualdieri, L.; Santagati, G.; Angelillo, I.F. Knowledge and attitudes toward HPV infection and vaccination among immigrants and refugees in Italy. *Vaccine* **2018**, *36*, 7536–7541. [CrossRef]
27. Pelullo, C.P.; Napolitano, F.; Di Giuseppe, G. Meningococcal disease and vaccination: Knowledge and acceptability among adolescents in Italy. *Hum. Vaccin. Immunother.* **2018**, *14*, 1197–1202. [CrossRef] [PubMed]
28. StataCorp. *Stata Statistical Software: Release 15*; StataCorp LLC: College Station, TX, USA, 2017.
29. Attwell, K.; Dube, E.; Gagneur, A.; Omer, S.B.; Suggs, L.S.; Thomson, A. Vaccine acceptance: Science, policy, and practice in a "post-fact" world. *Vaccine* **2019**, *37*, 677–682. [CrossRef] [PubMed]
30. Gagneur, A.; Lemaître, T.; Gosselin, V.; Farrands, A.; Carrier, N.; Petit, G.; Valiquette, L.; De Wals, P. A postpartum vaccination promotion intervention using motivational interviewing techniques improves short-term vaccine coverage: PromoVac study. *BMC Public Health* **2018**, *18*, 811. [CrossRef]
31. Kaufman, J.; Synnot, A.; Ryan, R.; Hill, S.; Horey, D.; Willis, N.; Lin, V.; Robinson, P. Face to face interventions for informing or educating parents about early childhood vaccination. *Cochrane Database Syst Rev.* **2013**, *5*, CD010038. [CrossRef] [PubMed]

32. Wangen, K.R.; Zhu, D.; Wang, J. Hepatitis B vaccination among 1997–2011 birth cohorts in rural China: The potential for further catch-up vaccination and factors associated with infant coverage rates. *Hum. Vaccin. Immunother.* **2019**, *15*, 228–234. [CrossRef]
33. Grandahl, M.; Paek, S.C.; Grisurapong, S.; Sherer, P.; Tydén, T.; Lundberg, P. Parents' knowledge, beliefs, and acceptance of the HPV vaccination in relation to their socio-demographics and religious beliefs: A cross-sectional study in Thailand. *PLoS ONE* **2018**, *13*, e0193054.
34. Li, T.; Wang, H.; Lu, Y.; Li, Q.; Chen, C.; Wang, D.; Li, M.; Li, Y.; Lu, J.; Chen, Z.; et al. Willingness and influential factors of parents to vaccinate their children with novel inactivated enterovirus 71 vaccines in Guangzhou, China. *Vaccine* **2018**, *36*, 3772–3778. [CrossRef]
35. Ragan, K.R.; Bednarczyk, R.A.; Butler, S.M.; Omer, S.B. Missed opportunities for catch-up human papillomavirus vaccination among university undergraduates: Identifying health decision-making behaviors and uptake barriers. *Vaccine* **2018**, *36*, 331–341. [CrossRef]
36. Wu, S.; Su, J.; Yang, P.; Zhang, H.; Li, H.; Chu, Y.; Hua, W.; Li, C.; Tang, Y.; Wang, Q. Factors associated with the uptake of seasonal influenza vaccination in older and younger adults: A large, population-based survey in Beijing, China. *BMJ Open* **2017**, *7*, e017459. [CrossRef] [PubMed]
37. Tsuchiya, Y.; Shida, N.; Izumi, S.; Ogasawara, M.; Kakinuma, W.; Tsujiuchi, T.; Machida, K. Factors associated with mothers not vaccinating their children against mumps in Japan. *Public Health* **2016**, *137*, 95–105. [CrossRef]
38. Campbell, H.; Edwards, A.; Letley, L.; Bedford, H.; Ramsay, M.; Yarwood, J. Changing attitudes to childhood immunisation in English parents. *Vaccine* **2017**, *35*, 2979–2985. [CrossRef] [PubMed]
39. Napolitano, F.; Napolitano, P.; Angelillo, I.F. Seasonal influenza vaccination in pregnant women: Knowledge, attitudes, and behaviors in Italy. *BMC Infect. Dis.* **2017**, *17*, 48. [CrossRef]
40. Greenfield, L.S.; Page, L.C.; Kay, M.; Li-Vollmer, M.; Breuner, C.C.; Duchin, J.S. Strategies for increasing adolescent immunizations in diverse ethnic communities. *J. Adolesc. Health* **2015**, *56*, S47–S53. [CrossRef]
41. Wheeler, M.; Buttenheim, A.M. Parental vaccine concerns, information source, and choice of alternative immunization schedules. *Hum. Vaccin. Immunother.* **2013**, *9*, 1782–1789. [CrossRef] [PubMed]
42. Gilkey, M.B.; Calo, W.A.; Marciniak, M.W.; Brewer, N.T. Parents who refuse or delay HPV vaccine: Differences in vaccination behavior, beliefs, and clinical communication preferences. *Hum. Vaccin. Immunother.* **2017**, *13*, 680–686. [CrossRef] [PubMed]

# First Detection of Rotavirus Group C in Asymptomatic Pigs of Smallholder Farms in East Africa

Joshua Oluoch Amimo [1,2,*], Eunice Magoma Machuka [2] and Edward Okoth [2]

[1] Department of Animal Production, Faculty of Veterinary Medicine, University of Nairobi, P.O. Box 29053, Nairobi 00625, Kenya
[2] Biosciences of East and Central Africa-International Livestock Research Institute, (BecA-ILRI) Hub, P.O. Box 30709, Nairobi 00100, Kenya; e.machuka@cgiar.org (E.M.M.); e.okoth@cgiar.org (E.O.)
* Correspondence: jamimo@uonbi.ac.ke

**Abstract:** Group C rotavirus (RVC) has been described to be a causative agent of gastroenteritis in humans and animals including pigs, cows, and dogs. Fecal samples collected from asymptomatic pigs in smallholder swine farms in Kenya and Uganda were screened for the presence of group C rotaviruses (RVC) using a reverse transcription-polymerase chain reaction assay. A total of 446 samples were tested and 37 were positive (8.3%). A significantly larger ($p < 0.05$) number of RVC-positive samples was detected in groups of older pigs (5–6 months) than in younger piglets (1–2 months). There were no significant differences in the RVC detection rate between the pigs that were full time housed/tethered and those that were free range combined with housing/tethering. After compiling these data with diagnostic results for group A rotaviruses (RVA), 13 RVC-positive samples were also positive for RVA. This study provides the first evidence that porcine group C rotavirus may be detected frequently in asymptomatic piglets (aged < 1–6 months) in East Africa. The occurrence of RVC in mixed infections with RVA and other enteric pathogens requires further research to investigate the pathogenic potential of RVC in pigs.

**Keywords:** smallholder pigs; rotavirus group C; East Africa

## 1. Introduction

Smallholder pig producers own the bulk of the pigs (>80%) in sub-Saharan Africa, and present the strongest influence to the swine industry in this region. These smallholder farms are characterized by low productivity compared to larger scale commercial farms in developed countries. The major constraints hampering the growth and development of the pig industry in the region is the high disease burden. In developing countries, one of the major causes of mortality among children (<5 years) and young piglets is diarrheal disease [1–3]. In the swine industry, piglets that suffer from Rotavirus RV diarrheal disease have stunted growth and some may die, resulting in high economic losses. Knowledge on RV prevalence in animals in East Africa is limited, with no information on non-group A rotaviruses, but it is suspected to be among the major causes of suckling and weaning piglet diarrheal disease and a concern for pork producers due to the resulting mortality, reduced growth, and high costs of treatment and control. Limited epidemiologic surveys globally suggest that group RVCs are widespread and enzootic in pig herds [4,5]. Outbreaks of diarrhea associated with RVCs have been documented in nursing, weaning, and post-weaning pigs [6–9], either alone or in mixed infections with other enteric pathogens. Collection of epidemiological and molecular data on RVCs in animals is crucial for a better understanding of their ecology, genetic/antigenic diversity, and zoonotic potential. Evidence for the zoonotic potential of porcine RVCs was revealed by analyses of archive fecal samples of children infected with porcine-like RVCs [10]. Detection of animal-like RVCs in humans requires detailed studies of the epidemiology and genetic diversity of animal RVCs, especially in regions where humans and animals or different animal species often live in close contact, making mixed infections more common. In this study, we investigated the presence of RVCs in smallholder swine herds in East Africa, where a total of 446 fecal samples from piglets aged 1 to 6 months were screened by using RVC-specific primers based on the VP6 gene described by Amimo et al. [6].

## 2. Results and Discussion

The information on the prevalence of porcine RVCs is very limited, especially in Africa, with no historic or current reports available, apart from the reports by Geyer et al. published nearly 30 years ago [11]. The absence of surveillance programs and appropriate diagnostic facilities for porcine RVC have resulted in a lack of data on its prevalence. In this study, we found an overall prevalence of RVC of 8.3% in 446 fecal samples (37/446) from western Kenya and eastern Uganda. Of the 37 samples which were positive, 35% (13/37) of them occurred in mixed infection with RVA. The results of RVA detection was discussed in detail by Amimo and colleagues in 2015 [12]. RVC was reported both in Uganda (7.7%) and Kenya (8.8%) in nearly equal proportions. The virus strain was also present in all the sub-counties studied; with Tororo sub-county (11.5%) having a higher detection rate and Busia sub-county (5.0%) in Uganda having the lowest rate (Table 1). Tororo region is characterized by a major town in the eastern part of Uganda with a high density of pigs compared to Busia area in Uganda, which could explain the high prevalence of RVC in Tororo. Based on the age group ($\leq 2$ months, 3 and 4 months, 5 and 6 months old), RVC prevalence was higher (11.6%) in the older pigs (5 and 6 months) than the nursing piglets (4.3%), as shown in Table 1. We also examined whether the management practices had effect on the RVC detection rate; we found that the difference was not statistically significant ($p > 0.05$), however, the prevalence was slightly higher in the piglets that were free range combined with tethering or housing (9.6%) compared with the piglets that were fully tethered or housed (7.3%). The study examined the effect of the herd size on the prevalence of RVC, and found that piglets in a herd of 6–10 pigs (10.8%) were more affected. Based on the month of sample collection, there was high prevalence of RVC in July (11.8%) and November (10.5%), however, there was no evidence of seasonal influence on RVC prevalence in the study region, since July is in the dry season and November is in the short rainy season. Nonetheless, we recommend a comprehensive study to elucidate the seasonal influence on RVC prevalence in the study area.

The prevalence reported here was lower than the 19.5% reported in the USA [6], 26.3% reported in S. Korea (Jeong et al., 2009), and 28.7% reported in Italy (Martella et al., 2007). However, the previous studies in Korea and Italy analyzed only samples from diarrheic pigs, whereas we used samples from non-diarrheic pigs. The study by Amimo and colleagues in the USA examined fecal samples from both symptomatic and asymptomatic piglets, and reported an overall porcine RVC prevalence of 19.5% with 8.5% in asymptomatic weaned pigs in USA, which is consistent with our results. The study reported high RVC prevalence (23.5%) in younger piglets (<30 days old). Similarly, Marthaler and colleagues reported 46% (53% using RT-qPCR) prevalence of RVC in 7520 pig fecal samples from the USA and Canada, and their results revealed that single RVC infection was very high (78%) in neonatal piglets (<3 days) and young piglets of 4–20 days (65%) compared to older pigs of 455 days (13%) [8,9]. In Brazil, Molinari et al. [13] also reported porcine RVC to be the most prevalent group in swine herd during a post-weaning diarrhea outbreak, occurring in single (34%) and mixed (44%) infections. In China, Peng et al. [14] also reported 16.65% prevalence of RCV in 793 fecal samples from diarrheic and non-diarrheic pigs from Lulong area. Porcine RVC has been also reported in pigs in Czech Republic (4.4%), Belgium (29%), and Germany (31%) [15–17].

Even though we sampled piglets older than 21 days, our results indicate that porcine RVC could be an important enteric pathogen in the study region, since many studies have described porcine RVC as an important enteric pathogen in nursing and weaned piglets. Further studies are therefore required to ascertain the pathogenic potential of RVC in the swine population in East Africa to be able to develop effective measures for the prevention and control of rotavirus infections in swine.

Table 1. Relative distribution of RVC in asymptomatic pigs in smallholder swine farms in East Africa during the study period.

| Details | Groups | N | Positive | Prevalence (%) |
|---|---|---|---|---|
| | Overall | 446 | 37 | 8.3 |
| Country | Kenya | 239 | 21 | 8.8 |
| | Uganda | 207 | 16 | 7.7 |
| Sub-Counties | Busia Kenya | 113 | 9 | 8.0 |
| | Teso, Kenya | 126 | 12 | 9.5 |
| | Busia Uganda | 120 | 6 | 5.0 |
| | Tororo Uganda | 87 | 10 | 11.5 |
| Age Group | Nursing (1 ≤ 3 months) | 47 | 2 | 4.3 |
| | Weaner (3 and 4 months) | 210 | 13 | 6.2 |
| | Weaner (5 and 6 months) | 189 | 22 | 11.6 |
| Management Systems | Free range with tethering/housing | 198 | 19 | 9.6 |
| | Full-time housing/tethering | 248 | 18 | 7.3 |
| Herd Size | <6 Pigs | 386 | 32 | 8.3 |
| | 6–10 Pigs | 37 | 4 | 10.8 |
| | >10 Pigs | 23 | 1 | 4.3 |
| Month of Collection | July 2012 | 51 | 6 | 11.8 |
| | August 2012 | 134 | 12 | 9.0 |
| | September 2012 | 22 | 0 | 0.0 |
| | October 2012 | 39 | 1 | 2.6 |
| | November 2012 | 153 | 16 | 10.5 |
| | February 2013 | 47 | 2 | 4.3 |

## 3. Materials and Methods

### 3.1. Fecal Sample Collection

A total of 446 fecal samples were collected from individual piglets aged 1–6 months from two sub-counties (Busia and Teso) in western Kenya and two sub-counties (Tororo and Busia) in eastern Uganda in the year 2012 (July to November) and February, 2013. In the study region, there are three seasons based on the rainfall pattern i.e., the long rainy season (March to May), the short rainy season (September to November), and the dry season (December to February, June to August). The detailed sampling procedure has been described by Amimo et al., 2014 and 2015 [12,18].

### 3.2. RNA Extraction and Detection of Rotavirus Group C

RNA was extracted from 250 μL of 10% (w/v) fecal suspensions in phosphate-buffered saline (PBS) using an RNeasy mini kit (Qiagen, CA, USA) according to the manufacturer's instructions. The total RNA recovered was suspended in 40 μL of nuclease free water and stored at −70 °C until used. Conventional RT-PCR was used for the detection of the RVCs with validated primer sets designed from the VP6 gene (giving 260bp PCR product), as described previously by Amimo et al. [6]. The RT-PCR assay was conducted using a one-step Qiagen RT-PCR kit (Qiagen, Valencia, CA, USA) according to the manufacturer's instructions, with minor modifications. The amplicons were analyzed in 2% agarose gel electrophoresis and visualized by ultraviolet illumination after staining with gel red™ nucleic acid gel stain (Biotium, Hayward, CA, USA). Cell-cultured porcine RVC prototype Cowden was used as positive control in all PCR reactions. A chi-square test was used to assess the relationship between several factors (country of origin, sub-counties, age group, management systems, and herd size) and the RVC detection using procedure frequency in the SAS computer program (SAS, 2002).

**Acknowledgments:** This research was supported by the BecA-ILRI Hub through the Africa Biosciences Challenge Fund (ABCF) program. The ABCF Program is funded by the Australian Department for Foreign Affairs and Trade (DFAT) through the BecA-CSIRO partnership; the Syngenta Foundation for Sustainable Agriculture (SFSA); the Bill & Melinda Gates Foundation (BMGF); the UK Department for International Development (DFID) and; the Swedish International Development Cooperation Agency (Sida). We thank the smallholder pig farmers in the study region for allowing us to sample their pigs for this study.

**Author Contributions:** J.O.A. and E.M.M. conducted laboratory work and drafted the manuscript; J.O.A. and E.O. developed study design, E.O. provided academic input and edited the manuscript.

## References

1. Othero, D.M.; Orago, A.S.S.; Groenewegen, T.; Kaseje, D.O.; Otengah, P.A. Home management of diarrhea among underfives in a rural community in kenya: Household perceptions and practices. *East Afr. J. Public Health* **2008**, *5*, 142–146. [CrossRef] [PubMed]
2. Tate, J.E.; Bunning, M.L.; Lott, L.; Lu, X.; Su, J.; Metzgar, D.; Brosch, L.; Panozzo, C.A.; Marconi, V.C.; Faix, D.J.; et al. Outbreak of severe respiratory disease associated with emergent human adenovirus serotype 14 at a us air force training facility in 2007. *J. Infect. Dis.* **2009**, *199*, 1419–1426. [CrossRef] [PubMed]
3. Wabacha, J.K.; Maribei, J.M.; Mulei, C.M.; Kyule, M.N.; Zessin, K.H.; Oluoch-Kosura, W. Health and production measures for smallholder pig production in kikuyu division, central kenya. *Prev. Vet. Med.* **2004**, *63*, 197–210. [CrossRef] [PubMed]
4. Saif, L.J.; Jiang, B. Nongroup A rotaviruses of humans and animals. *Curr. Top. Microbiol. Immunol.* **1994**, *185*, 339–371. [PubMed]
5. Tsunemitsu, H.; Jiang, B.; Saif, L.J. Detection of group C rotavirus antigens and antibodies in animals and humans by enzyme-linked immunosorbent assays. *J. Clin. Microbiol.* **1992**, *30*, 2129–2134. [PubMed]
6. Amimo, J.O.; Vlasova, A.N.; Saif, L.J. Prevalence and genetic heterogeneity of porcine group C rotaviruses in nursing and weaned piglets in Ohio, USA and identification of a potential new VP4 genotype. *Vet. Microbiol.* **2013**, *164*, 27–38. [CrossRef] [PubMed]
7. Kim, Y.; Chang, K.O.; Straw, B.; Saif, L.J. Characterization of group C rotaviruses associated with diarrhea outbreaks in feeder pigs. *J. Clin. Microbiol.* **1999**, *37*, 1484–1488. [PubMed]
8. Marthaler, D.; Homwong, N.; Rossow, K.; Culhane, M.; Goyal, S.; Collins, J.; Matthijnssens, J.; Ciarlet, M. Rapid detection and high occurrence of porcine rotavirus A, B, and C by RT-qPCR in diagnostic samples. *J. Virol. Methods* **2014**, *209*, 30–34. [CrossRef] [PubMed]
9. Marthaler, D.; Rossow, K.; Culhane, M.; Collins, J.; Goyal, S.; Ciarlet, M.; Matthijnssens, J. Identification, phylogenetic analysis and classification of porcine group C rotavirus VP7 sequences from the United States and Canada. *Virology* **2013**, *446*, 189–198. [CrossRef] [PubMed]
10. Gabbay, Y.B.; Borges, A.A.; Oliveira, D.S.; Linhares, A.C.; Mascarenhas, J.D.P.; Baraldi, C.R.M.; Simões, C.M.O.; Wang, Y.; Glass, R.I.; Jiang, B. Evidence for zoonotic transmission of group C rotaviruses among children in Belém, Brazil. *J. Med. Virol.* **2008**, *80*, 1666–1674. [CrossRef] [PubMed]
11. Geyer, A.; Sebata, T.; Peenze, I.; Steele, A.D. Group B and C porcine rotaviruses identified for the first time in South Africa. *J. S. Afr. Vet. Assoc.* **1996**, *67*, 115–116. [PubMed]
12. Amimo, J.O.; Junga, J.O.; Ogara, W.O.; Vlasova, A.N.; Njahira, M.N.; Maina, S.; Okoth, E.A.; Bishop, R.P.; Saif, L.J.; Djikeng, A. Detection and genetic characterization of porcine group A rotaviruses in asymptomatic pigs in smallholder farms in East Africa: Predominance of P[8] genotype resembling human strains. *Vet. Microbiol.* **2015**, *175*, 195–210. [CrossRef] [PubMed]
13. Molinari, B.L.; Possatti, F.; Lorenzetti, E.; Alfieri, A.F.; Alfieri, A.A. Unusual outbreak of post-weaning porcine diarrhea caused by single and mixed infections of rotavirus groups A, B, C, and H. *Vet. Microbiol.* **2016**, *193*, 125–132. [CrossRef] [PubMed]
14. Peng, R.; Li, D.D.; Cai, K.; Qin, J.J.; Wang, Y.X.; Lin, Q.; Guo, Y.Q.; Zhao, C.Y.; Duan, Z.J. The epidemiological characteristics of group C rotavirus in Lulong area and the analysis of diversity of VP6 gene. *Zhonghua Shi Yan He Lin Chuang Bing Du Xue Za Zhi* **2013**, *27*, 164–166. [PubMed]
15. Otto, P.H.; Rosenhain, S.; Elschner, M.C.; Hotzel, H.; Machnowska, P.; Trojnar, E.; Hoffmann, K.; Johne, R. Detection of rotavirus species A, B and C in domestic mammalian animals with diarrhoea and genotyping of bovine species A rotavirus strains. *Vet. Microbiol.* **2015**, *179*, 168–176. [CrossRef] [PubMed]

16. Smitalova, R.; Rodak, L.; Smid, B.; Psikal, I. Detection of nongroup A rotaviruses in fecal samples of pigs in the Czech Republic. *Vet. Med.* **2009**, *54*, 12–18.
17. Theuns, S.; Vyt, P.; Desmarets, L.M.; Roukaerts, I.D.; Heylen, E.; Zeller, M.; Matthijnssens, J.; Nauwynck, H.J. Presence and characterization of pig group A and C rotaviruses in feces of belgian diarrheic suckling piglets. *Virus Res.* **2016**, *213*, 172–183. [CrossRef] [PubMed]
18. Amimo, J.O.; Okoth, E.; Junga, J.O.; Ogara, W.O.; Njahira, M.N.; Wang, Q.; Vlasova, A.N.; Saif, L.J.; Djikeng, A. Molecular detection and genetic characterization of kobuviruses and astroviruses in asymptomatic local pigs in East Africa. *Archives Virol.* **2014**, *159*, 1313–1319. [CrossRef] [PubMed]

# Differences of Rotavirus Vaccine Effectiveness by Country: Likely Causes and Contributing Factors

**Ulrich Desselberger**

Department of Medicine, University of Cambridge, Addenbrooke's Hospital, Cambridge CB2 0QQ, UK; ud207@medschl.cam.ac.uk;

**Abstract:** Rotaviruses are a major cause of acute gastroenteritis in infants and young children worldwide and in many other mammalian and avian host species. Since 2006, two live-attenuated rotavirus vaccines, Rotarix® and RotaTeq®, have been licensed in >100 countries and are applied as part of extended program of vaccination (EPI) schemes of childhood vaccinations. Whereas the vaccines have been highly effective in high-income countries, they were shown to be considerably less potent in low- and middle-income countries. Rotavirus-associated disease was still the cause of death in >200,000 children of <5 years of age worldwide in 2013, and the mortality is concentrated in countries of sub-Saharan Africa and S.E. Asia. Various factors that have been identified or suggested as being involved in the differences of rotavirus vaccine effectiveness are reviewed here. Recognition of these factors will help to achieve gradual worldwide improvement of rotavirus vaccine effectiveness.

**Keywords:** rotavirus; vaccine efficacy; low income countries; malnutrition; avitaminoses; zinc deficiency; gut microbiome; microbial co-infections; immunological immaturity

## 1. Introduction

Rotaviruses (RVs) were discovered as a major cause of acute gastroenteritis (AGE) in infants and young children worldwide more than 40 years ago [1,2] and were also recognized as pathogenic agents in many mammalian and avian species [3]. Since 2006, two live attenuated RV vaccines (Rotarix®, RotaTeq®) have been licensed in >100 countries and are increasingly used in universal mass vaccination (UMV) programs [3,4]. While UMV against RV disease has been highly effective (80–90%—preventing severe RV-associated disease) in high income countries [3,4], their efficacy and effectiveness is much lower (40–60%) in low- and middle-income countries [5–7]. RV-associated disease still caused the death of over 200,000 children of <5 years of age worldwide in 2013 [8] and thus represents a major pediatric, public health and economic problem. Here, various factors are reviewed which do or may contribute to the differences in effectiveness of RV vaccines.

## 2. Rotavirus Structure and Classification

Rotaviruses are triple-layered particles containing 11 segments of genomic double-stranded (ds) RNA, which encode 6 structural proteins (VP1-VP4, VP6, VP7) and 5–6 non-structural proteins (NSP1-NSP5/6). With the exception of RNA segment 11, which codes for NSP5 and NSP6, all RNA segments are mono-cistronic (Figure 1). The viral genome, the RNA-dependent RNA polymerase (VP1) and the capping enzyme (VP3) are surrounded by an inner protein layer (VP2), forming a core. This in turn is surrounded by an intermediate layer (VP6), to form a dual-layered particle (DLP), and the DLP gains an outer layer, consisting of the VP7 protein and the spike-forming VP4, to become a triple-layered particle (TLP), the infectious virion [3,4] (Figure 1).

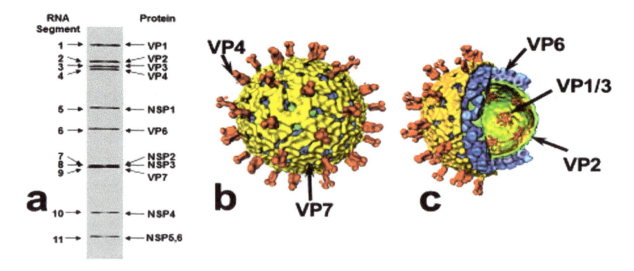

**Figure 1.** Structural organization of rotavirus. (**a**) Rotavirus dsRNA migration pattern by SDS-PAGE and gene-protein assignment (SA11 strain). (**b**) Surface representation and (**c**) cut-away of rotavirus structure (based on reconstructions from cryo-electron micrographs): VP4 spikes (red), VP7 outer layer (yellow), VP6 middle layer (blue), VP2 inner (core) layer (green), VP1/VP3 complexes, attached to the inside of the VP2 layer (red). Modified from: Pesavento JB, Estes MK and Prasad BVV. Structural organization of the genome in rotavirus. In: Viral Gastroenteritis, edited by U Desselberger and J Gray, pp. 115–127. Elsevier Science, Amsterdam, 2003 [9], where further details are described (with permission of authors; permission of publisher applied for).

Rotaviruses represent one of the 15 genera of the *Reoviridae* family. According to the serological reactivity and genetic variability of VP6 at least 10 groups/species (A- I; J) have been differentiated [10–12], and within species various genotypes encoding VP7 (G types) and VP4 (P types) have been observed. Furthermore, a comprehensive classification system defining genotypes of all 11 RNA segments of species A RVs (RVAs) has been developed [13]. Within RVAs, 28 G types, 39 P types and between 14 and 24 genotypes for the remaining nine RNA segments were recognized in 2015 [14]. Species A RVs are the main cause of human acute gastroenteritis (AGE).

## 3. Rotavirus Replication Cycle

Rotavirus TLPs first attach to sialo-glycans or histo-blood group antigens on the surface of susceptible host cells, followed by interactions with other cellular co-receptors, including integrins and Hsc70. Internalization of RV particles occurs by receptor-mediated endocytosis. Removal of the outer layer of TLPs in endosomes results in the release of DLPs into the cytoplasm from which (+)ssRNAs of all genomic segments are transcribed and released into the cytoplasm. These are either translated into viral proteins or act as templates for the dsRNA genomes of progeny virus. Once enough RV proteins have been synthesized, cytoplasmic inclusion bodies termed 'viroplasms' arise in which the viral RNA segments are assorted, packaged into new DLPs and replicated to dsRNA. The rotavirus NSP2 and NSP5 are essential components of viroplasms. The DLPs are released from viroplasms and bind to NSP4, which is inserted into the endoplasmic reticulum (ER), where it serves as an intracellular receptor mediating the transport of DLPs into the ER. NSP4 also acts as a viroporin, releasing $Ca^{2+}$ ions from intracellular stores, and has other pleiotropic properties. In the ER, DLPs acquire transient envelopes, which are lost as the outer capsid proteins VP4 and VP7 are assembled onto DLPs, resulting in the maturation of infectious TLPs. The progeny virions are released by cell lysis or, in polarized epithelial cells, by a non-classical vesicular transport mechanism (for further details see [3,4]).

## 4. Rotavirus Pathogenesis

Rotaviruses infect the mature enterocytes at the tips of the villous epithelium of the small intestine. Upon release of replicated viral progeny, epithelia are destroyed leading to an absorptive diarrhea. A crypt cell hyperplasia to replace the lost villous epithelium is accompanied by a secretory diarrhea component. The RV NSP4 acts as an enterotoxin [3], and the enteric nervous system is also involved in the emergence of diarrhea and vomiting [15,16]. The pathogenesis of RV AGE is multifactorial, and various RV gene products (VP3, VP4, VP7, NSP1, NSP2, NSP3 and NSP4) were found to be involved [3,4,17]. Human rotavirus-associated AGE is mainly caused by RVAs of highly variable genotypes, but also by species B rotaviruses (RVB; associated with diarrhea in adults in China) and species C rotaviruses (RVC, associated with some smaller disease outbreaks) [4].

## 5. Rotavirus Molecular Epidemiology

RVAs are transmitted via the faecal-oral route or by contaminated fomites, and clinical AGE occurs after an incubation period of 1–2 days. In the USA RVAs cause 5–10% of all cases of AGE in children <5 years of age [3]. In countries of temperate climate RVA-related outbreaks/epidemics take place during the winter months, and the genotype combinations P[8]G1, P[4]G12, P[8]G3, P[8]G4, P[8]G19, and P[8]G12 are found in the majority of clinical isolates [18,19]. In African, Asian and South American countries the genotype diversity is much higher, including P[8]G5 and P[6]G8 RVAs [20,21].

## 6. Immune Responses to Rotavirus Infection/Vaccination

Rotavirus infection elicits non-virus-specific innate and virus-specific acquired immune responses.

A. Innate immune responses (IIR). Upon rotavirus infection, the RNAs produced by actively transcribing DLPs are recognized by RIG-I and MDA-5 receptors, triggering the activation of transcription factors IRF-3 (Interferon [IFN] regulatory factor 3) and NF-κB. Those compounds migrate to the cell nucleus and stimulate IFN stimulatory genes (ISGs) and the production of IFN, which is secreted. Binding of IFN to other cells (which may or may not be infected) leads to activation of the transcription factors STAT1, STAT2 and IRF9, which in turn activate the transcription of ISGs and IFN in the nucleus, conveying an 'antiviral state' to the cell. NSP1, one of the non-structural gene products of RV, can block the IRF3/NF-κB pathway of the IIR, leading to the degradation of these compounds [22]. Furthermore, RV infection was observed to block the migration of STAT1, STAT2 and NF-κB to the nucleus, thus preventing host cell immune responses [23] (for further details, see [24]).

B. RV-specific humoral and cellular immune responses. Following rotavirus infection, virus-specific immune responses are elicited in B cells, which produce humoral antibodies, and in T cells, which recognize T-cell specific RV protein epitopes on the surface of infected cells in complexes with major histocompatibility (MHC) class I or class II antigens. The antibodies directed against VP7 and VP4 can neutralize *in vitro* and protect *in vivo* as shown by passive transfer experiments [25,26]. VP6-specific antibody can protect by 'intracellular neutralization' [27,28]. Passive transfer of RV-specific CD8+ T cells has also been shown to be protective [25].

For RVs, correlates of protection mainly consist of neutralizing antibodies and VP6 antibodies of the IgA class. However, the full correlates of protection against RV disease have not been identified [24,26,29].

## 7. Prevention of Rotavirus Disease by Vaccination

In 2006, two live attenuated RV vaccines were developed and licensed: Rotarix® and RotaTeq®. Rotarix® is a monovalent vaccine derived from a human G1P[8] isolate. RotaTeq® is pentavalent, consisting of a mixture of human bovine RV mono-reassortants, carrying the genes encoding the human G1, G2, G3, G4 and P[8] proteins in a genetic background of the bovine rotavirus Wi79 (G6P[5]). Both vaccines were found to be highly efficacious in phase III clinical trials [30,31] and have been included into the EPI scheme of childhood vaccination in >100 countries since 2006. Post-marketing studies showed both vaccines to be highly effective at population level [32–34]. The finding of 'herd immunity' in non-vaccinated children in contact with vaccines was a surprising but welcome 'side effect' [32,35].

## 8. Differences in Rotavirus Vaccine Effectiveness: Causes and Contributing Factors

Whereas vaccine effectiveness was high in high-income countries with protection rates against severe RV-disease at 80–90% [32–34], it was 30–50% lower in low- and middle-income countries, mainly in sub-Saharan Africa and S.E. Asia, where the vaccine is needed most [5–8]. In India, a human bovine natural reassortant vaccine consisting of the 116E RV strain (G9P8[11]) (originally isolated from asymptomatically infected neonates in India) was found to have an efficacy of 49–55% over two years against severe RV disease [36], i.e., to be of similar efficacy as Rotarix and RotaTeq in low income countries (see above), and is now being introduced for universal vaccination [37]. The reasons for the lower effectiveness of RV vaccination in low-income countries are at present not fully understood [24,26,38–40]. In the following, various factors by which the life of children in low-income countries differ from that in high-income countries will be reviewed.

### 8.1. Malnutrition

Malnutrition is associated with dysfunctions of innate and adaptive immunity [41] and therefore is a major factor negatively affecting vaccine efficacy and effectiveness in low- and middle-income countries [42]. Malnutrition has long been recognized as a determinant of adverse patient outcome in hospital [43]. Whereas some studies were uncertain about whether malnutrition decreased the efficacy of vaccination [44,45], more recently such a correlation was considered likely, in particular for RV vaccination [46,47]. Two components of malnutrition have attracted particular attention: zinc deficiency and avitaminoses.

### 8.1.1. Zinc Deficiency

Zinc deficiency alters immune functions [48] and is known to be a contributing factor to severe diarrhea [49]. Zinc deficiency is a major cause of childhood morbidity and mortality in low-income countries, in particular since it occurs in parallel with deficiencies of other micronutrients and animal proteins [49]. Environmental enteropathy (see below) perturbs zinc homeostasis in the gut [49]. Therefore, zinc supplementation reduces the incidence and severity of diarrhea, but is also considered to be part of a prevention strategy. The evaluation is complex: The zinc concentration in plasma is an indicator of zinc store status, and low concentration can indicate zinc deficiency (71% sensitivity), but this parameter is insensitive to early zinc depletion. Clinical symptoms of zinc deficiency are acne, dermatitis, alopecia, stomatitis, diarrhea, impaired immune responses, and hunger. In Bangladesh, lower zinc levels were found to be associated with an increased risk of developing RV disease [50]. A diarrhea-prevention program in Zambia, which included RV vaccination and zinc supplementation, led to a decrease of diarrhea-associated mortality of children of <5 years of age by 34% [51].

### 8.1.2. Avitaminoses

Sufficient concentrations of vitamins are vital for appropriate functions of the immune system [52]. In this context, vitamins A and D are of particular importance.

#### Vitamin A

Besides exerting various other functions, vitamin A is a key regulator of gut immunity (controlling mucosal homing of B and T cells, enhancing IgA antibody formation and secretion mediated by gut dendritic cells, maintaining integrity of mucosal surfaces, etc). Vitamin A deficiency (VAD) is found in 33% of all preschool children globally, but in 44% of them in Africa and 50% in SE Asia. Vitamin A supplementation reduces morbidity and mortality from diarrhea. There is good experimental evidence that prenatal VAD impairs the immune responses to RV vaccination. Gnotobiotic (gn) piglets with VAD have an imbalanced innate immune response to RV vaccination and upon challenge by human RV infection develop exacerbated disease, i.e., prolonged diarrhea, higher RV shedding, and are protected against RV disease to only 25%, compared to 100% of protection of vaccinated animals without VAD [53–55]. Vitamin A supplementation is recognized as a measure which increases vaccine efficiency/effectiveness [56].

Vitamin D

Apart from its effects on bone development and stability (deficiency causing rickets), vitamin D is important for the functioning of the immune system, since vitamin D deficiency (VDD) has been found to be associated with decreased immune responses to vaccines [57,58]. Low levels of vitamin D were observed to be associated with severe RV diarrhea compared to vitamin D adequate controls [59]. In gn piglets, vitamin D deficiency was shown to decrease the innate immune response to RV challenge, likely by activation of the RIG-I signalling pathway [60].

In a project jointly funded by Danish, Swedish and Bangladeshi agencies and research groups, using routine cost-benefit analyses, various health care measures were assessed for their benefit to the people of Bangladesh. It turned out that countering malnutrition of small children with micronutrient supplements (iodized salt, vitamin A, zinc) would generate a 19-fold benefit for each $1 spent [61].

*8.2. Gut Microbiota*

The gut microbiota of children in low-income countries are different from those of children in high- and middle-income countries: they are more diverse and more variable over time [62–64]. The composition of gut microbiota affects the immune system in different ways [65–69]. From work with gn pigs, there is good experimental evidence that the presence of gut commensals (probiotics) decreases the clinical symptoms of RV disease [70–74]. Intestinal commensals, e.g., *Lactobacillus rhamnosus GG*, *L acidophilus*, *L reuteri*, *Bifidobacterium lactis Bb12*, regulate the development of gut immunity and decrease the severity of viral gut infections. Colonisation of gn piglets with *LGG* and *Bb12* increased the immune response to RV vaccine (leading to 'immune homeostasis'), strengthened the tight junctions of ileum epithelium and resulted in less viral shedding and decreased diarrhea after RV infection, compared to non-colonized piglets. A significant correlation between the composition of the infant gut microbiome and response to RV vaccination was found in Ghana [75]. More generally, the composition of the gut microbiome is important for the pathogenesis of chronic inflammatory bowel diseases and other extra-intestinal infectious diseases [76–79]. In detail, the pathogenetic mechanisms remain to be explored, since the gut microbiome resides mainly in the large intestine. The gut microbiome is of such importance that a human intestinal tract chip was developed recording the temporal and qualitative dynamics of its composition [80].

Gn piglets can be transplanted with human gut microbiota (HGM) or pig gut microbiota (PGM). HGM-transplanted gn piglets show a switch from *Lactobacillus* spp (*Firmicutes*) to *Aeromonas*, *Erwinia*, *Klebsiella* (*Proteobacteria*) upon challenge with human RV. This change is prevented by pretreatment of piglets with *Lactobacillus rhamnosus* GG; the reasons for this remain unclear [81]. Selected gram-negative probiotics (e.g., *E. coli Nissle*) appear to be more effective than gram-positive probiotics (e.g., *Lactobacillus* spp) in enhancing protective immunity against RV in the gn piglet model [82]. Human enteric dysbiosis and its influence on RV immunity has now been modelled in gn pigs [83], and the effects of fecal transplantations on gut eubiosis is being studied [84].

*8.3. Co-Infections*

Similar to commensal gut microbiota [75], other infections can affect the outcome of RV vaccination. Thus, concurrent enterovirus infections were correlated with poor IgA seroconversion to RV1 in Bangladesh [85]. In Ecuador, co-infections with RVs and other enteric pathogens (*Giardia*, *E. coli*, *Shigella*) acted synergistically, with the pathogenicity of the individual microbe being enhanced [86,87].

Studies in Taiwan found that children infected with non-typhoid *Salmonella* spp had a greater risk of bacteremia [88] and prolonged hospitalization [89], when they were co-infected with RVs. Similarly, children infected with *Clostridium difficile* had more severe clinical symptoms when co-infected with RVs [90].

*8.4. Immaturity/Functional Reduction of the Infant's Immune System*

A newborn child's immune system (both innate and acquired) is immature and develops during infancy and childhood [91]. 'Intrinsic reduced immunogenicity' to RV vaccination and natural RV infection is a recognized condition in low-income countries, although it is not very well defined [38].

*8.5. Environmental Enteropathy*

Environmental enteropathy (EE) is characterized by anatomical and functional abnormalities in the small intestine of children living in low-income countries [92,93]. The response to RV vaccination is decreased in children presenting with biomarkers of EE [94,95].

*8.6. Passive Transfer of Maternal Antibodies*

8.6.1. Rotavirus Antibody Transferred to Infants in Breast Milk

Data from Africa [47,96], Europe [97] and the USA [98] did not show significant differences in RV vaccine efficacy, which depended on RV-specific antibodies passively transferred by mother's breast milk. Transient abstention from breastfeeding around the time of RV vaccination did not increase the efficacy of RV vaccination [99,100].

8.6.2. Transplacentally Acquired Maternal RV Specific Antibodies

Studies from Nicaragua [101], India [99,102] and South Africa [103] demonstrated that mother's RV-specific IgG levels before RV vaccination of their infants was negatively associated with infants' seroconversion after RV vaccination. A similar trend observed for vaccines in New Zealand lacked significance [104].

*8.7. Genetic Factors*

Rotaviruses bind to sialic acid residues or histo-blood group antigens (HBGAs) as cellular attachment receptors in a strain-specific manner [105–107]. The expression of HBGAs is genetically determined and developmentally regulated [107]. Genetic differences of HBGA expression may affect susceptibility of infection by different RV strains [108] and may impact the efficacy of RV vaccination [109]. More extensive data are required to answer the question of whether the expression of particular HBGAs of infants will determine their susceptibility to RV infections and interfere with the uptake of RV vaccines.

## 9. Outlook and Future Research

A number of health conditions, by which infants in low income countries differ from children in high income countries have been recognized as being important for the outcome of RV and other microbial infections and of vaccination with one of the licensed RV vaccines. The major problems are: malnutrition with deficiencies in micronutrients (zinc, vitamin A, vitamin D), connected with functional reduction of innate and acquired immune responses, and the gut microbiome which is of proven influence for disease severity and vaccine uptake. Maternal RV-specific antibodies are of variable importance for disease and vaccine outcome. Specific diarrhea prevention programs (supply of nutrients and micronutrients, such as vitamins, combined with RV vaccination) have been shown to be beneficial.

There are still many aspects requiring further research such as: the mechanisms by which micronutrients affect the immune system, the multifactorial influences of the gut microbiome on disease severity and vaccine take, a more detailed characterization of environmental enteropathy, the influence of host genetics on disease severity and outcome of vaccination, and further development of RV vaccines.

There is great optimism that recent achievements in basic virology will contribute to progress in these topics. First, RV replication in stem cell-derived human intestinal enteroid cultures [110] will help to advance many questions of viral replication and pathogenesis. Second, the availability of an entirely plasmid-based reverse genetics system for RVs [111] will help tackle research questions which before could not be addressed and will, besides many other topics, permit progress in the development of safer and widely cross-reactive RV vaccine candidates.

**Acknowledgments:** The author gratefully acknowledges discussion on the topic of this review with Beth D. Kirkpatrick and her research group at the University of Vermont, USA.

**Author Contributions:** U.D. wrote the review as a single author.

## References

1. Bishop, R.F.; Davidson, G.P.; Holmes, I.H.; Ruck, B.J. Virus particles in epithelial cells of duodenal mucosa from children with acute non-bacterial gastroenteritis. *Lancet* **1973**, *2*, 1281–1283. [CrossRef]
2. Flewett, T.H.; Bryden, A.S.; Davies, H. Virus particles in gastroenteritis. *Lancet* **1973**, *2*, 1497. [CrossRef]
3. Estes, M.K.; Greenberg, H.B. Rotaviruses. In *Fields Virology*, 6th ed.; Knipe, D.M., Howley, P.M., Cohen, J.I., Griffin, D.E., Lamb, R.A., Martin, M.A., Racaniello, V.R., Roizman, B., Eds.; Wolters Kluwer Health/Lippincott Williams & Wilkins: Philadelphia, PA, USA, 2013; pp. 1347–1401.
4. Desselberger, U. Rotaviruses. *Virus Res.* **2014**, *190*, 75–96. [CrossRef] [PubMed]
5. Armah, G.E.; Sow, S.O.; Breiman, R.F.; Dallas, M.J.; Tapia, M.D.; Feikin, D.R.; Binka, F.N.; Steele, A.D.; Laserson, K.F.; Ansah, N.A.; et al. Efficacy of pentavalent rotavirus vaccine against severe rotavirus gastroenteritis in infants in developing countries in sub-Saharan Africa: A randomised, double-blind, placebo-controlled trial. *Lancet* **2010**, *376*, 606–614. [CrossRef]
6. Madhi, S.A.; Cunliffe, N.A.; Steele, D.; Witte, D.; Kirsten, M.; Louw, C.; Ngwira, B.; Victor, J.C.; Gillard, P.H.; Cheuvart, B.B.; et al. Effect of human rotavirus vaccine on severe diarrhea in African infants. *N. Engl. J. Med.* **2010**, *362*, 289–298. [CrossRef] [PubMed]
7. Zaman, K.; Dang, D.A.; Victor, J.C.; Shin, S.; Yunus, M.; Dallas, M.J.; Podder, G.; Vu, D.T.; Le, T.P.; Luby, S.P.; et al. Efficacy of pentavalent rotavirus vaccine against severe rotavirus gastroenteritis in infants in developing countries in Asia: A randomised, double-blind, placebo-controlled trial. *Lancet* **2010**, *376*, 615–623. [CrossRef]
8. Tate, J.E.; Burton, A.H.; Boschi-Pinto, C.; Parashar, U.D. World Health Organization-Coordinated Global Rotavirus Surveillance Network. Global, regional, and national estimates of rotavirus mortality in children <5 years of age, 2000–2013. *Clin. Infect. Dis.* **2016**, *62* (Suppl. 2), S96–S105. [PubMed]
9. Pesavento, J.B.; Estes, M.K.; Prasad, B.V.V. Structural organization of the genome in rotavirus. In *Viral Gastroenteritis*; Desselberger, U., Gray, J., Eds.; Elsevier Science: Amsterdam, The Netherlands, 2003; pp. 115–127.
10. Matthijnssens, J.; Otto, P.H.; Ciarlet, M.; Desselberger, U.; Van Ranst, M.; Johne, R. VP6-sequence-based cutoff values as a criterion for rotavirus species demarcation. *Arch. Virol.* **2012**, *157*, 1177–1182. [CrossRef] [PubMed]
11. Mihalov-Kovács, E.; Gellért, Á.; Marton, S.; Farkas, S.L.; Fehér, E.; Oldal, M.; Jakab, F.; Martella, V.; Bányai, K. Candidate new rotavirus species in sheltered dogs, Hungary. *Emerg. Infect. Dis.* **2015**, *21*, 660–663. [CrossRef] [PubMed]
12. Bányai, K.; Kemenesi, G.; Budinski, I.; Földes, F.; Zana, B.; Marton, S.; Varga-Kugler, R.; Oldal, M.; Kurucz, K.; Jakab, F. Candidate new rotavirus species in Schreiber's bats, Serbia. *Infect. Genet. Evol.* **2017**, *48*, 19–26. [CrossRef] [PubMed]
13. Matthijnssens, J.; Ciarlet, M.; Heiman, E.; Arijs, I.; Delbeke, T.; McDonald, S.M.; Palombo, E.A.; Iturriza-Gómara, M.; Maes, P.; Patton, J.T.; et al. Full genome-based classification of rotaviruses reveals a common origin between human Wa-Like and porcine rotavirus strains and human DS-1-like and bovine rotavirus strains. *J. Virol.* **2008**, *82*, 3204–3219. [CrossRef] [PubMed]

14. Rega Institute, KU Leuven, Belgium. Available online: https://rega.kuleuven.be/cev/viralmetagenomics/virus-classification/7th-RCWG-meeting (accessed on 25 September 2017).
15. Lundgren, O.; Peregrin, A.T.; Persson, K.; Kordasti, S.; Uhnoo, I.; Svensson, L. Role of the enteric nervous system in the fluid and electrolyte secretion of rotavirus diarrhea. *Science* **2000**, *287*, 491–495. [CrossRef] [PubMed]
16. Hagbom, M.; Istrate, C.; Engblom, D.; Karlsson, T.; Rodriguez-Diaz, J.; Buesa, J.; Taylor, J.A.; Loitto, V.M.; Magnusson, K.E.; Ahlman, H.; et al. Rotavirus stimulates release of serotonin (5-HT) from human enterochromaffin cells and activates brain structures involved in nausea and vomiting. *PLoS Pathog.* **2011**, *7*, e1002115. [CrossRef] [PubMed]
17. Greenberg, H.B.; Estes, M.K. Rotaviruses: From pathogenesis to vaccination. *Gastroenterology* **2009**, *136*, 1939–1951. [CrossRef] [PubMed]
18. Santos, N.; Hoshino, Y. Global distribution of rotavirus serotypes/genotypes and its implication for the development and implementation of an effective rotavirus vaccine. *Rev. Med. Virol.* **2005**, *15*, 29–56. [CrossRef] [PubMed]
19. Iturriza-Gómara, M.; Dallman, T.; Bányai, K.; Böttiger, B.; Buesa, J.; Diedrich, S.; Fiore, L.; Johansen, K.; Koopmans, M.; Korsun, N.; et al. Rotavirus genotypes co-circulating in Europe between 2006 and 2009 as determined by EuroRotaNet, a pan-European collaborative strain surveillance network. *Epidemiol. Infect.* **2011**, *139*, 895–909. [CrossRef] [PubMed]
20. Todd, S.; Page, N.A.; Duncan Steele, A.; Peenze, I.; Cunliffe, N.A. Rotavirus strain types circulating in Africa: Review of studies published during 1997–2006. *J. Infect. Dis.* **2010**, *202*, S34–S42. [CrossRef] [PubMed]
21. Kang, G.; Desai, R.; Arora, R.; Chitamabar, S.; Naik, T.N.; Krishnan, T.; Deshpande, J.; Gupte, M.D.; Venkatasubramaniam, S.; Gentsch, J.R.; et al. Diversity of circulating rotavirus strains in children hospitalized with diarrhea in India, 2005–2009. *Vaccine* **2013**, *31*, 2879–2883. [CrossRef] [PubMed]
22. Graff, J.W.; Ettayebi, K.; Hardy, M.E. Rotavirus NSP1 inhibits NFkappaB activation by inducing proteasome-dependent degradation of beta-TrCP: A novel mechanism of IFN antagonism. *PLoS Pathog.* **2009**, *5*, e1000280. [CrossRef] [PubMed]
23. Holloway, G.; Truong, T.T.; Coulson, B.S. Rotavirus antagonizes cellular antiviral responses by inhibiting the nuclear accumulation of STAT1, STAT2, and NF-kappaB. *J. Virol.* **2009**, *83*, 4942–4951. [CrossRef] [PubMed]
24. Angel, J.; Franco, M.A.; Greenberg, H.B. Rotavirus immune responses and correlates of protection. *Curr. Opin. Virol.* **2012**, *2*, 419–425. [CrossRef] [PubMed]
25. Offit, P.A. Rotaviruses: Immunological determinants of protection against infection and disease. *Adv. Virus Res.* **1994**, *44*, 161–202. [PubMed]
26. Franco, M.A.; Angel, J.; Greenberg, H.B. Immunity and correlates of protection for rotavirus vaccines. *Vaccine* **2006**, *24*, 2718–2731. [CrossRef] [PubMed]
27. Burns, J.W.; Siadat-Pajouh, M.; Krishnaney, A.A.; Greenberg, H.B. Protective effect of rotavirus VP6-specific IgA monoclonal antibodies that lack neutralizing activity. *Science* **1996**, *272*, 104–107. [CrossRef] [PubMed]
28. Sapparapu, G.; Sims, A.L.; Aiyegbo, M.S.; Shaikh, F.Y.; Harth, E.M.; Crowe, J.E., Jr. Intracellular neutralization of a virus using a cell-penetrating molecular transporter. *Nanomedicine* **2014**, *9*, 1613–1624. [CrossRef] [PubMed]
29. Desselberger, U.; Huppertz, H.I. Immune responses to rotavirus infection and vaccination and associated correlates of protection. *J. Infect. Dis.* **2011**, *203*, 188–195. [CrossRef] [PubMed]
30. Ruiz-Palacios, G.M.; Pérez-Schael, I.; Velázquez, F.R.; Abate, H.; Breuer, T.; Clemens, S.C.; Cheuvart, B.; Espinoza, F.; Gillard, P.; Innis, B.L.; et al. Safety and efficacy of an attenuated vaccine against severe rotavirus gastroenteritis. *N. Engl. J. Med.* **2006**, *354*, 11–22. [CrossRef] [PubMed]
31. Vesikari, T.; Matson, D.O.; Dennehy, P.; Van Damme, P.; Santosham, M.; Rodriguez, Z.; Dallas, M.J.; Heyse, J.F.; Goveia, M.G.; Black, S.B.; et al. Safety and efficacy of a pentavalent human-bovine (WC3) reassortant rotavirus vaccine. *N. Engl. J. Med.* **2006**, *354*, 23–33. [CrossRef] [PubMed]
32. Leshem, E.; Moritz, R.E.; Curns, A.T.; Zhou, F.; Tate, J.E.; Lopman, B.A.; Parashar, U.D. Rotavirus vaccines and health care utilization for diarrhea in the United States (2007–2011). *Pediatrics* **2014**, *134*, 15–23. [CrossRef] [PubMed]
33. Rha, B.; Tate, J.E.; Payne, D.C.; Cortese, M.M.; Lopman, B.A.; Curns, A.T.; Parashar, U.D. Effectiveness and impact of rotavirus vaccines in the United States—2006–2012. *Expert Rev. Vaccines* **2014**, *13*, 365–376. [CrossRef] [PubMed]

34. Jonesteller, C.L.; Burnett, E.; Yen, C.; Tate, J.E.; Parashar, U.D. Effectiveness of Rotavirus Vaccination: A systematic review of the first decade of global post-licensure data, 2006–2016. *Clin. Infect. Dis.* **2017**. [CrossRef] [PubMed]
35. Pollard, S.L.; Malpica-Llanos, T.; Friberg, I.K.; Fischer-Walker, C.; Ashraf, S.; Walker, N. Estimating the herd immunity effect of rotavirus vaccine. *Vaccine* **2015**, *33*, 3795–3800. [CrossRef] [PubMed]
36. Bhandari, N.; Rongsen-Chandola, T.; Bavdekar, A.; John, J.; Antony, K.; Taneja, S.; Goyal, N.; Kawade, A.; Kang, G.; Rathore, S.S.; et al. Efficacy of a monovalent human-bovine (116E) rotavirus vaccine in Indian infants: A randomised, double-blind, placebo-controlled trial. *Lancet* **2014**, *383*, 2136–2143. [CrossRef]
37. Tate, J.E.; Arora, R.; Kang, G.; Parashar, U.D. Rotavirus vaccines at the threshold of implementation in India. *Natl. Med. J. India* **2014**, *27*, 245–248. [PubMed]
38. Lopman, B.A.; Pitzer, V.E.; Sarkar, R.; Gladstone, B.; Patel, M.; Glasser, J.; Gambhir, M.; Athison, C.; Grenfell, B.T.; Edmunds, W.J.; et al. Understanding reduced rotavirus vaccine efficacy in low socio-economic settings. *PLoS ONE* **2012**, *7*, e41720. [CrossRef] [PubMed]
39. Kirkpatrick, B.D.; Colgate, E.R.; Mychaleckyj, J.C.; Haque, R.; Dickson, D.M.; Carmolli, M.P.; Nayak, U.; Taniuchi, M.; Naylor, C.; Qadri, F.; et al. The "Performance of Rotavirus and Oral Polio Vaccines in Developing Countries" (PROVIDE) study: Description of methods of an interventional study designed to explore complex biologic problems. *Am. J. Trop. Med. Hyg.* **2015**, *92*, 744–751. [CrossRef] [PubMed]
40. Clarke, E.; Desselberger, U. Correlates of protection against human rotavirus disease and the factors influencing protection in low-income settings. *Mucosal Immunol.* **2015**, *8*, 1–17. [CrossRef] [PubMed]
41. Prendergast, A.J. Malnutrition and vaccination in developing countries. *Philos. Trans. R. Soc. Lond. B Biol. Sci.* **2015**, *370*. [CrossRef] [PubMed]
42. Hoest, C.; Seidman, J.C.; Pan, W.; Ambikapathi, R.; Kang, G.; Kosek, M.; Knobler, S.; Mason, C.J.; Miller, M.; MAL-ED Network Investigators. Evaluating associations between vaccine response and malnutrition, gut function, and enteric infections in the MAL-ED cohort study: Methods and challenges. *Clin. Infect. Dis.* **2014**, *59* (Suppl. 4), S273–S279. [CrossRef] [PubMed]
43. Stratton, R.J.; Elia, M. Deprivation linked to malnutrition risk and mortality in hospital. *Br. J. Nutr.* **2006**, *96*, 870–876. [CrossRef] [PubMed]
44. Perez-Schael, I.; Salinas, B.; Tomat, M.; Linhares, A.C.; Guerrero, M.L.; Ruiz-Palacios, G.M.; Bouckenooghe, A.; Yarzabal, J.P. Efficacy of the human rotavirus vaccine RIX4414 in malnourished children. *J. Infect. Dis.* **2007**, *196*, 537–540. [CrossRef] [PubMed]
45. Savy, M.; Edmond, K.; Fine, P.E.; Hall, A.; Hennig, B.J.; Moore, S.E.; Mulholland, K.; Schaible, U.; Prentice, A.M. Landscape analysis of interactions between nutrition and vaccine responses in children. *J. Nutr.* **2009**, *139*, 2154S–2218S. [CrossRef] [PubMed]
46. Gastañaduy, P.A.; Contreras-Roldán, I.; Bernart, C.; López, B.; Benoit, S.R.; Xuya, M.; Muñoz, F.; Desai, R.; Quaye, O.; Tam, K.I.; et al. Effectiveness of Monovalent and Pentavalent Rotavirus Vaccines in Guatemala. *Clin. Infect. Dis.* **2016**, *62* (Suppl. 2), S121–S126. [CrossRef] [PubMed]
47. Gruber, J.F.; Hille, D.A.; Liu, G.F.; Kaplan, S.S.; Nelson, M.; Goveia, M.G.; Mast, T.C. Heterogeneity of Rotavirus Vaccine Efficacy Among Infants in Developing Countries. *Pediatr. Infect. Dis. J.* **2017**, *36*, 72–78. [CrossRef] [PubMed]
48. Ibs, K.H.; Rink, L. Zinc-altered immune function. *J. Nutr.* **2003**, *133*, 1452S–1456S. [PubMed]
49. Young, G.P.; Mortimer, E.K.; Gopalsamy, G.L.; Alpers, D.H.; Binder, H.J.; Manary, M.J.; Ramakrishna, B.S.; Brown, I.L.; Brewer, T.G. Zinc deficiency in children with environmental enteropathy-development of new strategies: Report from an expert workshop. *Am. J. Clin. Nutr.* **2014**, *100*, 1198–1207. [CrossRef] [PubMed]
50. Colgate, E.R.; Haque, R.; Dickson, D.M.; Carmolli, M.P.; Mychaleckyj, J.C.; Nayak, U.; Qadri, F.; Alam, M.; Walsh, M.C.; Diehl, S.A.; et al. Delayed Dosing of Oral Rotavirus Vaccine Demonstrates Decreased Risk of Rotavirus Gastroenteritis Associated With Serum Zinc: A Randomized Controlled Trial. *Clin. Infect. Dis.* **2016**, *63*, 634–641. [CrossRef] [PubMed]
51. Bosomprah, S.; Beach, L.B.; Beres, L.K.; Newman, J.; Kapasa, K.; Rudd, C.; Njobvu, L.; Guffey, B.; Hubbard, S.; Foo, K.; et al. Findings from a comprehensive diarrhoea prevention and treatment programme in Lusaka, Zambia. *BMC Public Health* **2016**, *16*, 475. [CrossRef] [PubMed]
52. Mora, J.R.; Iwata, M.; von Andrian, U.H. Vitamin effects on the immune system: Vitamins A and D take centre stage. *Nat. Rev. Immunol.* **2008**, *8*, 685–698. [CrossRef] [PubMed]

53. Vlasova, A.N.; Chattha, K.S.; Kandasamy, S.; Siegismund, C.S.; Saif, L.J. Prenatally acquired vitamin A deficiency alters innate immune responses to human rotavirus in a gnotobiotic pig model. *J. Immunol.* **2013**, *190*, 4742–4753. [CrossRef] [PubMed]
54. Chattha, K.S.; Kandasamy, S.; Vlasova, A.N.; Saif, L.J. Vitamin A deficiency impairs adaptive B and T cell responses to a prototype monovalent attenuated human rotavirus vaccine and virulent human rotavirus challenge in a gnotobiotic piglet model. *PLoS ONE* **2013**, *8*, e82966. [CrossRef] [PubMed]
55. Kandasamy, S.; Chattha, K.S.; Vlasova, A.N.; Saif, L.J. Prenatal vitamin A deficiency impairs adaptive immune responses to pentavalent rotavirus vaccine (RotaTeq®) in a neonatal gnotobiotic pig model. *Vaccine* **2014**, *32*, 816–824. [CrossRef] [PubMed]
56. Jensen, K.J.; Ndure, J.; Plebanski, M.; Flanagan, K.L. Heterologous and sex differential effects of administering vitamin A supplementation with vaccines. *Trans. R. Soc. Trop. Med. Hyg.* **2015**, *109*, 36–45. [CrossRef] [PubMed]
57. Zitt, E.; Sprenger-Mähr, H.; Knoll, F.; Neyer, U.; Lhotta, K. Vitamin D deficiency is associated with poor response to active hepatitis B immunisation in patients with chronic kidney disease. *Vaccine* **2012**, *30*, 931–935. [CrossRef] [PubMed]
58. Surman, S.L.; Penkert, R.R.; Jones, B.G.; Sealy, R.E.; Hurwitz, J.L. Vitamin Supplementation at the Time of Immunization with a Cold-Adapted Influenza Virus Vaccine Corrects Poor Mucosal Antibody Responses in Mice Deficient for Vitamins A and D. *Clin. Vaccine Immunol.* **2016**, *23*, 219–227. [CrossRef] [PubMed]
59. Bucak, I.H.; Ozturk, A.B.; Almis, H.; Cevik, M.Ö.; Tekin, M.; Konca, Ç.; Turgut, M.; Bulbul, M. Is there a relationship between low vitamin D and rotaviral diarrhea? *Pediatr. Int.* **2016**, *58*, 270–273. [CrossRef] [PubMed]
60. Zhao, Y.; Yu, B.; Mao, X.; He, J.; Huang, Z.; Zheng, P.; Yu, J.; Han, G.; Liang, X.; Chen, D. Dietary vitamin D supplementation attenuates immune responses of pigs challenged with rotavirus potentially through the retinoic acid-inducible gene I signalling pathway. *Br. J. Nutr.* **2014**, *112*, 381–389. [CrossRef] [PubMed]
61. Lomberg, B. Making government smarter. How to set national priorities. *For. Aff.* **2017**, *96*, 90–98.
62. Dethlefsen, L.; McFall-Ngai, M.; Relman, D.A. An ecological and evolutionary perspective on human-microbe mutualism and disease. *Nature* **2007**, *449*, 811–818. [CrossRef] [PubMed]
63. Lin, A.; Bik, E.M.; Costello, E.K.; Dethlefsen, L.; Haque, R.; Relman, D.A.; Singh, U. Distinct distal gut microbiome diversity and composition in healthy children from Bangladesh and the United States. *PLoS ONE* **2013**, *8*, e53838. [CrossRef] [PubMed]
64. Azad, M.B.; Konya, T.; Maughan, H.; Guttman, D.S.; Field, C.J.; Chari, R.S.; Sears, M.R.; Becker, A.B.; Scott, J.A.; Kozyrskyj, A.L.; et al. Gut microbiota of healthy Canadian infants: Profiles by mode of delivery and infant diet at 4 months. *Can. Med. Assoc. J.* **2013**, *185*, 385–394. [CrossRef] [PubMed]
65. Chinen, T.; Rudensky, A.Y. The effects of commensal microbiota on immune cell subsets and inflammatory responses. *Immunol. Rev.* **2012**, *245*, 45–55. [CrossRef] [PubMed]
66. Gallo, R.L.; Hooper, L.V. Epithelial antimicrobial defence of the skin and intestine. *Nat. Rev. Immunol.* **2012**, *12*, 503–516. [CrossRef] [PubMed]
67. Kamada, N.; Chen, G.Y.; Inohara, N.; Núñez, G. Control of pathogens and pathobionts by the gut microbiota. *Nat. Immunol.* **2013**, *14*, 685–690. [CrossRef] [PubMed]
68. Kamada, N.; Seo, S.U.; Chen, G.Y.; Núñez, G. Role of the gut microbiota in immunity and inflammatory disease. *Nat. Rev. Immunol.* **2013**, *13*, 321–335. [CrossRef] [PubMed]
69. Praharaj, I.; John, S.M.; Bandyopadhyay, R.; Kang, G. Probiotics, antibiotics and the immune responses to vaccines. *Philos. Trans. R. Soc. Lond. B Biol. Sci.* **2015**, *370*. [CrossRef] [PubMed]
70. Zhang, W.; Azevedo, M.S.; Wen, K.; Gonzalez, A.; Saif, L.J.; Li, G.; Yousef, A.E.; Yuan, L. Probiotic Lactobacillus acidophilus enhances the immunogenicity of an oral rotavirus vaccine in gnotobiotic pigs. *Vaccine* **2008**, *26*, 3655–3661. [CrossRef] [PubMed]
71. Vlasova, A.N.; Chattha, K.S.; Kandasamy, S.; Liu, Z.; Esseili, M.; Shao, L.; Rajashekara, G.; Saif, L.J. Lactobacilli and bifidobacteria promote immune homeostasis by modulating innate immune responses to human rotavirus in neonatal gnotobiotic pigs. *PLoS ONE* **2013**, *8*, e76962. [CrossRef] [PubMed]
72. Chattha, K.S.; Vlasova, A.N.; Kandasamy, S.; Rajashekara, G.; Saif, L.J. Divergent immunomodulating effects of probiotics on T cell responses to oral attenuated human rotavirus vaccine and virulent human rotavirus infection in a neonatal gnotobiotic piglet disease model. *J. Immunol.* **2013**, *191*, 2446–2456. [CrossRef] [PubMed]

73. Liu, F.; Li, G.; Wen, K.; Wu, S.; Zhang, Y.; Bui, T.; Yang, X.; Kocher, J.; Sun, J.; Jortner, B.; et al. Lactobacillus rhamnosus GG on rotavirus-induced injury of ileal epithelium in gnotobiotic pigs. *J. Pediatr. Gastroenterol. Nutr.* **2013**, *57*, 750–758. [CrossRef] [PubMed]
74. Kandasamy, S.; Chattha, K.S.; Vlasova, A.N.; Rajashekara, G.; Saif, L.J. Lactobacilli and Bifidobacteria enhance mucosal B cell responses and differentially modulate systemic antibody responses to an oral human rotavirus vaccine in a neonatal gnotobiotic pig disease model. *Gut Microbes* **2014**, *5*, 639–651. [CrossRef] [PubMed]
75. Harris, V.C.; Armah, G.; Fuentes, S.; Korpela, K.E.; Parashar, U.; Victor, J.C.; Tate, J.; de Weerth, C.; Giaquinto, C.; Wiersinga, W.J.; et al. Significant correlation between the infant gut microbiome and rotavirus vaccine response in rural Ghana. *J. Infect. Dis.* **2017**, *215*, 34–41. [CrossRef] [PubMed]
76. Virgin, H.W. The virome in mammalian physiology and disease. *Cell* **2014**, *157*, 142–150. [CrossRef] [PubMed]
77. Norman, J.M.; Handley, S.A.; Virgin, H.W. Kingdom-agnostic metagenomics and the importance of complete characterization of enteric microbial communities. *Gastroenterology* **2014**, *146*, 1459–1469. [CrossRef] [PubMed]
78. Wang, W.; Jovel, J.; Halloran, B.; Wine, E.; Patterson, J.; Ford, G.; O'Keefe, S.; Meng, B.; Song, D.; Zhang, Y.; et al. Metagenomic analysis of microbiome in colon tissue from subjects with inflammatory bowel diseases reveals interplay of viruses and bacteria. *Inflamm. Bowel Dis.* **2015**, *21*, 1419–1427. [CrossRef] [PubMed]
79. Harris, V.C.; Haak, B.W.; Boele van Hensbroek, M.; Wiersinga, W.J. The Intestinal Microbiome in Infectious Diseases: The Clinical Relevance of a Rapidly Emerging Field. *Open Forum Infect. Dis.* **2017**, *4*, ofx144. [CrossRef] [PubMed]
80. Rajilić-Stojanović, M.; Heilig, H.G.; Molenaar, D.; Kajander, K.; Surakka, A.; Smidt, H.; de Vos, W.M. Development and application of the human intestinal tract chip, a phylogenetic microarray: Analysis of universally conserved phylotypes in the abundant microbiota of young and elderly adults. *Environ. Microbiol.* **2009**, *11*, 1736–1751. [CrossRef] [PubMed]
81. Zhang, H.; Wang, H.; Shepherd, M.; Wen, K.; Li, G.; Yang, X.; Kocher, J.; Giri-Rachman, E.; Dickerman, A.; Settlage, R.; et al. Probiotics and virulent human rotavirus modulate the transplanted human gut microbiota in gnotobiotic pigs. *Gut Pathog.* **2014**, *6*, 39. [CrossRef] [PubMed]
82. Kandasamy, S.; Vlasova, A.N.; Fischer, D.D.; Chattha, K.S.; Shao, L.; Kumar, A.; Langel, S.N.; Rauf, A.; Huang, H.C.; Rajashekara, G.; et al. Unraveling the Differences between Gram-Positive and Gram-Negative Probiotics in Modulating Protective Immunity to Enteric Infections. *Front. Immunol.* **2017**, *8*, 334. [CrossRef] [PubMed]
83. Twitchell, E.L.; Tin, C.; Wen, K.; Zhang, H.; Becker-Dreps, S.; Azcarate-Peril, M.A.; Vilchez, S.; Li, G.; Ramesh, A.; Weiss, M.; et al. Modeling human enteric dysbiosis and rotavirus immunity in gnotobiotic pigs. *Gut Pathog.* **2016**, *8*, 51. [CrossRef] [PubMed]
84. Gallo, A.; Passaro, G.; Gasbarrini, A.; Landolfi, R.; Montalto, M. Modulation of microbiota as treatment for intestinal inflammatory disorders: An uptodate. *World J. Gastroenterol.* **2016**, *22*, 7186–7202. [CrossRef] [PubMed]
85. Taniuchi, M.; Platts-Mills, J.A.; Begum, S.; Uddin, M.J.; Sobuz, S.U.; Liu, J.; Kirkpatrick, B.D.; Colgate, E.R.; Carmolli, M.P.; Dickson, D.M.; et al. Impact of enterovirus and other enteric pathogens on oral polio and rotavirus vaccine performance in Bangladeshi infants. *Vaccine* **2016**, *34*, 3068–3075. [CrossRef] [PubMed]
86. Bhavnani, D.; Goldstick, J.E.; Cevallos, W.; Trueba, G.; Eisenberg, J.N.S. Synergistic effects between rotavirus and coinfecting pathogens on diarrheal disease: Evidence from a community-based study in Northwestern Ecuador. *Am. J. Epidemiol.* **2012**, *176*, 387–395. [CrossRef] [PubMed]
87. Vasco, G.; Trueba, G.; Atherton, R.; Calvopiña, M.; Cevallos, W.; Andrade, T.; Eguiguren, M.; Eisenberg, J.N. Identifying etiological agents causing diarrhea in low income Ecuadorian communities. *Am. J. Trop. Med. Hyg.* **2014**, *91*, 563–569. [CrossRef] [PubMed]
88. Hung, T.Y.; Liu, M.C.; Hsu, C.F.; Lin, Y.C. Rotavirus infection increases the risk of bacteremia in children with nontyphoid Salmonella gastroenteritis. *Eur. J. Clin. Microbiol. Infect. Dis.* **2009**, *28*, 425–428. [CrossRef] [PubMed]
89. Lee, W.T.; Lin, P.C.; Lin, L.C.; Chen, H.L.; Yang, R.C. Salmonella/rotavirus coinfection in hospitalized children. *Kaohsiung J. Med. Sci.* **2012**, *28*, 595–600. [CrossRef] [PubMed]

90. Valentini, D.; Vittucci, A.C.; Grandin, A.; Tozzi, A.E.; Russo, C.; Onori, M.; Menichella, D.; Bartuli, A.; Villani, A. Coinfection in acute gastroenteritis predicts a more severe clinical course in children. *Eur. J. Clin. Microbiol. Infect. Dis.* **2013**, *32*, 909–915. [CrossRef] [PubMed]
91. Simon, A.K.; Hollander, G.A.; McMichael, A. Evolution of the immune system in humans from infancy to old age. *Proc. Biol. Sci.* **2015**, *282*, 20143085. [CrossRef] [PubMed]
92. Campbell, D.I.; Murch, S.H.; Elia, M.; Sullivan, P.B.; Sanyang, M.S.; Jobarteh, B.; Lunn, P.G. Chronic T cell-mediated enteropathy in rural west African children: Relationship with nutritional status and small bowel function. *Pediatr. Res.* **2003**, *54*, 306–311. [CrossRef] [PubMed]
93. Campbell, D.I.; Elia, M.; Lunn, P.G. Growth faltering in rural Gambian infants is associated with impaired small intestinal barrier function, leading to endotoxemia and systemic inflammation. *J. Nutr.* **2003**, *133*, 1332–1338. [PubMed]
94. Naylor, C.; Lu, M.; Haque, R.; Mondal, D.; Buonomo, E.; Nayak, U.; Mychaleckyj, J.C.; Kirkpatrick, B.; Colgate, R.; Carmolli, M.; et al. Environmental enteropathy, oral vaccine failure and growth faltering in infants in Bangladesh. *EBioMedicine* **2015**, *2*, 1759–1766. [CrossRef] [PubMed]
95. Becker-Dreps, S.; Vilchez, S.; Bucardo, F.; Twitchell, E.; Choi, W.S.; Hudgens, M.G.; Perez, J.; Yuan, L. The association between fecal biomarkers of environmental enteropathy and rotavirus vaccine response in Nicaraguan infants. *Pediatr. Infect. Dis. J.* **2017**, *36*, 412–416. [CrossRef] [PubMed]
96. Goveia, M.G.; DiNubile, M.J.; Dallas, M.J.; Heaton, P.; Kuter, B. Efficacy of pentavalent human-bovine (WC3) reassortant rotavirus vaccine based on breastfeeding frequency. *Pediatr. Infect. Dis. J.* **2008**, *27*, 656–658. [CrossRef] [PubMed]
97. Vesikari, T.; Prymula, R.; Schuster, V.; Tejedor, J.C.; Cohen, R.; Bouckenooghe, A.; Damaso, S.; Han, H.H. Efficacy and immunogenicity of live-attenuated human rotavirus vaccine in breast-fed and formula-fed European infants. *Pediatr. Infect. Dis. J.* **2012**, *31*, 509–513. [CrossRef] [PubMed]
98. Rennels, M.B.; Wasserman, S.S.; Glass, R.I.; Keane, V.A. Comparison of immunogenicity and efficacy of rhesus rotavirus reassortant vaccines in breastfed and nonbreastfed children. US Rotavirus Vaccine Efficacy Group. *Pediatrics* **1995**, *96*, 1132–1136. [PubMed]
99. Rongsen-Chandola, T.; Strand, T.A.; Goyal, N.; Flem, E.; Rathore, S.S.; Arya, A.; Winje, B.A.; Lazarus, R.; Shanmugasundaram, E.; Babji, S.; et al. Effect of withholding breastfeeding on the immune response to a live oral rotavirus vaccine in North Indian infants. *Vaccine* **2014**, *32* (Suppl. 1), A134–A139. [CrossRef] [PubMed]
100. Groome, M.J.; Moon, S.S.; Velasquez, D.; Jones, S.; Koen, A.; van Niekerk, N.; Jiang, B.; Parashar, U.D.; Madhi, S.A. Effect of breastfeeding on immunogenicity of oral live-attenuated human rotavirus vaccine: A randomized trial in HIV-uninfected infants in Soweto, South Africa. *Bull. World Health Organ.* **2014**, *92*, 238–245. [CrossRef] [PubMed]
101. Becker-Dreps, S.; Vilchez, S.; Velasquez, D.; Moon, S.S.; Hudgens, M.G.; Zambrana, L.E.; Jiang, B. Rotavirus-specific IgG antibodies from mothers' serum may inhibit infant immune responses to the pentavalent rotavirus vaccine. *Pediatr. Infect. Dis. J.* **2015**, *34*, 115–116. [CrossRef] [PubMed]
102. Appaiahgari, M.B.; Glass, R.; Singh, S.; Taneja, S.; Rongsen-Chandola, T.; Bhandari, N.; Mishra, S.; Vrati, S. Transplacental rotavirus IgG interferes with immune response to live oral rotavirus vaccine ORV-116E in Indian infants. *Vaccine* **2014**, *32*, 651–656. [CrossRef] [PubMed]
103. Moon, S.S.; Groome, M.J.; Velasquez, D.E.; Parashar, U.D.; Jones, S.; Koen, A.; van Niekerk, N.; Jiang, B.; Madhi, S.A. Prevaccination rotavirus serum IgG and IgA are associated with lower immunogenicity of live, oral human rotavirus vaccine in South African infants. *Clin. Infect. Dis.* **2016**, *62*, 157–165. [CrossRef] [PubMed]
104. Chen, M.Y.; Kirkwood, C.D.; Bines, J.; Cowley, D.; Pavlic, D.; Lee, K.J.; Orsini, F.; Watts, E.; Barnes, G.; Danchin, M. Rotavirus specific maternal antibodies and immune response to RV3-BB neonatal rotavirus vaccine in New Zealand. *Hum. Vaccines Immunother.* **2017**, *13*, 1126–1135. [CrossRef] [PubMed]
105. Hu, L.; Crawford, S.E.; Czako, R.; Cortes-Penfield, N.W.; Smith, D.F.; Le Pendu, J.; Estes, M.K.; Prasad, B.V. Cell attachment protein VP8* of a human rotavirus specifically interacts with A-type histo-blood group antigen. *Nature* **2012**, *485*, 256–259. [CrossRef] [PubMed]
106. Imbert-Marcille, B.M.; Barbé, L.; Dupé, M.; Le Moullac-Vaidye, B.; Besse, B.; Peltier, C.; Ruvoën-Clouet, N.; Le Pendu, J. A FUT2 gene common polymorphism determines resistance to rotavirus A of the P[8] genotype. *J. Infect. Dis.* **2014**, *209*, 1227–1230. [CrossRef] [PubMed]

107. Ramani, S.; Hu, L.; Venkataram Prasad, B.V.; Estes, M.K. Diversity in Rotavirus-Host Glycan Interactions: A "Sweet" Spectrum. *Cell. Mol. Gastroenterol. Hepatol.* **2016**, *2*, 263–273. [CrossRef] [PubMed]
108. Nordgren, J.; Sharma, S.; Bucardo, F.; Nasir, W.; Günaydın, G.; Ouermi, D.; Nitiema, L.W.; Becker-Dreps, S.; Simpore, J.; Hammarström, L.; et al. Both Lewis and secretor status mediate susceptibility to rotavirus infections in a rotavirus genotype-dependent manner. *Clin. Infect. Dis.* **2014**, *59*, 1567–1573. [CrossRef] [PubMed]
109. Kazi, A.M.; Cortese, M.M.; Yu, Y.; Lopman, B.; Morrow, A.L.; Fleming, J.A.; McNeal, M.M.; Steele, A.D.; Parashar, U.D.; Zaidi, A.K.M.; et al. Secretor and Salivary ABO Blood Group Antigen Status Predict Rotavirus Vaccine Take in Infants. *J. Infect. Dis.* **2017**, *215*, 786–789. [CrossRef] [PubMed]
110. Saxena, K.; Blutt, S.E.; Ettayebi, K.; Zeng, X.L.; Broughman, J.R.; Crawford, S.E.; Karandikar, U.C.; Sastri, N.P.; Conner, M.E.; Opekun, A.R.; et al. Human Intestinal Enteroids: A New Model to Study Human Rotavirus Infection, Host Restriction, and Pathophysiology. *J. Virol.* **2015**, *90*, 43–56. [CrossRef] [PubMed]
111. Kanai, Y.; Komoto, S.; Kawagishi, T.; Nouda, R.; Nagasawa, N.; Onishi, M.; Matsuura, Y.; Taniguchi, K.; Kobayashi, T. Entirely plasmid-based reverse genetics system for rotaviruses. *Proc. Natl. Acad. Sci. USA* **2017**, *114*, 2349–2354. [CrossRef] [PubMed]

# Genome Characterization of a Pathogenic Porcine Rotavirus B Strain Identified in Buryat Republic, Russia in 2015

Konstantin P. Alekseev [1,2,*,†], Aleksey A. Penin [3,4,5,6], Alexey N. Mukhin [1], Kizkhalum M. Khametova [7], Tatyana V. Grebennikova [1], Anton G. Yuzhakov [1,2], Anna S. Moskvina [7], Maria I. Musienko [7], Sergey A. Raev [2,7], Alexandr M. Mishin [7], Alexandr P. Kotelnikov [7], Oleg A. Verkhovsky [7], Taras I. Aliper [1,2], Eugeny A. Nepoklonov [8], Diana M. Herrera-Ibata [9], Frances K. Shepherd [10,†] and Douglas G. Marthaler [9,*]

1. N. F. Gamaleya National Research Center for Epidemiology and Microbiology, Gamaleya Str. 18, Moscow 123098, Russia; amuhin@yahoo.com (A.N.M.); t_grebennikova@mail.ru (T.V.G.); anton_oskol@mail.ru (A.G.Y.); aliper@narvac.com (T.I.A.)
2. Federal State Budget Scientific Institution "Federal Scientific Centre VIEV", Moscow 109428, Russia; raevsergey@mail.ru
3. A. N. Belozersky Institute of Physico-Chemical Biology, Lomonosov Moscow State University, Moscow 119991, Russia; alekseypenin@gmail.com
4. Institute for Information Transmission Problems of the Russian Academy of Sciences, Moscow 127051, Russia
5. Laboratory of Extreme Biology, Institute of Fundamental Biology and Medicine, Kazan Federal University, Kazan 420021, Russia
6. Department of Genetics, Faculty of Biology, Lomonosov Moscow State University, Moscow 119991, Russia
7. Independent Non-Profit Organization "Diagnostic and Prevention Research Institute for Human and Animal Diseases", Moscow 123098, Russia; kizkhalum@yandex.ru (K.M.K.); annamoskvina17@gmail.com (A.S.M.); m_vovk@list.ru (M.I.M.); doktor-mishin@mail.ru (A.M.M.); apkotelnikov@yandex.ru (A.P.K.); info@dpri.ru (O.A.V.)
8. The Ministry of Agriculture of the Russian Federation, Orlikov Pereulok 1/11, Moscow 107139, Russia; pr.nepoklonova@mcx.ru
9. Veterinary Diagnostic Laboratory, College of Veterinary Medicine, Kansas State University, 1800 Denison Ave, Manhattan, KS 66502, USA; dianaherrera@vet.k-state.edu
10. Department of Veterinary and Biomedical Sciences, College of Veterinary Medicine, University of Minnesota, St. Paul, MN 55108, USA; sheph085@umn.edu

* Correspondence: kalekseev@hotmail.com (K.P.A.); dmarth027@vet.k-state.edu (D.G.M.);
† These authors equally contributed to the study.

**Abstract:** An outbreak of enteric disease of unknown etiology with 60% morbidity and 8% mortality in weaning piglets occurred in November 2015 on a farm in Buryat Republic, Russia. Metagenomic sequencing revealed the presence of rotavirus B in feces from diseased piglets while no other pathogens were identified. Clinical disease was reproduced in experimentally infected piglets, yielding the 11 RVB gene segments for strain Buryat15, with an RVB genotype constellation of G12-P[4]-I13-R4-C4-M4-A8-N10-T4-E4-H7. This genotype constellation has also been identified in the United States. While the Buryat15 VP7 protein lacked unique amino acid differences in the predicted neutralizing epitopes compared to the previously published swine RVB G12 strains, this report of RVB in Russian swine increases our epidemiological knowledge on the global prevalence and genetic diversity of RVB.

**Keywords:** porcine group B rotavirus; RVB; gastrointestinal disease; porcine enteric disease; phylogenetic analysis

## 1. Introduction

Rotaviruses (RVs) were first isolated in 1973 from children in Australia [1,2]. After the identification in swine two years later [3], RVs were recognized as the major etiological agents of acute viral gastroenteritis in humans and domesticated livestock worldwide [4–6]. Belonging to the *Reoviridae* family, the RV genome is composed of 11 double stranded RNA segments [7]. Eight RV species (RVA-RVH) and two tentative species (RVI and RVJ) have been identified by sequence-based classification of inner capsid protein 6 (VP6) [8–10]. RVA, RVB, RVC and RVH have been detected in both humans and animals while RVD-RVG, RVI, and RVJ have only been found in animals. Five out of ten RV species have been described in pigs (RVA, RVB, RVC, RVE, and RVH) [11–13].

Of the RV species, RVA is most common and well characterized both in animals and humans due to its high prevalence and pathogenicity. Porcine RVA was isolated in 1975 [3] followed by identification of swine RVC [14] and RVB [15,16]. A recent two-year study found RVB in 31.8% of diarrheic samples from North American swine, indicating higher detection of RVB than previously observed [16,17]. Similar detection rates of porcine RVB (25.9%) have been identified in Japan [18]. Although identified at lower rates than in North America and Japan, swine RVB has also been detected in Europe, South Africa, India, and Brazil [19–22].

Despite unexpectedly high detection rates of RVB in swine, RVB pathogenesis has only been established in gnotobiotic and caesarian-derived colostrum-deprived piglets [16,23]. The inability to cultivate RVB and limited whole genome sequence data has hampered an understanding of transmission and evolution within pigs. In order to fill these knowledge gaps, this study used metagenomic sequencing to identify porcine RVB from an enteric outbreak in a farm from southern Siberia, determined its disease-causing ability using experimental inoculation experiments, and studied its phylogenetic relationship with previously characterized swine RVB strains.

## 2. Results

During late autumn 2015, an outbreak of enteric disease occurred in three-day old suckling piglets on a farm located in Buryat Republic, Russia. Approximately 60% of litters had watery diarrhea (lasting 3–5 days), and the mortality rate was approximately 8%. The surviving piglets had reduced weight gain and a delay of being sent to market. Fecal and intestinal samples from infected piglets were submitted to the Diagnostic and Prevention Research Institute for Human and Animal Diseases to identify the cause of the disease. The samples tested negative for TGEV (Transmissible Gastroenteritis Virus), RVA, ASFV (African Swine Fever Virus), PCV-2 (Porcine Circovirus Type 2), CSFV (Classical Swine Fever Virus), and PRCV (Porcine Respiratory Coronavirus) using ELISA and PCR commercial kits from Vetbiochim (Moscow, Russia). Fecal samples were passaged on Vero, ST, and PK-15. Cell culture was halted after six blind passages since the cytopathic effect (CPE) was not observed. The fecal and intestinal samples were negative for bacterial pathogens on blood agar plates. Since a pathogen was not identified as the causative agent of disease, the purified RNA from the intestinal samples were submitted for Next Generation Sequencing (NGS). De novo assembly of the reads generated two contigs, which upon BLAST (NCBI) analysis yielded 83% and 86% nucleotide identities to the VP3 and VP4 genes of porcine RVB strain LS00011_Ohio, respectively. No other pathogens were detected in the NGS data.

A piglet was infected with the filtered fecal material and commingled with a mock-inoculated piglet to investigate the etiology and transmission associated with porcine RVB strain Buryat15. The fecal infected piglet developed diarrhea within 12 h while the mock-inoculated piglet developed diarrhea 24 h post-inoculation (PI) due to being commingled with the infected piglet. The small and large intestinal homogenates from the two pigs tested negative by the previously described commercial ELISA and PCR kits from Vetbiochim. Passage of the small and large intestinal homogenates in the Vero, ST, and PK-15 cells lacked CPE after six passages. Testing of the intestinal homogenates by NGS identified the addition of nine gene segments of RVB strain Buryat15. NGS did not identify any other pathogens in the intestinal homogenates.

The eleven gene segments of Buryat15 had the highest nucleotide identities with genes of RVB available through GenBank and were assigned a genotype constellation of G12-P[4]-I13-R4-C4-M4-A8-N10-T4-E4-H7 based on the whole RVB genome nucleotide cutoff values proposed by Shepherd et al. (manuscript in review). Thus, phylogenetic analysis focused on comparison with strains of porcine origin. Phylogenetic analysis of strain Buryat15 revealed a porcine ancestry of mixed geographic origins (Figure 1A–K).

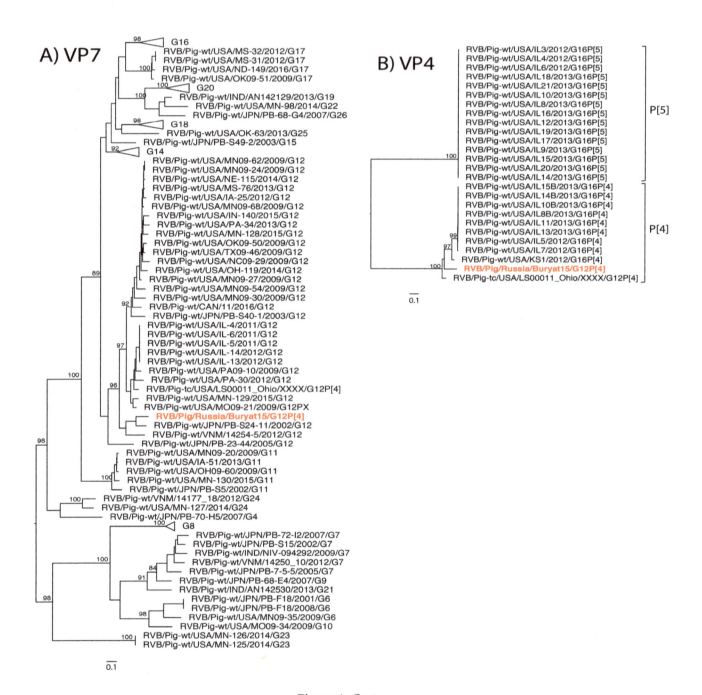

**Figure 1.** *Cont.*

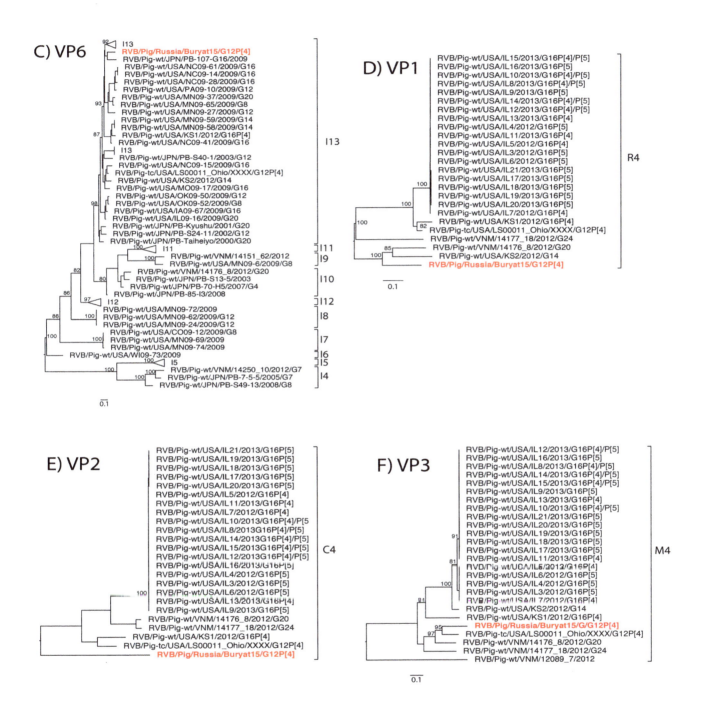

Figure 1. Cont.

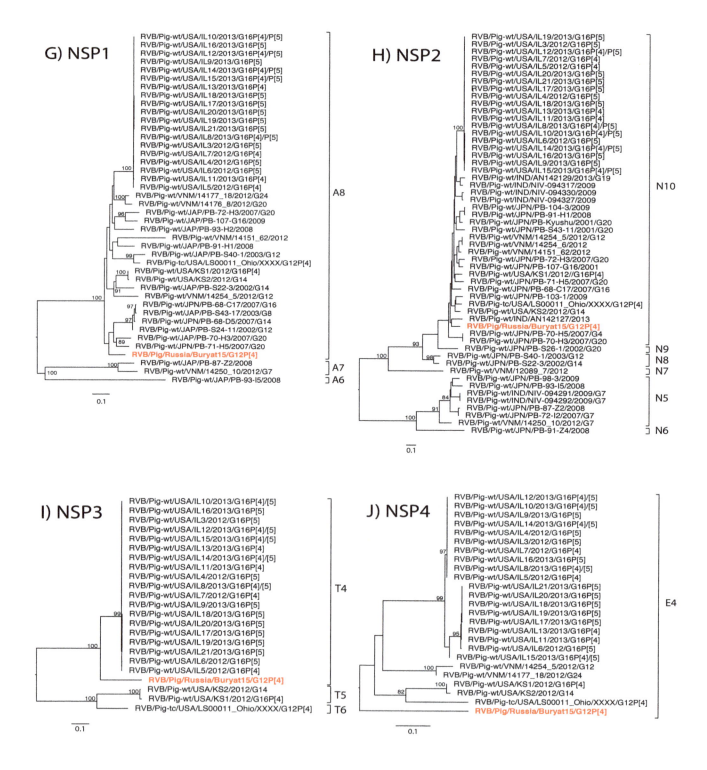

**Figure 1.** *Cont.*

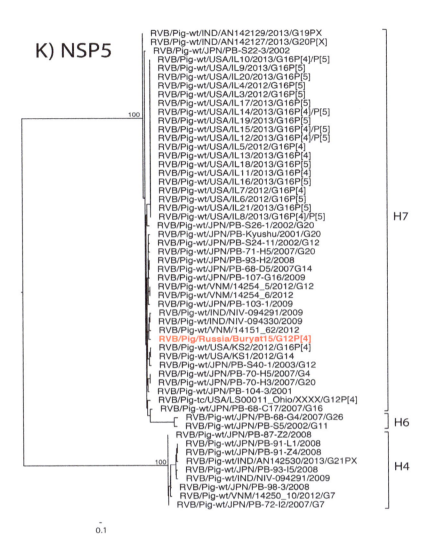

**Figure 1.** Phylogenetic trees for the 11 gene segments of swine RVB (**A–K**) with bootstrap values represented at the nodes (500 replicates). Bootstrap values below 80% are not shown. Selected genotype clades were clasped and represented by triangles. Russian strain Buryat15 is represented in bolded red. Scale bars represent 10 nucleotide changes per nucleotide site. Genotypes are labeled with brackets for all strains except VP7, where G genotypes are listed in the strain name.

The VP7 gene shared close common ancestors with Japanese strains while the NSP2 gene was most closely related to a porcine strain from India. The VP6 gene branched with Japanese strain PB-107-G16, but both fell within a larger clade of United States strains. The NSP5 gene was most closely related to the cogent gene of a porcine strain from Vietnam. The VP1 gene shared a clade with swine RVB strains from Vietnam and United States. The NSP3 gene shared a large clade with swine RVB strains from the United States. The tissue culture adapted strain USA/LS00011_Ohio was closely related to the Buryat15 VP3 gene segment. The VP4, VP2, and NSP4 genes from Buryat15 lacked close neighbors in the phylogenetic trees.

To explore the antigenic diversity of Buryat15, the VP7 amino acid identities were compared to previously characterized swine RVB strains of the G12 genotype at predicted antigenic sites [24] (Table 1). Buryat15 has an asparagine at the hypervariable residue 65, which is only shared by RVB strains isolated in Illinois, USA. Strains Buryat15 and Japanese PB-S24-11 have a glutamic acid at residue 91 while all the RVB strains have an alanine residue.

**Table 1.** Comparison of the predicted antigenic sites on VP7 [24] for swine RVB G12 strains. Dots represent the same residues compared to the consensus, determined by the majority amino acid residue of the alignment.

| Predicted Epitope Location | 33 | 34 | 36 | 37 | 39 | 40 | 65 | 66 | 67 | 89 | 90 | 91 | 92 | 130 | 158 | 159 | 160 | 161 | 179 | 180 | 181 |
|---|---|---|---|---|---|---|---|---|---|---|---|---|---|---|---|---|---|---|---|---|---|
| Consensus | D | D | N | D | K | Q | X | N | Y | K | Y | A | Y | D | P | D | R | R | S | N | N |
| Russia/Buryat15/2015 | . | . | . | . | . | . | N | . | . | . | . | . | . | . | . | . | . | . | . | . | . |
| JPN/PB-S24-11/2002 | . | . | . | . | E | . | D | . | . | . | . | E | . | . | . | . | . | . | . | . | . |
| JPN/PB-S40-1/2003 | . | . | . | E | . | . | V | . | . | . | . | E | . | . | . | . | . | . | . | . | . |
| CAN/11/2016 | . | . | T | . | . | . | D | S | . | . | . | . | . | . | . | . | . | . | . | . | . |
| USA/PA-30/2012 | . | . | T | . | . | K | D | Q | . | . | . | . | . | . | . | N | . | . | . | . | . |
| USA/MN-129/2015 | . | . | T | . | . | K | D | . | . | . | . | . | . | . | . | . | . | . | . | . | . |
| USA/MN-128/2015 | . | . | . | . | . | . | E | . | . | . | . | . | . | . | . | N | . | . | . | . | . |
| USA/IL-13/2012 | . | . | T | . | . | K | N | D | . | . | . | . | . | . | . | . | . | . | . | . | . |
| USA/IL-5/2011 | . | . | T | . | . | K | N | D | . | . | . | . | . | . | . | . | . | . | . | . | . |
| USA/IL-6/2011 | . | . | T | . | . | K | N | D | . | . | . | . | . | . | . | . | . | . | . | . | . |
| USA/IL-4/2011 | . | . | T | . | . | K | N | D | . | . | . | . | . | . | . | . | . | . | . | . | . |
| USA/IL-14/2012 | . | . | T | . | . | K | N | D | . | . | . | . | . | . | . | . | . | . | . | . | . |
| USA/IN-140/2015 | . | . | . | . | . | . | G | . | . | . | . | . | . | . | . | . | . | . | . | . | . |
| USA/OH-119/2014 | . | . | . | . | . | . | Q | . | . | . | . | . | . | . | . | N | . | . | . | . | . |
| USA/PA-34/2013 | . | . | . | . | . | . | E | . | . | . | . | . | . | . | . | N | . | . | . | . | . |
| USA/IA-25/2012 | . | . | . | . | . | . | D | . | . | . | . | . | . | . | . | N | . | . | . | . | . |
| USA/NE-115/2014 | . | . | . | . | . | . | E | . | . | . | . | . | . | . | . | . | . | . | . | . | . |
| USA/MS-76/2013 | . | . | . | . | . | . | E | . | . | . | . | . | . | . | . | . | . | . | . | . | . |
| USA/PA09-10/2009 | . | . | T | . | . | K | D | . | . | . | . | . | . | . | . | N | . | . | . | . | . |
| USA/MO09-21/2009 | . | . | T | . | . | K | D | . | . | . | . | . | . | . | . | . | . | . | . | . | . |
| USA/OK09-50/2009 | . | . | . | . | . | . | E | . | . | . | . | . | . | . | . | . | . | . | . | . | . |
| USA/MN09-54/2009 | . | . | . | . | . | . | Q | . | . | . | . | . | . | . | . | . | . | . | . | S | . |
| USA/MN09-30/2009 | . | . | . | . | . | . | I | . | . | . | . | . | . | . | . | . | . | . | . | . | . |
| USA/MN09-27/2009 | . | . | . | . | . | . | Q | . | . | . | . | . | . | . | . | . | . | . | . | . | . |
| USA/MN09-24/2009 | . | . | . | . | . | . | E | . | . | . | . | . | . | . | . | N | . | . | . | . | . |
| USA/MN09-68/2009 | . | . | . | . | . | . | E | . | . | . | . | . | . | . | . | N | . | . | . | . | . |
| USA/LS00011_Ohio/XXXX | . | . | T | . | . | K | S | D | . | . | . | . | . | . | . | . | . | . | . | . | . |

## 3. Discussion

Limited information is available for non-RVA species in human and domesticated livestock from Russia. A single manuscript described RVC in humans from the Novosibirsk and Omsk regions of Russia [25] while RVB in Russia has so far not been reported. Until recently, RVB was not considered an important pathogen in pigs, although early research demonstrated pathogenesis of RVB in gnotobiotic piglets [16]. While RVC infections are common in neonatal piglets, outbreaks of RVB in neonatal piglets are not typically reported as RVB infections are predominantly identified in older pigs [11]. Our results indicate that RVB is capable of causing enteric disease in conventionally raised, neonatal piglets and highlight the ability of RVB to cause and replicate clinical disease in piglets. These results further improve our understanding of the complexity associated with RVB as a swine pathogen.

The clinical disease reproduced by in conventionally raised piglets induced severe watery diarrhea 12 h PI. While the samples were negative for other bacterial and viral pathogens by traditional detection methods and NGS, it is still possible that RVB infection may cause disease in concert with other RV species or bacteria. However, several factors suggest RVB was the causative agent of enteric disease in the piglets. First, no other pathogens were identified in the NGS data, suggesting that RVB was the main disease-causing pathogen in the sample. Moreover, the purified fecal sample used to infect the piglet did not contain bacteria, and RVB RNA was detected in the mock-inoculated, commingled piglet, suggesting transmission of RVB. However, IHC staining or in situ hybridization is necessary to confirm this hypothesis and were not available at the time of the study.

RVB strains from different host species are genetically different from one another [26–28], which was consistent with our analysis since Buryat15 had the highest nucleotide identity with swine RVB strains. The long branches with Buryat15 in the VP2, VP4, and NSP4 phylogenetic trees indicate a lack of information on the genetic diversity of porcine RVB strains. The Buryat15 gene segments clustered closely with porcine RVB strains from different countries including Vietnam, India, Japan, and the United States. Reassortment is a common event within RV species [27,29–31], and swine RVB strains from India and the United States share recent common ancestors with Japanese porcine RVB strains [20,31]. A similar genetic relationship between Japanese and North American swine RVC has been demonstrated as well [32].

The genotype constellation of Buryat15 has not been identified in swine before but is closely related to constellations previously identified in swine from the United States (Shepherd et al., manuscript in review). Buryat15 and tissue culture strain LS00011_Ohio share the same genotypes for all genes except for NSP3 (T4 versus T6, respectively) while Buryat15 and United States strains IL11, IL13, IL5, and IL7 share genotypes for all genes besides VP7. The Russian strain was also related to United States swine based on its similarity at the predicted antigenic site to swine RVB strains from the USA [24]. However, the number of RVB gene segments available for comparison is limited, especially for several of the NSP gene segments, and a finer resolution of RVB evolution and antigenic diversity may be obtained with sequencing additional RVB strains.

Although the NGS data strongly suggest that RVB was responsible for the diarrhea outbreak in the Buryat Republic, immunofluorescent staining for the RVB antigens and in situ hybridization of the nucleic acid in fixed enterocytes from clinical and experimental animals would confirm infection and viral replication. Nevertheless, this study demonstrates the ability of an RVB strain to cause disease within conventionally raised piglets and illustrates the potential of reassortment within the evolutionary history of RVB in swine. Future epidemiological studies should be performed to continue characterizing the prevalence and diversity of Russian and global RVB strains in swine.

## 4. Materials and Methods

In November 2015, severe watery diarrhea was reported in newborn piglets (3–5 days of age). Samples were submitted to Diagnostic and Prevention Research Institute for Human and Animal Diseases for diagnostic testing. ELISA and PCR diagnostic kits were used to detect the following: TGEV and RVA, ELISA; ASFV, ELISA and PCR; PCV2, PCR; CSFV, PCR; and TGEV/PRCV,

PCR; were used according to manufacturer recommendation (Vetbiochim, Moscow, Russia). RNA extraction was performed with GeneJET Viral DNA/RNA Purification Kit (Thermo Scientific, Waltham, MA, USA). Once RVB was identified by NGS, subsequent samples were tested using RVB primers by PCR (VP4-I-823-842-F: CGTATCCAAAGCCAACGGGA and VP4-I-1008-1028-R: TGGGCCCTTATTTTCCAGTGT), which were designed using the primer-BLAST online software and Buryat15 VP4 sequence KU744407. Synthesis of cDNA was performed according to a random primer protocol using RevertAid H Minus First Strand cDNA Synthesis Kit (Thermo Scientific). PCR was carried out using True-Start DNA polymerase with 10 mM dNTPs mix (Thermo Scientific) according to the manufacturer's protocols.

Fecal samples from diarrheic piglets were diluted 1:10 in minimal essential medium (MEM) containing 1% actinomycin and 1% non-essential amino acids (Gibco, Grand Island, NY, USA) and clarified by centrifugation. Supernatants were filtered through 0.8 μm, 0.45 μm and 0.2 μm syringe filters sequentially, serial diluted, and added to five-day old monolayers of Vero, Swine testicular cells (ST) and porcine kidney 15 (PK-15). Six blind passages were performed with the cell lines and supernatants were saved at −70 °C.

To establish pathogenicity of the unknown virus, a single ten-day-old conventionally raised piglet was infected with 0.2 μm filtered, 1:10 diluted fecal sample while a single piglet was mock-infected with MEM. The two piglets were comingled to demonstrate transmission of pathological agent between piglets under experimental conditions. The sample was tested for the absence of bacterial contamination by seeding the filtered dilutions on blood agar plates. Piglets were monitored every 30 min for clinical signs of diarrhea. The piglets were sacrificed after the onset of diarrhea, and intestinal samples were collected.

For NGS, previously extracted RNA underwent cDNA synthesis according to random primer protocol was performed on RevertAid H Minus First Strand cDNA Synthesis Kit (Thermo scientific). PCR was carried out using True-Start DNA polymerase with 10 mM dNTPs mix and 10 pmol specific primers per reaction (Thermo Scientific), according to manufacturer's protocols. TruSeq Stranded Total RNA Library Prep Kit was used with 1 μg total RNA for the construction of libraries according to the manufacturer's protocol. For rRNA-depleted library, rRNA was removed from 2.5 μg total RNA using Ribo-Zero rRNA Removal Kit (mixture 1:1 Human/Mouse/Rat probe and Bacteria probe), according to the manufacturer's protocol (with probe concentration for epidemiology kit protocol). All cDNA libraries were sequenced using an Illumina HiSeq2000 (Illumina, San Diego, CA, USA), producing $101 \times 7 \times 101$ bp paired-end reads with multiplexing. Reads were trimmed using default parameters with CLC Genomics Workbench 8.5.1 (Qiagen Bioinformatics, Redwood City, CA, USA). Trimmed reads were de novo assembled using a word size of 64, bubble size of 100, and minimum contig length of 300. The contigs were subject to the BLASTN search. RVB sequences were deposited into GenBank with the accession numbers KU744406 (VP3), KU744407 (VP4), KX869730-KX869737 (VP1, VP6, VP7, NSP1-NSP5), and MH093644 (VP2).

The newly generated RVB sequences were aligned using MUSCLE in Geneious (version 9.6.1, Newark, NJ, USA) [33] with porcine RVB sequences that had at least 80% of the open reading frame available in GenBank (Supplementary Tables S1–S11). Maximum likelihood phylogenetic trees were made with the RAxML method using a Generalized Time Reversible gamma model of nucleotide substitution and 500 bootstrap replicates. The swine RVB G12 strains were translated and aligned with Buryat15 to compare the 21 predicted antigenic sites of RVB VP7 [24].

**Acknowledgments:** The local Ethical and Animal Welfare Committee of the Federal State Budget Scientific Institution "Federal Scientific Centre VIEV", (Moscow, Russia) approved the animal experiment. Sequencing and data processing were funded through the Russian Science Foundation grant project No. 14-50-00029.

**Author Contributions:** K.P.A. wrote the original draft, generated RVB primers and submitted sequences to GenBank, A.A.P. generated raw NGS data and performed preliminary data analysis, A.N.M. handled original sample, made preparation for RNA extraction, piglet and cell culture inoculation, performed piglet inoculation study, K.M.K. performed virus adaptation to cell culture study, T.V.G. coordinated the molecular biology part of the study, A.G.Y. performed PCR testing for different pathogens and carried out part of the sequence analysis, A.S.M. performed RVB PCR testing, M.I.M. provided the study with cell cultures, S.A.R. original sample ELISA testing, participated in the cell culture adaptation study and contributed to the experimental design, A.M.M. and A.P.K. communicated with the farm and collected the material, O.A.V., T.I.A. and E.A.N. designed and conceived the experiment, D.M.H.I. generated the RVB sequences, F.K.S. and D.G.M. revised original draft substantially and performed analysis of NGS data, and F.K.S. performed phylogenetic analysis and antigenic site comparisons for the manuscript.

## References

1. Bishop, R.; Davidson, G.P.; Holmes, I.H.; Ruck, B.J. Virus particles in epithelial cells of duodenal mucosa from children with acute non-bacterial gastroenteritis. *Lancet* **1973**, *302*, 1281–1283. [CrossRef]
2. Flewett, T.H.; Bryden, A.S.; Davies, H. Virus particles in gastroenteritis. *Lancet* **1973**, *2*, 1497. [CrossRef]
3. Rodger, S.M.; Craven, J.A.; Williams, I. Demonstration of Reovirus-like Particles in Intestinal Contents of Piglets with Diarrhoea. *Aust. Vet. J.* **1975**, *51*, 536. [CrossRef] [PubMed]
4. Flewett, T.H.; Bryden, A.S.; Davies, H.; Woode, G.N.; Bridger, J.C.; Derrick, J.M. Relation between viruses from acute gastroenteritis of children and newborn calves. *Lancet* **1974**, *304*, 61–63. [CrossRef]
5. Flewett, T.H.; Woode, G.N. The rotaviruses. *Arch. Virol.* **1978**, *57*, 1–25. [CrossRef] [PubMed]
6. Janke, B.H.; Nelson, J.K.; Benfield, D.A.; Nelson, E.A. Relative prevalence of typical and atypical strains among rotaviruses from diarrheic pigs in conventional swine herds. *J. Vet. Diagn. Investig.* **1990**, *2*, 308–311. [CrossRef] [PubMed]
7. Estes, M.K.; Greenberg, H.B. Rotaviruses. In *Fields Virology*, 6th ed.; Wolters Kluwer Health/Lippincott Williams & Wilkins: Philadelphia, PA, USA, 2013; pp. 1347–1401.
8. Matthijnssens, J.; Otto, P.H.; Ciarlet, M.; Desselberger, U.; Van Ranst, M.; Johne, R. VP6-sequence-based cutoff values as a criterion for rotavirus species demarcation. *Arch. Virol.* **2012**, *157*, 1177–1182. [CrossRef] [PubMed]
9. Bányai, K.; Kemenesi, G.; Budinski, I.; Földes, F.; Zana, B.; Marton, S.; Varga-Kugler, R.; Oldal, M.; Kurucz, K.; Jakab, F. Candidate new rotavirus species in Schreiber's bats, Serbia. *Infect. Genet. Evol.* **2016**, *48*, 19–26. [CrossRef] [PubMed]
10. Mihalov-Kovács, E.; Gellért, Á.; Marton, S.; Farkas, S.L.; Fehér, E.; Oldal, M.; Jakab, F.; Martella, V.; Bányai, K. Candidate new rotavirus species in sheltered dogs, Hungary. *Emerg. Infect. Dis.* **2015**, *21*, 660–663. [CrossRef] [PubMed]
11. Marthaler, D.; Homwong, N.; Rossow, K.; Culhane, M.; Goyal, S.; Collins, J.; Matthijnssens, J.; Ciarlet, M. Rapid detection and high occurrence of porcine rotavirus A, B, and C by RT-qPCR in diagnostic samples. *J. Virol. Methods* **2014**, *209*, 30–34. [CrossRef] [PubMed]
12. Marthaler, D.; Rossow, K.; Culhane, M.; Goyal, S.; Collins, J.; Matthijnssens, J.; Nelson, M.; Ciarlet, M. Widespread Rotavirus H in Commercially Raised Pigs, United States. *Emerg. Infect. Dis.* **2014**, *20*, 1203–1206. [CrossRef] [PubMed]
13. Pedley, S.; Bridger, J.C.; Chasey, D.; McCrae, M.A. Definition of two new groups of atypical rotaviruses. *J. Gen. Virol.* **1986**, *67 Pt 1*, 131–137. [CrossRef] [PubMed]
14. Saif, L.J.; Bohl, E.H.; Theil, K.W.; Cross, R.F.; House, J.A. Rotavirus-like, calicivirus-like, and 23-nm virus-like particles associated with diarrhea in young pigs. *J. Clin. Microbiol.* **1980**, *12*, 105–111. [PubMed]
15. Bridger, J.C.; Brown, J.F. Prevalence of antibody to typical and atypical rotaviruses in pigs. *Vet. Rec.* **1985**, *116*, 50. [CrossRef] [PubMed]
16. Theil, K.W.; Saif, L.J.; Moorhead, P.D.; Whitmoyer, R.E. Porcine Rotavirus-Like Virus (Group B Rotavirus): Characterization and Pathogenicity for Gnotobiotic Pigs. *J. Clin. Microbiol.* **1985**, *21*, 340–345. [PubMed]
17. Homwong, N.; Diaz, A.; Rossow, S.; Ciarlet, M.; Marthaler, D. Three-Level Mixed-Effects Logistic Regression Analysis Reveals Complex Epidemiology of Swine Rotaviruses in Diagnostic Samples from North America. *PLoS ONE* **2016**, *11*, e0154734. [CrossRef] [PubMed]
18. Kuga, K.; Miyazaki, A.; Suzuki, T.; Takagi, M.; Hattori, N.; Katsuda, K.; Mase, M.; Sugiyama, M.;

Tsunemitsu, H. Genetic diversity and classification of the outer capsid glycoprotein VP7 of porcine group B rotaviruses. *Arch. Virol.* **2009**, *154*, 1785. [CrossRef] [PubMed]
19. Otto, P.H.; Rosenhain, S.; Elschner, M.C.; Hotzel, H.; Machnowska, P.; Trojnar, E.; Hoffmann, K.; Johne, R. Detection of rotavirus species A, B and C in domestic mammalian animals with diarrhoea and genotyping of bovine species A rotavirus strains. *Vet. Microbiol.* **2015**, *179*, 168–176. [CrossRef] [PubMed]
20. Lahon, A.; Ingle, V.C.; Birade, H.S.; Raut, C.G.; Chitambar, S.D. Molecular characterization of group B rotavirus circulating in pigs from India: Identification of a strain bearing a novel VP7 genotype, G21. *Vet. Microbiol.* **2014**, *174*, 342–352. [CrossRef] [PubMed]
21. Molinari, B.L.D.; Possatti, F.; Lorenzetti, E.; Alfieri, A.F.; Alfieri, A.A. Unusual outbreak of post-weaning porcine diarrhea caused by single and mixed infections of rotavirus groups A, B, C, and H. *Vet. Microbiol.* **2016**, *193*, 125–132. [CrossRef] [PubMed]
22. Geyer, A.; Sebata, T.; Peenze, I.; Steele, A.D. Group B and C porcine rotaviruses identified for the first time in South Africa. *J. S. Afr. Vet. Assoc.* **1996**, *67*, 115–116. [PubMed]
23. Madson, D. Comparative Analysis: The Pathogenesis of Disease Induced in Piglets by Group A, B and C Rotaviruses, Singularly or Concurrently. Available online: https://www.pork.org/research/comparative-analysis-the-pathogenesis-of-disease-induced-in-piglets-by-group-a-b-and-c-rotaviruses-singularly-or-concurrently/ (accessed on 1 January 2013).
24. Shepherd, F.K.; Murtaugh, M.P.; Chen, F.; Culhane, M.R.; Marthaler, D.G. Longitudinal Surveillance of Porcine Rotavirus B Strains from the United States and Canada and In Silico Identification of Antigenically Important Sites. *Pathogens* **2017**, *6*, 64. [CrossRef] [PubMed]
25. Zhirakovskaia, E.; Tikunov, A.; Klemesheva, V.; Loginovskikh, N.; Netesov, S.; Tikunova, N. First genetic characterization of rotavirus C in Russia. *Infect. Genet. Evol. J. Mol. Epidemiol. Evol. Genet. Infect. Dis.* **2016**, *39*, 1–8. [CrossRef] [PubMed]
26. Suzuki, T.; Soma, J.; Miyazaki, A.; Tsunemitsu, H. Phylogenetic analysis of nonstructural protein 5 (NSP5) gene sequences in porcine rotavirus B strains. *Infect. Genet. Evol.* **2012**, *12*, 1661–1668. [CrossRef] [PubMed]
27. Suzuki, T.; Soma, J.; Kuga, K.; Miyazaki, A.; Tsunemitsu, H. Sequence and phylogenetic analyses of nonstructural protein 2 genes of species B porcine rotaviruses detected in Japan during 2001–2009. *Virus Res.* **2012**, *165*, 46–51. [CrossRef] [PubMed]
28. Marthaler, D.; Rossow, K.; Gramer, M.; Collins, J.; Goyal, S.; Tsunemitsu, H.; Kuga, K.; Suzuki, T.; Ciarlet, M.; Matthijnssens, J. Detection of substantial porcine group B rotavirus genetic diversity in the United States, resulting in a modified classification proposal for G genotypes. *Virology* **2012**, *433*, 85–96. [CrossRef] [PubMed]
29. Bwogi, J.; Jere, K.C.; Karamagi, C.; Byarugaba, D.K.; Namuwulya, P.; Baliraine, F.N.; Desselberger, U.; Iturriza-Gomara, M. Whole genome analysis of selected human and animal rotaviruses identified in Uganda from 2012 to 2014 reveals complex genome reassortment events between human, bovine, caprine and porcine strains. *PLoS ONE* **2017**, *12*. [CrossRef] [PubMed]
30. Aung, M.S.; Nahar, S.; Aida, S.; Paul, S.K.; Hossain, M.A.; Ahmed, S.; Haque, N.; Ghosh, S.; Malik, Y.S.; Urushibara, N.; et al. Distribution of two distinct rotavirus B (RVB) strains in the north-central Bangladesh and evidence for reassortment event among human RVB revealed by whole genomic analysis. *Infect. Genet. Evol.* **2017**, *47*, 77–86. [CrossRef] [PubMed]
31. Marthaler, D.; Suzuki, T.; Rossow, K.; Culhane, M.; Collins, J.; Goyal, S.; Tsunemitsu, H.; Ciarlet, M.; Matthijnssens, J. VP6 genetic diversity, reassortment, intragenic recombination and classification of rotavirus B in American and Japanese pigs. *Vet. Microbiol.* **2014**, *172*, 359–366. [CrossRef] [PubMed]
32. Suzuki, T.; Hasebe, A.; Miyazaki, A.; Tsunemitsu, H. Analysis of genetic divergence among strains of porcine rotavirus C, with focus on VP4 and VP7 genotypes in Japan. *Virus Res.* **2015**, *197*, 26–34. [CrossRef] [PubMed]
33. Kearse, M.; Moir, R.; Wilson, A.; Stones-Havas, S.; Cheung, M.; Sturrock, S.; Buxton, S.; Cooper, A.; Markowitz, S.; Duran, C.; et al. Geneious Basic: An integrated and extendable desktop software platform for the organization and analysis of sequence data. *Bioinform. Oxf. Engl.* **2012**, *28*, 1647–1649. [CrossRef] [PubMed]

# Rotavirus Burden, Genetic Diversity and Impact of Vaccine in Children under Five in Tanzania

Joseph J. Malakalinga [1,2], Gerald Misinzo [2], George M. Msalya [3] and Rudovick R. Kazwala [4,*]

1. Food and Microbiology Laboratory, Tanzania Bureau of Standards, Ubungo Area, Morogoro Road/Sam Nujoma Road, P.O. Box 9524, Dar es Salaam, Tanzania; joseph.malakalinga@sacids.org
2. Southern African Centre for Infectious Disease Surveillance (SACIDS), Africa Centre of Excellence for Infectious Diseases of Humans and Animals in Eastern and Southern Africa (ACE), Sokoine University of Agriculture (SUA), P.O. Box 3297, Chuo Kikuu, SUA, Morogoro, Tanzania; gerald.misinzo@sacids.org
3. Department of Animal, Aquaculture and Range Sciences, College of Agriculture, Sokoine University of Agriculture, P.O. Box 3004, Morogoro, Tanzania; msalya@sua.ac.tz
4. Department of Veterinary Medicine and Public Health, College of Veterinary Medicine and Biomedical Sciences, Sokoine University of Agriculture, P.O. Box 3021, Morogoro, Tanzania
* Correspondence: kazwala@sua.ac.tz

**Abstract:** In Tanzania, rotavirus infections are responsible for 72% of diarrhea deaths in children under five. The Rotarix vaccine was introduced in early 2013 to mitigate rotavirus infections. Understanding the disease burden and virus genotype trends over time is important for assessing the impact of rotavirus vaccine in Tanzania. When assessing the data for this review, we found that deaths of children under five declined after vaccine introduction, from 8171/11,391 (72% of diarrhea deaths) in 2008 to 2552/7087 (36% of diarrhea deaths) in 2013. Prior to vaccination, the prevalence of rotavirus infections in children under five was 18.1–43.4%, 9.8–51%, and 29–41% in Dar es Salaam, Mwanza and Tanga, respectively, and after the introduction of vaccines, these percentages declined to 17.4–23.5%, 16–19%, and 10–29%, respectively. Rotaviruses in Tanzania are highly diverse, and include genotypes of animal origin in children under five. Of the genotypes, 10%, 28%, and 7% of the strains are untypable in Dar es Salaam, Tanga, and Zanzibar, respectively. Mixed rotavirus genotype infection accounts for 31%, 29%, and 12% of genotypes in Mwanza, Tanga and Zanzibar, respectively. The vaccine effectiveness ranges between 53% and 75% in Mwanza, Manyara and Zanzibar. Rotavirus vaccination has successfully reduced the rotavirus burden in Tanzania; however, further studies are needed to better understand the relationship between the wildtype strain and the vaccine strain as well as the zoonotic potential of rotavirus in the post-vaccine era.

**Keywords:** rotavirus; genetic diversity; diarrhoea; vaccine effectiveness; Tanzania

## 1. Introduction

Rotavirus group A (RVA) is the major causative agent of diarrhea. A recent analysis at the global, regional, and national levels using a standard year (2013) and a standard list of 186 countries revealed that in children under 5 years of age, rotavirus deaths ranged from 197,000 to 233,000, with almost half of these deaths occurring in sub-Saharan Africa [1,2]. Rotavirus infection can be controlled by improved sanitation, good hygiene, and vaccination, with vaccination being the most promising control method [1,3,4]. Rotavirus is a double-stranded RNA (dsRNA) virus belonging to the family *Reoviridae*. The genome consists of 11 segments of dsRNA. Six of the segments encode for six structural viral proteins (*VP*), namely, *VP1*, *VP2*, *VP3*, *VP4*, *VP6*, and *VP7* [5]. The remaining five segments encode for six non-structural proteins (*NSPs*), namely, *NSP1*, *NSP2*, *NSP3*, *NSP4*, *NSP5*, and *NSP6* [5]. *VP4* and *VP7* play a role in genotype-specific induced immunity and are targets for vaccine development and production [6–8]. It is believed that accumulated point mutations in the segments encoding for *VP4* and *VP7* are associated with the acquisition of different or novel antigenic properties that help the rotavirus strain to escape host neutralization antibodies induced by the vaccine and lead to the generation of virus diversification [9,10]. Similarly, the presence of glycosylation sites in the RotaTeq vaccine *VP7* at amino acid residue 238 is associated with a reduction in immunogenicity of the 7-1a epitope [10]. The glycosylation of amino acid residue 238 has also been reported to reduce the neutralization of animal RVA by monoclonal antibodies and hyper-immune sera [10–12]. Therefore, monitoring changes in circulating rotavirus strains over time is an essential method for assessing vaccine effectiveness. Furthermore, rotavirus is categorized into six groups, A to H, based on the *VP6* gene nucleotide sequence classification [13]. Groups A to C have been shown to infect both humans and animals [5,13,14]. Members of Rotavirus Group A are classified according to their glycoprotein (G) structures, namely, G (G1, G2, G3, ... , Gn) genotypes, and their protein cleavage (P), namely, P (P[1], P[2], P[3], ... , P[n]) genotypes [5,15]. Currently, 36 G genotypes and 51 P genotypes have been identified in humans and animals worldwide [16]. Globally, the most common G and P genotype combinations include G1P[8], G2P[4], G3P[8], G4P[8], and G9P[8], with G1P[8] being the most prevalent [17–19]. In Africa, the most common rotavirus genotype combinations detected between 2006 and 2015 were G1P[8], G2P[4], G9P[8], G2P[6], G12P[8], and G3P[6], with G1P[8] and G2P[4] being the most dominant [20–22]. Unusual genotypes included G1P[4], G2P[8], G9P[4], G12P[4], G8P[6], G8P[8], G12P[6], and G12P[8] [20–22]. This degree of diversity in rotavirus strains may have implications for vaccine effectiveness; thus, continuous genotype monitoring is important for monitoring vaccine impact, improvement, and development. Recently, a new classification system was developed by the Rotavirus Classification Working Group (RCWG), which involves the sequencing of all 11 RNA segments (whole-genome sequencing) and locating genotypes based on the percentage nucleotide sequence identity cutoff value from each segment (Gx–Px–Ix–Rx–Cx–Mx–Ax–Nx–Tx–Ex–Hx, where x stands for numbers such as 1, 2, 3, ... , n) [23]. Along with phylogenetic analysis, whole-genome sequencing provides broad viral factor information, such as regarding origin, evolutionary relationships, interspecies transmission, antigenic shift (reassortment), antigenic drift (accumulated point mutation), and gene rearrangements [7,23]. All of these events contribute to the genetic diversity of the human rotavirus, which leads to reduced vaccine effectiveness [10,15,21,24]. Therefore, an understanding of genetic diversity within the country after vaccine introduction is necessary for the design of effective control programs.

Two rotavirus vaccines have been internationally licensed, Rotarix (GlaxoSmithKline Biologicals, Rue de l'Institut, Rixensart, Belgium) and RotaTeq (Merck and Co., Inc., Kenilworth, NJ, USA). Both vaccines were found to be efficacious and safe, with high efficacy (range: 85–100%) in developed countries [25,26] and moderate efficacy (range: 39.1–61.2%) in developing countries [27,28]. By 2017, rotavirus vaccines had been introduced in 92 countries worldwide, with 32 of those countries being in Africa [29]. Despite the moderate vaccine efficacy in sub-Saharan Africa, it is expected that a decline in efficacy will result from changes in rotavirus strain patterns after vaccine introduction [30]. To evaluate vaccine performance, it is important to assess the disease burden and rotavirus genotype trends both before and after the introduction of vaccination to a country. This is necessary in order to assess vaccine performance and to aid decision making in areas such as the need to extend coverage for a particular vaccine strain, the replacement of vaccines, or the need for development of new vaccines that can provide effective disease control.

In Tanzania, the Rotarix vaccine (RV1) was introduced in 2012 and implemented in the national immunization program in January 2013 [21,31]. The level of vaccine coverage was 85% 97%, 98%, 96%, and 100% in 2013, 2014, 2015, 2016, and 2017, respectively [32]. Several studies were conducted to determine the prevalence and genetic diversity of rotavirus in children under five before and after rotavirus vaccine introduction [20–22,31,33–44]. The purpose of this review article is to elucidate the genetic diversity of rotavirus, potential changes in strain type and the change in rotavirus burden after the introduction of the rotavirus vaccine in Tanzania.

## 2. Trends of Rotavirus Infection and Impact of the Rotavirus Vaccine in Tanzania

In Tanzania, diarrhea is responsible for 9% (11,391/113,471) of deaths in children under five [28,45]. In 2008, rotavirus alone accounted for one-third of diarrhea-related hospitalization and over 72% (8171/11,391) of diarrhea-related deaths in children under five in Tanzania [28,45,46]. The prevalence of RVA infection based on the detection of the RVA antigen in fecal samples from children under five in Tanzania has been reported to range from 9.5% to 51% (Figure 1), with most cases occurring in children under two years of age [20,33–36,40,42]. A study in Mwanza in 2009 showed that children with rotavirus infection had prolonged hospital stays of 3.66 days compared to 2.5 days for children without rotavirus infection [42]. Prolonged hospital stays have an economic impact on parents in terms of the cost of treatment and the time spent at hospital. To mitigate the rotavirus infection burden, Rotarix vaccine was incorporated into the national vaccination program of Tanzania in January 2013 [31]. In the first year after introduction, the number of rotavirus-related deaths declined from 8171 to 2552 in children aged under five [4]. The prevalence of rotavirus infections in children aged under five with diarrhea ranged from 9.8% to 51% before vaccine introduction, and this declined to 9–37% after vaccine introduction, showing the positive impact of the vaccine. However, other factors such as improved sanitation and hygiene may also have contributed to this decline of prevalence. Based on an enzyme immunoassay (EIA) for the detection of RVA in fecal samples, a hospital-based study found a reduction in the prevalence of RVA infection in children under five years of age from 58% pre-vaccination to 18% post-vaccination in the Mwanza region and from 37% to 16% in the Tanga region of Tanzania [37]. The same study reported a reduction in the prevalence of RVA infection in the post-vaccination period from 26% in 2014 to 18% in 2015 in Mbeya [37]. In Dar es Salaam, based on EIA for the detection of RVA in fecal samples, the prevalence of RVA in children under five declined from 18.1–43.4% in the pre-vaccination period to 17–23.5% during the post-vaccination period (Figure 1), whereas the prevalence of RVA in Mwanza declined from 9.8–51% [36,37,43] to 16–19% [37]. Similar findings were observed in Tanga, where the prevalence of RVA declined from 29–41% [20,37] to 10–29% [37]. These results are complemented by other similar case control studies conducted in the post-vaccination era, which found a 44.9% reduction in rotavirus hospitalization in Manyara in 2015 [47] and reductions of 40%, 46%, and 69% in Zanzibar in 2013, 2014, and 2015, respectively [33]. The progressive reduction in rotavirus hospitalizations in Zanzibar, Mbeya, Dodoma and Moshi could be attributed to the increasing coverage of the rotavirus vaccine. This suggests that vaccine performance can be improved by maximizing coverage, both in the study regions and elsewhere in Tanzania. No pre- and post-vaccination data are available for the other 24 regions and the impact of vaccine introduction is therefore unknown in these regions. Hence, further studies with the aim of assessing the impact of vaccine introduction in these regions are necessary, as most of the regions are geographically and seasonally different. The findings from previous studies show that the Rotarix vaccine has had a positive impact on the reduction of rotavirus deaths, virus positivity and hospitalizations due to diarrhea. Similarly, a reduction in the rotavirus burden has been reported in neighboring countries such as Malawi [48,49] and Rwanda [50].

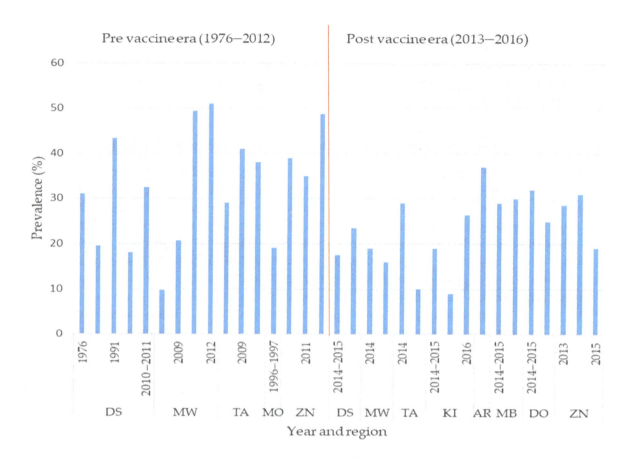

**Figure 1.** Histogram presentation of regional studies showing the rotavirus prevalence in children under five with diarrhea in Tanzania in pre vaccine era (1976–2012) and post vaccine era (2013–2015) (DS = Dar es Salaam, MW = Mwanza, TA = Tanga, MO = Morogoro, ZN = Zanzibar, KI = Kilimanjaro, AR = Arusha, MB = Mbeya).

The difference in RVA prevalence between studies may be explained by seasonal variation. We observed a higher prevalence of RVA in studies conducted during the cool/dry season than those conducted in the hot/rainy season (Figure 2). These findings suggest that the rotavirus prevalence in the tropics is higher during the cool/dry season compared to the hot/rainy season [51]. For example, the prevalence of RVA based on the latex agglutination test (LAT) for the detection of the RVA antigen from children's faeces in Morogoro was 23.5% (82/348) in the dry/cool season (July–September) and 3.8% (4/103) in the rainy/hot season (February–May) (Figure 2). A similar finding was observed in Dar es Salaam, where a higher prevalence of RVA was found in studies conducted in the cool/dry season (43%, n = 99, May and August) [41] than in the hot/rainy season (19.5%, n = 89, January–February) based on the LAT [39] (Figure 2). In the same region, based on EIA, the prevalence of RVA was found to be higher in the dry/cool season (23.9%, May–August) [31] than in the rainy/hot season (17.1%, November–February [31]; 18.1%, n = 270, December–February [40]) (Figure 2). In Mwanza, based on EIA, a higher prevalence (29%, n = 197) of RVA was observed in the dry/cool season (May–July) and a lower prevalence (0–2%, n = 197) was observed in the rainy/hot season (November–April) [37]. In same region, the rainy/hot season (February–May) was shown to have a lower prevalence of RVA 9.8%

(n = 805) based on EIA [43]. However, in the same Mwanza region, a higher prevalence of 50.2% was observed in the rainy season (November–April) compared with 44.6% in the dry season (May–October), although the difference was not statistically significant [36]. In Tanga, a higher prevalence was observed in the dry/cool season (May and October) compared with the rainy/hot season (November–April) in 2009, 2014, and 2015 both before and after vaccine introduction, even though no seasonal variation was observed in 2011 [37]. Generally, the prevalence of RVA seems to be higher during the dry/cool season in the study regions (Figure 2).

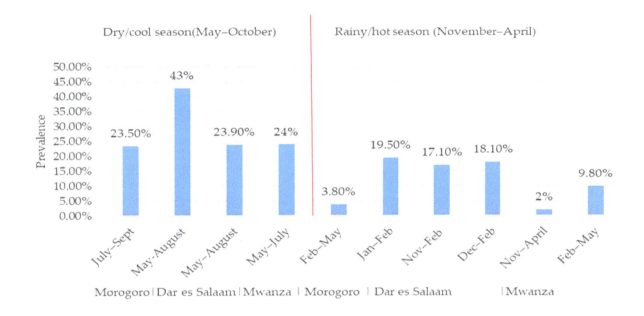

**Figure 2.** Rotavirus prevalence variation in children under five in Tanzania during dry/cool and rainy/hot season.

The impact of vaccine introduction on seasonal peaks of RVA cases has been clearly observed in Mwanza, Tanga, Zanzibar and Manyara, with a seasonal peak delay of 1–4 months observed after vaccine introduction (Figure 3). Similar findings in the delay of the seasonal peak after vaccine introduction have been reported in the United States [52]. Before vaccine introduction, the peak months were May 2009 and August 2011 in Tanga, May 2012 in Mwanza, May–July of 2010–2012 in Manyara and July 2010 and May of 2011–2012 in Zanzibar [33,37,47]. After vaccine introduction, the peaks in rotavirus cases were delayed for 1–4 months towards the end of the year; in Tanga, the peak was in September of 2014–2015; in Mwanza, it was in July 2014 and July and August of 2015; in Manyara, it was in August–October of 2013–2015 and in Zanzibar, it was in June and July of 2013, September 2014 and October 2015 [33,37]. This information on the changes in seasonal peaks after vaccine introduction is crucial for the timing of rotavirus investigations. However, continual surveillance is necessary across the country to confirm these changes.

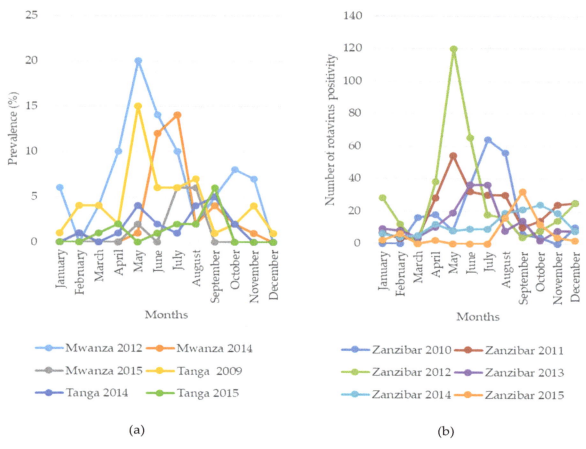

**Figure 3.** Seasonal pattern and peak months of rotavirus positivity before (2009–2012) and after (2014–2015) vaccine introduction in mainland (**a**) Tanzania and (**b**) Zanzibar.

In addition, based on EIA, studies in Mwanza, Manyara and Zanzibar have shown that the vaccine effectiveness (VE) against rotavirus hospitalization in Tanzania ranges from 53% to 75%, with an average effectiveness of 61% for two doses of Rotarix vaccine (RV1) in children aged 5–23 months of age (Table 1). This is a moderate level of vaccine effectiveness; therefore, having a way to improve vaccine effectiveness could improve the performance of the vaccine in terms of reducing the number of rotavirus diarrhea hospitalizations and deaths. The performance of the vaccine may also be improved by increasing the vaccine strain coverage, developing a new, more effective vaccine and the transmission of animal strain to humans could be avoided by carrying out animal vaccination, which is not currently practiced in Tanzania. Other ways to improve vaccine performance include the use of zinc supplementation or the antisecretory agent racecadotril, adjusting the duration of breastfeeding, improving nutrition, and carrying out alternate dosing schedules [30]. The VE has only been determined in two (Mwanza and Manyara) out of the 25 regions in mainland Tanzania, as well as in Zanzibar. Mwanza and Manyara are found in northern Tanzania, while Zanzibar is an island in eastern Tanzania [53]. These regions represent the northern part of mainland Tanzania; therefore, further studies across the country are necessary to generate generalizable findings on vaccine effectiveness to allow for accurate decision making. The vaccine effectiveness in Tanzania is similar to that of bordering and other African countries, with a VE of 58.3% in Malawi [48], 56% in Zambia [54], 54% in Botswana [55], and 57% in South Africa [56]. The moderate vaccine effectiveness observed in Tanzania and other bordering countries may be attributed to the wide rotavirus strain diversity in Africa, infection with multiple genotypes at once, the high rate of mutation in the rotavirus genome, and the close proximity of inhabitants to animals [57,58]. This highlights the need to understand the shared and evolutionary relationships among rotaviruses circulating between humans and animals in most African countries, including Tanzania, where little is known regarding rotavirus infection in animals and humans, particularly in rural areas where inhabitants live in close proximity to animals. In addition, rotavirus can be carried asymptomatically [59], and 7.7–15% of children in Dar es Salaam were found to be carriers [41]. Asymptomatic carriers of rotavirus may act as reservoirs for the infection of susceptible individuals [40,42]. Therefore, the role of asymptomatic individuals in the propagation of rotavirus infection needs to be investigated in Tanzania.

Table 1. Rotarix vaccine effectiveness (case control studies) in Tanzanian regions in children aged 5–23 months and the impact of the vaccine on the reduction of hospitalizations.

| Region | Reference | Diagnostic Technique | Settings, Year of Study | Rotavirus Vaccine Dosage Comparison | VE (95% CI) |
|---|---|---|---|---|---|
| Zanzibar | [1] | EIA | Single hospital, December 2012–2015 | 2 doses vs. 0 doses | 57 (14–78) |
| Manyara | [47] | EIA | Single hospital, August–December 2015 | 2 doses vs. 0 doses<br>2 doses vs. 0 doses | 74.8 (−8.2 to 94.1) 85.1 (26.5–97.0) |
| Mwanza | [28] | RT-PCR | Multiple hospitals, May 2015 | 2 doses vs. 0 doses<br>≥1 dose vs. 0 doses | 49 (−30 to 80)<br>53 (−14 to 81) |

EIA = enzyme immunoassay, RT-PCR = reverse transcription polymerase chain reaction.

Overall, studies have shown that the Rotarix vaccine has successfully reduced the number of rotavirus diarrhea cases, hospitalizations and deaths and has changed the seasonal patterns of rotavirus in the studied regions in Tanzania. However, further studies are needed across the country to form generalizable conclusions. Almost all available studies were hospital-based and located in urban and peri-urban areas. Hence, there is a need for more information from rural areas; future studies should therefore involve participants from communities and dispensary/health centers in rural areas.

## 3. Trends in Rotavirus Genetic Diversity in Tanzania

In Tanzania, there is high diversity in RVA strains circulating among children under five years of age (Table 2). Studies from the years 2002–2018 reported circulating genotypes including G1P[8], G2P[4], G1P[6], G1P[4], G3P[8], G3P[6], G8P[4], G8P[6], G8P[8], G4P[4], G4P[6], G9P[8] and G12P[6], along with untypable and mixed strains (Table 2). The high observed strain diversity may be one of the reasons for vaccine effectiveness being only moderate in Tanzania. Strain diversity has been shown to hinder vaccine performance in terms of both effectiveness and efficacy in Africa [24]. In Dar es Salaam, Mwanza and Tanga, G1P[8] was the predominant genotype (24–75.1% of detected strains) both before and after vaccine introduction, followed by G2P[4] (8–50%) and G1P[6] (0.5–17%) (Table 2). G1P[8] is the most dominant of the detected genotypes, accounting for 24–64.7% of genotypes [20–22,31] before vaccine introduction and 41–75.1% after vaccine introduction [21]. Variation in the prevalence of rotavirus genotypes was observed in Dar es Salaam between 2005–2006 and 2010–2012, when G9P[8] accounted for 80% of the detected genotypes compared to 10% for G1P[8] in 2005–2006 [40]. A shift was observed in 2010 to 2011, when G1P[8] accounted for 64.7% of the detected genotypes compared to 0.5% from G9P[8] [31]. In another study, conducted in children aged under five years of age in Mwanza, Tanga, Mbeya, Dodoma, Kilimanjaro and Dar es Salaam, G2P[4] was shown to dominate, accounting for 50% of the genotypes compared to 15.63% G1P[8] and 15.63% G3P[6] [37]. Domination of G2P[4] over G1P[8] after vaccine introduction was reported in Tanga, Mwanza, Moshi, Mbeya, Dar es Salaam and Dodoma between 2009 and 2015 [48], which may have implications for vaccine effectiveness in these regions, as Rotarix vaccine is more efficacious against G1P[8] (68.3%) compared to the G2P[4] strain (49.3%) [60]. It is difficult to conclude whether G1P[8] is being suppressed in these regions due to the Rotarix vaccine, as G1P[8] is the main component of the vaccine cocktail. However, it is common for the rotavirus strain prevalence to fluctuate year after year—a certain genotype may dominate in one season and be completely absent in the next season [61–63]. The variation in rotavirus genotypes in Tanzania highlights the need for continuous monitoring of rotavirus genotypes to assess vaccine effectiveness, detect non-vaccine genotypes, and develop effective local multistrain vaccines.

Table 2. Regional rotavirus genotype distribution in Tanzania, showing the most to the least prevalent genotypes per given study.

| Region | Ref | Year | n | G1P[8] | G2P[4] | G9P[8] | G12P[6] | G12P[8] | G1P[4] | G8P[4] | G8P[6] | G4P[6] | G4P[4] | G3P[6] | G3P[8] | G8P[8] | G1P[6] | Untypeable | Mixed genotypes |
|---|---|---|---|---|---|---|---|---|---|---|---|---|---|---|---|---|---|---|---|
| Dar es Salaam | [48] | 2005–2006 | 49 | 10% | 0 | 90.7% | 0 | 0 | 0 | 0 | 0 | 0 | 0 | 0 | 0 | 0 | 5% | 10% | 0 |
| | [47] | 2010–2011 | 211 | 64.7% | 0 | 0.5% | 11.1% | 0 | 3.7% | 14.2% | 3.2% | 1.1% | 1.1% | 0 | 0 | 0 | 0.5% | 0 | 0 |
| Tanga | [49] | 2007–2008 | 32 | 34% | 0 | 3% | 0 | 0 | 0 | 0 | 0 | 0 | 0 | 0 | 0 | 0 | 3% | 28% | 31% |
| Mwanza | [25] | 2010–2011. | 100 | 24% | 2% | 0 | 0 | 0 | 0 | 7% | 4% | 0 | 0 | 0 | 0 | 6% | 17% | 0 | 29% |
| Zanzibar | [1] | 2010–2015 | 101 | 52% | 8% | 0 | 0 | 2% | 0 | 0 | 3% | 0 | 0 | 16% | 0 | 0 | 1% | 7% | 12% |
| ND | [28] | 2009–2015 | 32 | 15.63% | 50% | 0 | 0 | 0 | 3.1% | 0 | 0 | 0 | 0 | 15.6% | 3.1% | 0 | 3.1% | 6.3% | 9.3% |
| ND | [62] | 2010 | – | 31.4% | – | – | – | – | – | – | – | – | – | – | – | – | – | – | – |
| ND | [62] | 2011 | – | 25.8% | – | – | – | – | – | – | – | – | – | – | – | – | – | – | – |
| ND | [62] | 2014 | – | 41.1% | – | – | – | – | – | – | – | – | – | – | – | – | – | – | – |
| ND | [62] | 2015 | – | 75.1% | – | – | – | – | – | – | – | – | – | – | – | – | – | – | – |
| East Africa | [63] | 2007–2011 | – | 23% | 8% | 12% | 0 | 4% | 0 | 4% | 5% | 0 | 0 | 4% | 0 | 0 | 4% | 0 | 0 |

ND: Not determined to region level; "–": Data unavailable.

Despite the moderate vaccine effectiveness in Tanzania, very little is known about the relationship between the circulating strain and vaccine strains in Tanzania. Only one study prior to vaccine introduction sequenced the antigenic region (*VP7* and *VP4*), and a distant relationship was observed between the data on the vaccine strains in GenBank and the circulating strain in Dar es Salaam [31]. This provides a potential clue regarding the vaccine performance in the region, as the circulating strain might have been antigenically different to the vaccine strains. Due to the segmented genome structure of rotavirus, circulating strains may evolve rapidly through accumulating point mutations, reassortment, gene rearrangement, or due to vaccine pressure, thus driving an increase in rotavirus genetic diversity [10,15,21]. This kind of rotavirus evolution may lead to the emergence of new or novel strains that may escape neutralization antibodies [10,15]. Additionally, the parental strain of the Rotarix vaccine strain introduced in Tanzania was isolated 31 years ago in the United States [64]. Since RVA can accumulate point mutations in its antigenic regions, it is possible that the antigenic region of the circulating strain differs from those of the strains in the vaccine, thus allowing it to evade neutralization antibodies. This scenario is supported by the evidence of a moderate vaccine effectiveness of 54% in Mwanza and 53% in Zanzibar [21,33]. Also, there is evidence of vaccinated individuals shedding RVA strains in Arusha and Kilimanjaro [35,38]; however, it has not been determined whether the strains being shed are vaccine strains or circulating strains. Therefore, it is very important to ascertain the genetic relationship between circulating rotavirus strains from distinct geographical locations as compared with the strains in the vaccine used in Tanzania and elsewhere in this post-vaccine era.

In addition, high percentages of untypable, mixed genotype infections, atypical/unusual (G1P[4]) and classical animal origin genotypes (such as G8P[6], G4P[6] and G3P[6]) have been detected in studies conducted in Zanzibar, Mwanza, Dar es Salaam, Mbeya, Dodoma and Tanga (Table 2). The occurrence of animal origin genotypes in humans may indicate direct interspecies transmission or the occurrence of reassortment events between human and animal rotaviruses in Tanzania, which needs to be further clarified. The existence of atypical/unusual G1P[4] genotypes is believed to have arisen through inter-genogroup or inter-genotype reassortment between Wa- and DS–1-like strains [21,65] and untypable RVA strains are also thought to have originated from animals [65–67]. Therefore, understanding the zoonotic potential of livestock RVA is of particular interest in Tanzania as, currently, the potential sharing of RVA genotypes between humans and animals remains unknown. In the rural areas of developing countries, including Tanzania, people live in close proximity to animals and sanitation, and hygiene may be poor, thus increasing the risk of zoonotic rotavirus infection [68]. Infected animals or humans shed over 10 billion infectious rotavirus particles per gram/milliliter stool [69], thus contaminating environmental objects. Rotaviruses are very stable in the environment and can withstand harsh conditions for several weeks on surfaces and water (portable and recreational water) [70]. Fecal–oral transmission can occur from person to person, or through contact with an infected animal, fecal–contaminated fomites, hands, food and water. Zoonotic rotavirus transfer may occur either by direct transmission from animals to humans or through the exchange of RNA segments, such as through reassortment [71,72]. Strains such as G6, G8, G5, G10, G11, P[1], P[2], P[3], P[5], P[7] and P[12] are commonly detected in animals, and G2, G3, G4, and G9, P[6], are common in both humans and animals [71]. The classic animal strains G8P[6], G4P[6] and G3P[6] have been detected in children under five in Tanzania [33,36,37,40]; however, the studies did not further investigate whether the infections were due to direct interspecies transmission or reassortment events or both. Direct transmission of rotaviruses from animals to humans has been suspected in children with acute diarrhea in Thailand (infected with G10P[14]), Italy (infected with G10P[14] and G8P[14]), Cameroon (infected with G5P[7]) and Nigeria (infected with G8P[1]) [73–75]. Reassortment between human and animal strains may increase the human-to-human transmission of the resultant reassortant strain [76]. Unusual reassortant strains, such as the G6P[8] strain, have been detected in Bangladesh [27].

The observed mixed genotype infections may facilitate reassortment events, which is one of the mechanisms for increasing rotavirus strain diversity [7,21,77]. Due to the segmented nature of rotaviruses, there is the possibility of segment exchange in mixed genotype infections. This kind of rotavirus evolution may generate reassortant strains with novel antigenic properties that are capable of fast spread in human populations [76]. Since there is evidence of untypable, mixed infection strains and strains of animal origin circulating in humans in Tanzania (Table 2), there is a need to understand the zoonotic potential and reassortment events of the circulating rotavirus strains to allow for the effective design and implementation of strategic intervention programs, including the reduction or limitation of strain diversity in human rotaviruses. Understanding the occurrences of these phenomena cannot be achieved by RT-PCR genotyping alone; rather, sequencing is needed of antigenic regions such as *VP4* and *VP7*, or whole-genome sequencing of selected strains including those of animal origin and unusual, untypable, and mixed genotype infection strains. Therefore, after PCR genotyping, sequencing may be important for tracking changes over time as the virus evolves [77,78], to enable comprehension of the rotavirus vaccine performance or effectiveness.

Overall, there have been no major changes in rotavirus strain patterns. G1P[8] was predominant in the pre-vaccine period, and is still the predominant strain after vaccine introduction. However, continuous strain surveillance is crucial to allow for a clear understanding of the impact of the vaccine on RVA genotype patterns, as well as the early identification of emerging, unusual and novel genotypes not covered by the vaccine. Also, it would be beneficial for Tanzania and other African countries to develop their own vaccines based on the local circulating strains.

## 4. Conclusions

The Rotarix vaccine successfully reduced the rotavirus burden in Tanzania; however, due to the moderate vaccine effectiveness, we recommend that further studies be carried out to determine the vaccine effectiveness across the country and to clarify the genetic and antigenic relationships between the circulating rotavirus strains and the strains in the vaccine. In Tanzania, very little is known about the genetic composition of circulating rotavirus strains, and we therefore suggest that whole-genome sequencing be performed on selected circulating rotavirus strains from distinct geographical locations in order to understand viral factors and mechanisms associated with rotavirus genetic diversity in Tanzania. As only a few studies have been conducted on rotavirus genotypes after vaccine introduction, further studies are needed in order to better understand the impact of the vaccine on rotavirus strain patterns and to identify novel, reassortant, unusual and untypable strains that are present in the post-vaccine era in Tanzania.

**Author Contributions:** Conceptualization, J.J.M., G.M.M. and R.R.K.; Writing—original draft preparation, J.J.M.; Writing—review & editing, J.J.M., G.M., G.M.M. and R.R.K.; Supervision, G.M., G.M.M. and R.R.K.

**Acknowledgments:** The authors would like to acknowledge the SACIDS Africa Centre of Excellence for Infectious Diseases of Human and Animals in Eastern and Southern Africa for providing the doctoral scholarship to J.J.M and College of Veterinary Medicine and Biomedical Sciences of Sokoine University of Agriculture. The authors also acknowledge Annette Rouge for her technical support.

## References

1. Tate, J.E.; Burton, A.H.; Boschi-Pinto, C.; Parashar, U.D.; World Health Organization–Coordinated Global Rotavirus Surveillance Network; Agocs, M.; Serhan, F.; de Oliveira, L.; Mwenda, J.M.; Mihigo, R.; et al. Global, regional, and national estimates of rotavirus mortality in children <5 years of age, 2000–2013. *Clin. Infect. Dis.* **2016**, *62*, 96–105. [CrossRef] [PubMed]
2. Troeger, C.; Forouzanfar, M.; Rao, P.C.; Khalil, I.; Brown, A.; Reiner, R.C., Jr.; Fullman, N.; Thompson, R.L.; Abajobir, A.; Ahmed, M.; et al. Estimates of global, regional, and national morbidity, mortality, and aetiologies of diarrhoeal diseases: A systematic analysis for the Global Burden of Disease Study 2015. *Lancet. Infect. Dis.* **2017**, *17*, 909–948. [CrossRef]
3. Fischer, T.K.; Viboud, C.; Parashar, U.; Malek, M.; Steiner, C.; Glass, R.; Simonsen, L. Hospitalizations and deaths from diarrhea and rotavirus among children <5 years of age in the United States, 1993–2003. *J. Infect. Dis.* **2007**, *195*, 1117–1125. [PubMed]

4. WHO. Immunization, Vaccines and Biologicals. Rotavirus. Last Updated on December, 2018. Available online: https://www.who.int/immunization/diseases/rotavirus/en/ (accessed on 20 February 2019).
5. Estes, M.K.; Kapikian, A.Z. Rotaviruses. *Fields Virol.* **2007**, *2*, 1917–1974.
6. Gentsch, J.R.; Laird, A.R.; Bielfelt, B.; Griffin, D.D.; Bányai, K.; Ramachandran, M.; Jain, V.; Cunliffe, N.A.; Nakagomi, O.; Kirkwood, C.D.; et al. Serotype diversity and reassortment between human and animal rotavirus strains: Implications for rotavirus vaccine programs. *J. Infect. Dis.* **2005**, *192*, 146–159. [CrossRef] [PubMed]
7. Matthijnssens, J.; Ciarlet, M.; Heiman, E.; Arijs, I.; Delbeke, T.; McDonald, S.M.; Palombo, E.A.; Iturriza-Gómara, M.; Maes, P.; Patton, J.T.; et al. Full genome-based classification of rotaviruses reveals a common origin between human Wa-Like and porcine rotavirus strains and human DS-1-like and bovine rotavirus strains. *J. Virol.* **2008**, *82*, 3204–3219. [CrossRef]
8. Park, S.I.; Matthijnssens, J.; Saif, L.J.; Kim, H.J.; Park, J.G.; Alfajaro, M.M.; Kim, D.S.; Son, K.Y.; Yang, D.K.; Hyun, B.H.; et al. Reassortment among bovine, porcine and human rotavirus strains results in G8P [7] and G6P [7] strains isolated from cattle in South Korea. *Veter Microbiol.* **2011**, *152*, 55–66. [CrossRef]
9. Arista, S.; Giammanco, G.M.; De Grazia, S.; Ramirez, S.; Biundo, C.L.; Colomba, C.; Cascio, A.; Martella, V. Heterogeneity and temporal dynamics of evolution of G1 human rotaviruses in a settled population. *J. Virol.* **2006**, *80*, 10724–10733. [CrossRef]
10. Zeller, M.; Patton, J.T.; Heylen, E.; De Coster, S.; Ciarlet, M.; Van Ranst, M.; Matthijnssens, J. Genetic analyses reveal differences in the VP7 and VP4 antigenic epitopes between human rotaviruses circulating in Belgium and rotaviruses in Rotarix and RotaTeq. *J. Clin. Microbiol.* **2012**, *50*, 966–976. [CrossRef]
11. Ciarlet, M.; Hoshino, Y.; Liprandi, F. Single point mutations may affect the serotype reactivity of serotype G11 porcine rotavirus strains: A widening spectrum? *J. Virol.* **1997**, *71*, 8213–8220.
12. Ciarlet, M.; Reggeti, F.; Piña, C.I.; Liprandi, F. Equine rotaviruses with G14 serotype specificity circulate among Venezuelan horses. *J. Clin. Microbiol.* **1994**, *32*, 2609–2612. [PubMed]
13. Matthijnssens, J.; Otto, P.H.; Ciarlet, M.; Desselberger, U.; Van Ranst, M.; Johne, R. VP6-sequence-based cutoff values as a criterion for rotavirus species demarcation. *Arch. Virol.* **2012**, *157*, 1177–1182. [CrossRef] [PubMed]
14. Matthijnssens, J.; Martella, V.; Van Ranst, M. Genomic evolution, host-species barrier, reassortment and classification of rotaviruses. *Futur. Virol.* **2010**, *5*, 385–390. [CrossRef]
15. Kirkwood, C.D. Genetic and antigenic diversity of human rotaviruses: Potential impact on vaccination programs. *J. Infect. Dis.* **2010**, *202*, 43–48. [CrossRef] [PubMed]
16. RCWG. List of Accepted Genotypes. 2018. Available online: https://rega.kuleuven.be/cev/viralmetagenomics/virus-classification/rcwg (accessed on 9 September 2018).
17. Matthijnssens, J.; Bilcke, J.; Ciarlet, M.; Martella, V.; Bányai, K.; Ranst, M.V. Rotavirus disease and vaccination: Impact on genotype diversity. *Futur. Microbiol.* **2009**, *4*, 1303–1316. [CrossRef] [PubMed]
18. Rahman, M.; Matthijnssens, J.; Yang, X.; Delbeke, T.; Arijs, I.; Taniguchi, K.; Iturriza-Gómara, M.; Iftekharuddin, N.; Azim, T.; Van Ranst, M. Evolutionary history and global spread of the emerging G12 human rotaviruses. *J. Virol.* **2007**, *81*, 2382–2390. [CrossRef]
19. Santos, N.; Hoshino, Y. Global distribution of rotavirus serotypes/genotypes and its implication for the development and implementation of an effective rotavirus vaccine. *Rev. Med. Virol.* **2005**, *15*, 29–56. [CrossRef]
20. Mwenda, J.M.; Ntoto, K.M.; Abebe, A.; Enweronu-Laryea, C.; Amina, I.; Mchomvu, J.; Kisakye, A.; Mpabalwani, E.M.; Pazvakavambwa, I.; Armah, G.E.; et al. Burden and epidemiology of rotavirus diarrhea in selected African countries: Preliminary results from the African Rotavirus Surveillance Network. *J. Infect. Dis.* **2010**, *202*, 5–11. [CrossRef]
21. Seheri, L.M.; Magagula, N.B.; Peenze, I.; Rakau, K.; Ndadza, A.; Mwenda, J.M.; Weldegebriel, G.; Steele, A.D.; Mphahlele, M.J. Rotavirus strain diversity in Eastern and Southern African countries before and after vaccine introduction. *Vaccine* **2018**, *36*, 7222–7230. [CrossRef]
22. Seheri, M.; Nemarude, L.; Peenze, I.; Netshifhefhe, L.; Nyaga, M.M.; Ngobeni, H.G.; Maphalala, G.; Maake, L.L.; Steele, A.D.; Mwenda, J.M.; et al. Update of rotavirus strains circulating in Africa from 2007 through 2011. *Pediatric Infect. Dis. J.* **2014**, *33*, 76–84. [CrossRef]
23. Matthijnssens, J.; Ciarlet, M.; Rahman, M.; Attoui, H.; Bányai, K.; Estes, M.K.; Gentsch, J.R.; Iturriza-Gómara, M.; Kirkwood, C.D.; Martella, V.; et al. Recommendations for the classification of

group A rotaviruses using all 11 genomic RNA segments. *Arch. Virol.* **2008**, *153*, 1621–1629. [CrossRef] [PubMed]
24. Nyaga, M.M.; Stucker, K.M.; Esona, M.D.; Jere, K.C.; Mwinyi, B.; Shonhai, A.; Tsolenyanu, E.; Mulindwa, A.; Chibumbya, J.N.; Adolfine, H.; et al. Whole-genome analyses of DS-1-like human G2P [4] and G8P [4] rotavirus strains from Eastern, Western and Southern Africa. *Virus Genes* **2014**, *49*, 196–207. [CrossRef] [PubMed]
25. Block, S.L.; Vesikari, T.; Goveia, M.G.; Rivers, S.B.; Adeyi, B.A.; Dallas, M.J.; Bauder, J.; Boslego, J.W.; Heaton, P.M. Efficacy, immunogenicity, and safety of a pentavalent human-bovine (WC3) reassortant rotavirus vaccine at the end of shelf life. *Pediatrics* **2007**, *119*, 11–18. [CrossRef] [PubMed]
26. Vesikari, T.; Matson, D.O.; Dennehy, P.; Van Damme, P.; Santosham, M.; Rodriguez, Z.; Dallas, M.J.; Heyse, J.F.; Goveia, M.G.; Black, S.B.; et al. Safety and efficacy of a pentavalent human–bovine (WC3) reassortant rotavirus vaccine. *N. Engl. J. Med.* **2006**, *354*, 23–33. [CrossRef]
27. Afrad, M.H.; Matthijnssens, J.; Moni, S.; Kabir, F.; Ashrafi, A.; Rahman, M.Z.; Faruque, A.S.; Azim, T.; Rahman, M. Genetic characterization of a rare bovine-like human VP4 mono-reassortant G6P [8] rotavirus strain detected from an infant in Bangladesh. *Infect. Genet. Evol.* **2013**, *19*, 120–126. [CrossRef]
28. Liu, L.; Johnson, H.L.; Cousens, S.; Perin, J.; Scott, S.; Lawn, J.E.; Rudan, I.; Campbell, H.; Cibulskis, R.; Li, M.; et al. Global, regional, and national causes of child mortality: An updated systematic analysis for 2010 with time trends since 2000. *Lancet* **2012**, *379*, 2151–2161. [CrossRef]
29. WHO. Global Health Observatory Data Repository, Rotavirus Immunization Coverage Estimates by Country. 2018. Available online: http://apps.who.int/gho/data/node.main.ROTACnfiltertable\T1\textbar{}resettable (accessed on 2 November 2018).
30. Shah, M.P.; Tate, J.E.; Mwenda, J.M.; Steele, A.D.; Parashar, U.D. Estimated reductions in hospitalizations and deaths from childhood diarrhea following implementation of rotavirus vaccination in Africa. *Exp. Rev. Vaccines* **2017**, *16*, 987–995. [CrossRef]
31. Moyo, S.J.; Blomberg, B.; Hanevik, K.; Kommedal, O.; Vainio, K.; Maselle, S.Y.; Langeland, N. Genetic diversity of circulating rotavirus strains in Tanzania prior to the introduction of vaccination. *PLoS ONE* **2014**, *9*, 97562. [CrossRef]
32. WHO. United Republic of Tanzania: WHO and UNICEF Estimates of Immunization Coverage: 2017 Revision. 2017. Available online: http://apps.who.int/immunization_monitoring/globalsummary/wucoveragecountrylist.html (accessed on 13 July 2019).
33. Abeid, K.A.; Jani, B.; Cortese, M.M.; Kamugisha, C.; Mwenda, J.M.; Pandu, A.S.; Msaada, K.A.; Mohamed, A.S.; Khamis, A.U.; Parashar, U.D.; et al. Monovalent rotavirus vaccine effectiveness and impact on rotavirus hospitalizations in Zanzibar, Tanzania: Data from the first 3 years after introduction. *J. Infect. Dis.* **2016**, *215*, 183–191. [CrossRef]
34. Brookfield, D.S.K.; Cosgrove, B.P.; Bell, E.J.; Madeley, C.R. Viruses demonstrated in children in Tanzania: Studies in diarrhoea and measles. *J. Infect.* **1979**, *1*, 249–255. [CrossRef]
35. Gachanja, E.; Buza, J.; Petrucka, P. Molecular Detection of Group A Rotavirus in Children under Five in Urban and Peri-Urban Arusha, Tanzania. *J. Adv. Med. Med Res.* **2016**, *12*, 1–9. [CrossRef]
36. Hokororo, A.; Kidenya, B.R.; Seni, J.; Mapaseka, S.; Mphahlele, J.; Mshana, S.E. 2Predominance of rotavirus G1 [P8] genotype among under-five children with gastroenteritis in Mwanza, Tanzania. *J. Trop. Pediatric* **2014**, *60*, 393–396. [CrossRef] [PubMed]
37. Jani, B.; Hokororo, A.; Mchomvu, J.; Cortese, M.M.; Kamugisha, C.; Mujuni, D.; Kallovya, D.; Parashar, U.D.; Mwenda, J.M.; Lyimo, D.; et al. Detection of rotavirus before and after monovalent rotavirus vaccine introduction and vaccine effectiveness among children in mainland Tanzania. *Vaccine* **2018**, *36*, 7149–7156. [CrossRef] [PubMed]
38. Mchaile, D.N.; Philemon, R.N.; Kabika, S.; Albogast, E.; Morijo, K.J.; Kifaro, E.; Mmbaga, B.T. Prevalence and genotypes of Rotavirus among children under 5 years presenting with diarrhoea in Moshi, Tanzania: A hospital-based cross sectional study. *BMC Res. Notes* **2017**, *10*, 542. [CrossRef]
39. Mhalu, F.S.; Myrmel, H.; Msengi, A.; Haukenes, G. Prevalence of infection with rotavirus and enteric adenoviruses among children in Tanzania. *NIPH Ann.* **1988**, *11*, 3–7.
40. Moyo, S.J.; Gro, N.; Kirsti, V.; Matee, M.I.; Kitundu, J.; Maselle, S.Y.; Langeland, N.; Myrmel, H. Prevalence of enteropathogenic viruses and molecular characterization of group A rotavirus among children with diarrhea in Dar es Salaam Tanzania. *BMC Public Health* **2007**, *7*, 359. [CrossRef]

41. Sam, N.E.; Haukenes, G.; Szilvay, A.M.; Mhalu, F. Rotavirus infection in Tanzania: A virological, epidemiological and clinical study among young children. *APMIS* **1992**, *100*, 790–796. [CrossRef]
42. Temu, A.; Kamugisha, E.; Mwizamholya, D.L.; Hokororo, A.; Seni, J.; Mshana, S.E. Prevalence and factors associated with Group A rotavirus infection among children with acute diarrhea in Mwanza, Tanzania. *J. Infect. Dev. Ctries.* **2012**, *6*, 508–515. [CrossRef]
43. Temu, M.M.; Changalucha, J.M.; Mngara, J.T.; Steele, A.D. Prevalence of rotavirus infections and strain types detected among under-five children presenting with diarrhoea at selected MCH clinics in Mwanza City, Tanzania. *Tanzan. J. Health Res.* **2002**, *4*, 30–32. [CrossRef]
44. Vargas, M.; Gascon, J.; Casals, C.; Schellenberg, D.; Urassa, H.; Kahigwa, E.; Ruiz, J.; Vila, J. Etiology of diarrhea in children less than five years of age in Ifakara, Tanzania. *Am. J. Trop. Med. Hyg.* **2004**, *70*, 536–539. [CrossRef]
45. PATH. Rotavirus Disease and Vaccines in Tanzania. 2012. Available online: https://www.path.org/resources/rotavirus-disease-and-vaccines-in-tanzania/ (accessed on 22 September 2018).
46. WHO. 2008 Rotavirus Deaths, under 5 Years of Age, as of 31 January 2012. Available online: https://www.who.int/immunization/monitoring_surveillance/burden/estimates/rotavirus/en (accessed on 12 November 2018).
47. Platts-Mills, J.A.; Amour, C.; Gratz, J.; Nshama, R.; Walongo, T.; Mujaga, B.; Maro, A.; McMurry, T.L.; Liu, J.; Mduma, E.; et al. Impact of rotavirus vaccine introduction and postintroduction etiology of diarrhea requiring hospital admission in Haydom, Tanzania, a rural African setting. *Clin. Infect. Dis.* **2017**, *65*, 1144–1151. [CrossRef] [PubMed]
48. Bar-Zeev, N.; Jere, K.C.; Bennett, A.; Pollock, L.; Tate, J.E.; Nakagomi, O.; Iturriza-Gomara, M.; Costello, A.; Mwansambo, C.; Parashar, U.D.; et al. Population impact and effectiveness of monovalent rotavirus vaccination in urban Malawian children 3 years after vaccine introduction: Ecological and case-control analyses. *Clin. Infect. Dis.* **2016**, *62*, S213–S219. [CrossRef] [PubMed]
49. Bar-Zeev, N.; Kapanda, L.; Tate, J.E.; Jere, K.C.; Iturriza-Gomara, M.; Nakagomi, O.; Mwansambo, C.; Costello, A.; Parashar, U.D.; Heyderman, R.S.; et al. Effectiveness of a monovalent rotavirus vaccine in infants in Malawi after programmatic roll-out: An observational and case-control study. *Lancet Infect. Dis.* **2015**, *15*, 422–428. [CrossRef]
50. Ngabo, F.; Tate, J.E.; Gatera, M.; Rugambwa, C.; Donnen, P.; Lepage, P.; Mwenda, J.M.; Binagwaho, A.; Parashar, U.D. Effect of pentavalent rotavirus vaccine introduction on hospital admissions for diarrhoea and rotavirus in children in Rwanda: A time-series analysis. *Lancet Glob. Health* **2016**, *4*, 129–136. [CrossRef]
51. Levy, K.; Hubbard, A.E.; Eisenberg, J.N. Seasonality of rotavirus disease in the tropics: A systematic review and meta-analysis. *Int. J. Epidemiol.* **2009**, *38*, 1487–1496. [CrossRef] [PubMed]
52. Tate, J.E.; Panozzo, C.A.; Payne, D.C.; Patel, M.M.; Cortese, M.M.; Fowlkes, A.L.; Parashar, U.D. Decline and Change in Seasonality of US Rotavirus Activity After the Introduction of Rotavirus Vaccine. *Am. Acad. Pediatrics* **2009**, *123*, 465–471. [CrossRef]
53. National Bureau of Statistics. 2015–16 Tanzania Demographic and Health Survey and Malaria Indicator Survey (TDHS-MIS) Report. Available online: https://www.nbs.go.tz/index.php/en/census-surveys/health-statistics/demographic-and-health-survey-dhs (accessed on 21 July 2019).
54. Beres, L.K.; Tate, J.E.; Njobvu, L.; Chibwe, B.; Rudd, C.; Guffey, M.B.; Stringer, J.S.; Parashar, U.D.; Chilengi, R.A. preliminary assessment of rotavirus vaccine effectiveness in Zambia. *Clin. Infect. Dis.* **2016**, *62*, 175–182. [CrossRef]
55. Gastañaduy, P.A.; Steenhoff, A.P.; Mokomane, M.; Esona, M.D.; Bowen, M.D.; Jibril, H.; Pernica, J.M.; Mazhani, L.; Smieja, M.; Tate, J.E.; et al. Effectiveness of monovalent rotavirus vaccine after programmatic implementation in Botswana: A multisite prospective case-control study. *Clin. Infect. Dis.* **2016**, *62*, 161–167. [CrossRef]
56. Groome, M.J.; Page, N.; Cortese, M.M.; Moyes, J.; Zar, H.J.; Kapongo, C.N.; Mulligan, C.; Diedericks, R.; Cohen, C.; Fleming, J.A.; et al. Effectiveness of monovalent human rotavirus vaccine against admission to hospital for acute rotavirus diarrhoea in South African children: A case-control study. *Lancet Infect. Dis.* **2014**, *14*, 1096–1104. [CrossRef]
57. Bányai, K.; Gentsch, J.R.; Schipp, R.; Jakab, F.; Meleg, E.; Mihály, I.; Szücs, G. Dominating prevalence of P [8], G1 and P [8], G9 rotavirus strains among children admitted to hospital between 2000 and 2003 in Budapest, Hungary. *J. Med. Virol.* **2005**, *76*, 414–423. [CrossRef]

58. Sharma, S.; Paul, V.K.; Bhan, M.K.; Ray, P. Genomic characterization of nontypeable rotaviruses and detection of a rare G8 strain in Delhi, India. *J. Clin. Microbiol.* **2009**, *47*, 3998–4005. [CrossRef] [PubMed]
59. Cortese, M.M.; Parashar, U.D. Prevention of rotavirus gastroenteritis among infants and children: Recommendations of the Advisory Committee on Immunization Practices (ACIP). *Morb. Mortal. Wkly. Rep. Recomm. Rep.* **2009**, *58*, 1–25.
60. Steele, A.D.; Neuzil, K.M.; Cunliffe, N.A.; Madhi, S.A.; Bos, P.; Ngwira, B.; Witte, D.; Todd, S.; Louw, C.; Kirsten, M.; et al. Human rotavirus vaccine Rotarix™ provides protection against diverse circulating rotavirus strains in African infants: A randomized controlled trial. *BMC Infect. Dis.* **2012**, *12*, 213. [CrossRef] [PubMed]
61. De Grazia, S.; Ramirez, S.; Giammanco, G.M.; Colomba, C.; Martella, V.; Biundo, C.L.; Mazzola, R.; Arista, S. Diversity of human rotaviruses detected in Sicily, Italy, over a 5-year period (2001–2005). *Arch. Virol.* **2007**, *152*, 833–837. [CrossRef]
62. Martella, V.; Bányai, K.; Matthijnssens, J.; Buonavoglia, C.; Ciarlet, M. Zoonotic aspects of rotaviruses. *Vet. Microbiol.* **2010**, *140*, 246–255. [CrossRef]
63. Rahman, M.; Matthijnssens, J.; Goegebuer, T.; De Leener, K.; Vanderwegen, L.; van der Donck, I.; Van Hoovels, L.; De Vos, S.; Azim, T.; Van Ranst, M. Predominance of rotavirus G9 genotype in children hospitalized for rotavirus gastroenteritis in Belgium during 1999–2003. *J. Clin. Virol.* **2005**, *33*, 1–6. [CrossRef]
64. Ward, R.L.; Bernstein, D.I.; Plotkin, S. Rotarix: A rotavirus vaccine for the world. *Clin. Infect. Dis.* **2009**, *48*, 222–228. [CrossRef]
65. Banyai, K.; Mijatovic-Rustempasic, S.; Hull, J.J.; Esona, M.D.; Freeman, M.M.; Frace, A.M.; Bowen, M.D.; Gentsch, J.R. Sequencing and phylogenetic analysis of the coding region of six common rotavirus strains: Evidence for intragenogroup reassortment among co-circulating G1P [8] and G2P [4] strains from the United States. *J. Med. Virol.* **2011**, *83*, 532–539. [CrossRef]
66. Martella, V.; Bányai, K.; Ciarlet, M.; Iturriza-Gómara, M.; Lorusso, E.; De Grazia, S.; Arista, S.; Decaro, N.; Elia, G.; Cavalli, A.; et al. Relationships among porcine and human P [6] rotaviruses: Evidence that the different human P [6] lineages have originated from multiple interspecies transmission events. *Virology* **2006**, *344*, 509–519. [CrossRef]
67. Papp, H.; László, B.; Jakab, F.; Ganesh, B.; De Grazia, S.; Matthijnssens, J.; Ciarlet, M.; Martella, V.; Bányai, K. Review of group A rotavirus strains reported in swine and cattle. *Vet. Microbiol.* **2013**, *165*, 190–199. [CrossRef]
68. Assenga, J.A.; Matemba, L.E.; Muller, S.K.; Mhamphi, G.G.; Kazwala, R.R. Predominant leptospiral serogroups circulating among humans, livestock and wildlife in Katavi-Rukwa ecosystem, Tanzania. *PLoS Negl. Trop. Dis.* **2015**, *9*, e0003607. [CrossRef] [PubMed]
69. Bishop, R.F. Natural history of human rotavirus infection. *Arch. Virol. Suppl.* **1996**, *12*, 119–128. [PubMed]
70. Ansari, S.A.; Springthorpe, V.S.; Sattar, S.A. Survival and vehicular spread of human rotaviruses: Possible relation to seasonality of outbreaks. *Rev. Infect. Dis.* **1991**, *13*, 448–461. [CrossRef] [PubMed]
71. Matthijnssens, J.; De Grazia, S.; Piessens, J.; Heylen, E.; Zeller, M.; Giammanco, G.M.; Bányai, K.; Buonavoglia, C.; Ciarlet, M.; Martella, V.; et al. Multiple reassortment and interspecies transmission events contribute to the diversity of feline, canine and feline/canine-like human group A rotavirus strains. *Infect. Genet. Evol.* **2011**, *11*, 1396–1406. [CrossRef]
72. Komoto, S.; Adah, M.I.; Ide, T.; Yoshikawa, T.; Taniguchi, K. Whole genomic analysis of human and bovine G8P [1] rotavirus strains isolated in Nigeria provides evidence for direct bovine-to-human interspecies transmission. *Infect. Genet. Evol.* **2016**, *43*, 424–433. [CrossRef]
73. Medici, M.C.; Tummolo, F.; Bonica, M.B.; Heylen, E.; Zeller, M.; Calderaro, A.; Matthijnssens, J. Genetic diversity in three bovine-like human G8P [14] and G10P [14] rotaviruses suggests independent interspecies transmission events. *J. Gen. Virol.* **2015**, *96*, 1161–1168. [CrossRef]
74. Tacharoenmuang, R.; Komoto, S.; Guntapong, R.; Ide, T.; Singchai, P.; Upachai, S.; Fukuda, S.; Yoshida, Y.; Murata, T.; Yoshikawa, T.; et al. Characterization of a G10P [14] rotavirus strain from a diarrheic child in Thailand: Evidence for bovine-to-human zoonotic transmission. *Infect. Genet. Evol.* **2018**, *63*, 43–57. [CrossRef]
75. Dóró, R.; Farkas, S.L.; Martella, V.; Bányai, K. Zoonotic transmission of rotavirus: Surveillance and control. *Expert Rev. Anti-Infect. Ther.* **2015**, *13*, 1337–1350. [CrossRef]
76. Medici, M.C.; Abelli, L.A.; Vito, M.; Monica, M.; Eleonora, L.; Canio, B.; Giuseppe, D.; Carlo, C.

Characterization of inter-genogroup reassortant rotavirus strains detected in hospitalized children in Italy. *J. Med. Virol.* **2007**, *79*, 1406–1412. [CrossRef]
77. Iturriza-Gómara, M.; Cubitt, D.; Desselberger, U.; Gray, J. Amino acid substitution within the VP7 protein of G2 rotavirus strains associated with failure to serotype. *J. Clin. Microbiol.* **2001**, *39*, 3796–3798. [CrossRef]
78. Iturriza-Gómara, M.; Kang, G.; Gray, J. Rotavirus genotyping: Keeping up with an evolving population of human rotaviruses. *J. Clin. Virol.* **2004**, *31*, 259–265. [CrossRef] [PubMed]

# Histo-Blood Group Antigens in Children with Symptomatic Rotavirus Infection

Raúl Pérez-Ortín, Susana Vila-Vicent, Noelia Carmona-Vicente, Cristina Santiso-Bellón, Jesús Rodríguez-Díaz[ID] and Javier Buesa *[ID]

Department of Microbiology, School of Medicine, University of Valencia and Clinical Microbiology Service, Hospital Clínico Universitario de Valencia, Instituto de Investigación INCLIVA, 46010 Valencia, Spain; raul.perez@clinicalapau.es (R.P.-O.); susana.vila@uv.es (S.V.-V.); noelia.carmona@uv.es (N.C.-V.); cristina.santiso@hotmail.com (C.S.-B.); jesus.rodriguez@uv.es (J.R.-D.)
* Correspondence: javier.buesa@uv.es

**Abstract:** Group A rotaviruses are a major cause of acute gastroenteritis in children. The diversity and unequal geographical prevalence of rotavirus genotypes have been linked to histo-blood group antigens (HBGAs) in different human populations. In order to evaluate the role of HBGAs in rotavirus infections in our population, secretor status (FUT2+), ABO blood group, and Lewis antigens were determined in children attended for rotavirus gastroenteritis in Valencia, Spain. During three consecutive years (2013–2015), stool and saliva samples were collected from 133 children with rotavirus infection. Infecting viral genotypes and HBGAs were determined in patients and compared to a control group and data from blood donors. Rotavirus G9P[8] was the most prevalent strain (49.6%), followed by G1P[8] (20.3%) and G12P[8] (14.3%). Rotavirus infected predominantly secretor (99%) and Lewis b positive (91.7%) children. Children with blood group A and AB were significantly more prone to rotavirus gastroenteritis than those with blood group O. Our results confirm that a HBGA genetic background is linked to rotavirus P[8] susceptibility. Rotavirus P[8] symptomatic infection is manifestly more frequent in secretor-positive (FUT2+) than in non-secretor individuals, although no differences between rotavirus G genotypes were found.

**Keywords:** rotavirus; histo-blood group antigens (HBGAs); secretor; Lewis; ABO group antigens; susceptibility; gastroenteritis

---

## 1. Introduction

Group A rotaviruses are the main cause of acute gastroenteritis in infants and young children worldwide, with similar prevalence in developed and developing countries. However, the most severe cases and higher mortality rates occur in developing countries [1]. The World Health Organization (WHO) recommends the use of rotavirus vaccines in all national immunization programs, particularly in South and Southeastern Asia and sub-Saharan Africa [2]. Two oral, live-attenuated rotavirus vaccines (Rotarix and RotaTeq) are available internationally, both considered safe and effective in preventing gastrointestinal disease. However, the efficiency of rotavirus vaccines has been reported to be lower in African children [3,4]. Malnutrition, concomitant infections, simultaneous administration with oral poliovirus vaccine, rotavirus strain diversity, and genetic host factors have been proposed to explain these differences. In addition, the intestinal microbiome may contribute to alter the immune response to rotavirus vaccines [5,6]. It was reported that human rotaviruses recognize the different host histo-blood group antigens (HBGAs) of individuals in a type-specific manner [7–9]. HBGAs are complex carbohydrates located on the surface of red blood cells and mucosal epithelia and in body fluids such as saliva, intestinal secretions, milk, and blood as soluble oligosaccharides [10–12]. These antigens are genetically determined and depend on an individual's ABO, secretor, and Lewis status. Recent epidemiological studies indicate that histo-blood group antigens (HBGAs) act as susceptibility factors for the globally dominant P[4], P[6], and P[8] genotypes of human strains of rotavirus A, that recognize fucosylated HBGAs through their spike protein VP8* [13–15].

The gene responsible for the secretor phenotype, *FUT2*, encodes an α(1,2)fucosyltransferase that produces the carbohydrate H found on the surface of epithelial cells and in mucosal secretions [16]. The Lewis gene (*FUT3*) codes for an α(1,3/4)fucosyltransferase that transfers fucose to the subterminal βGlcNac unit of precursor chains [17]. Rotavirus P[6] mainly infects Lewis-negative children, a phenotype more common in African populations, providing a plausible explanation for the relatively high frequency of the P[6] genotype in Africa and in some Latin American countries [8,18–20]. It was hypothesized that resistance to P[8] strains in Lewis-negative children could be an important contributing factor to the low rotavirus vaccine efficacy in sub-Saharan Africa [8]. However, secretor genotyping in other studies showed that P[8] rotaviruses infect both secretor and non-secretor individuals and that infection correlated with the presence of Lewis antigen [21].

The aim of this study was to evaluate the HBGA profile (ABO, secretor, and Lewis status) in rotavirus-infected children in Valencia, Spain and to investigate potential associations between rotavirus P/G genotypes and HBGA patterns in patients.

## 2. Materials and Methods

### 2.1. Study Population and Specimens

Stool and saliva samples were collected from 133 children under 5 years of age with rotavirus infection between January 2013 and December 2015. Children were attended at the pediatric clinics and emergency room of the Hospital Clínico Universitario of Valencia (Department of Health No. 5). This study was conducted with the approval of the Ethics Committee of the Hospital (code F-CE-GEva-15; 26 March 2015), and informed written consent was obtained from patients' parents/tutors before sample collection. Only patients with signed consent were enrolled. To compare the genetic background of the rotavirus-infected children with non-infected counterparts, the distribution of ABO blood groups, H type 1 (*FUT2*), and Lewis antigens were assessed in a control group of 50 healthy children of the same ages and geographic locations. Data from blood donors ($n$ = 283,399 individuals) were also obtained from the Transfusion Center of the Autonomous Region of Valencia (Dr. Emma Castro Izaguirre, personal communication).

### 2.2. Rotavirus Detection and Genotyping

Rotaviruses were detected by immunochromatographic assay (Rotavirus–Adenovirus Certest Biotec, Zaragoza, Spain) and rotavirus G (VP7) and P (VP4) genotypes were determined by a semi-nested multiplex RT-PCR method. For this purpose, a 10%–20% suspension of stool sample was prepared in phosphate buffered saline and subsequent viral RNA extraction was performed using TRIzol (Life Technologies, Carlsbad, CA, USA). Rotavirus G and P genotyping was carried out by RT-PCR following the standardized procedures of the EuroRotaNet network (www.eurorota.net) [22].

### 2.3. Determination of Histo-Blood Group Antigens in Saliva

Lewis (Le$^a$ and Le$^b$) antigens and ABO group phenotypes were analyzed in saliva samples by enzyme-linked immunosorbent assay (ELISA), essentially as previously described [23]. Polystyrene microtiter plates (Costar, Corning, NY, USA) were coated with previously boiled saliva diluted 1:500 in coating buffer (0.1 M carbonate–bicarbonate buffer, pH 9.6) and incubated for 2 h at 37 °C followed by

4 °C overnight. Plates were washed with phosphate-buffered saline (PBS) containing 0.05% Tween-20 (PBS-T) and blocked with 3% bovine serum albumin (BSA) in PBS. Monoclonal antibodies anti-A and anti-B (Diagast, Loos, France), anti-Le$^a$ and anti-Le$^b$ (Covance, Dedham, MA, USA), were diluted 1:100 in PBS with 1% BSA and incubated for 1 h at 37 °C. After three washes, horseradish peroxidase goat anti-mouse IgG (Sigma Immunochemicals, St. Louis, MO, USA) diluted 1:2000 in PBS–BSA was added, and incubated for 1 h at 37 °C. After three washes, reactions were developed with o-phenylenediamine dihydrochloride (OPD-Fast) (Sigma, St. Louis, MO, USA), stopped with 2M H$_2$SO$_4$, and recorded at 492 nm. The cutoff value was defined as a threefold increase in absorbance value compared to two negative control samples.

*2.4. Genotypic Characterization of the FUT2 Gene (Secretor Status)*

Saliva DNA was extracted with a commercial kit (JetFlex Genomic DNA Purification kit, Genomed, Vilnius, Lithuania) and PCR analysis was performed as previously described [16,24]. The secretor genotype (*FUT2*) was characterized by PCR with saliva-extracted DNA and AvaII (Thermo Fisher Scientific, Vilnius, Lithuania) digestion of the amplimers [24,25], to be able to differentiate homozygous and heterozygous alleles for the inactivating mutation G428A in the *FUT2* gene [26].

*2.5. Statistical Analysis*

Categorical data were analyzed using the $X^2$ test or, when $n < 5$, the Fisher exact test with two-tailed significance was used. Odds ratios (OR) and 95% confidence intervals (CIs) were also calculated. *P* values lower than 0.05 were considered statistically significant. Data were statistically analyzed using R Core Team (2015) v 3.2.2. software.

## 3. Results

*3.1. Study Population and Sample Collection*

This study was conducted with pediatric patients from the health area served by the Hospital Clínico Universitario of Valencia. The total population attended by this hospital was 345,498, of which 20,091 (5.82%) were children under 5 years of age. Patient ages ranged from 13 days to 5 years, average 22 months. Most children (84.2%) were under 3 years of age, 62 were female (46.6%; 95% CI: 37.9–55.5), and 71 were male (53.4%; 95% CI: 44.5–62.1). A control group composed of 50 healthy children, 24 boys (48%; 95% CI: 33.7–62.6) and 26 girls (52%; 95% CI: 37.4–66.3) with similar demographic characteristics to the patient group was included for comparison.

*3.2. Rotavirus Genotypes*

Most children were infected with one genotype (90.2%), 10 (7.5%) children had mixed infections with two genotypes, and in 3 (2.3%) patients the infecting genotype could not be determined. Rotavirus G9P[8] was the most prevalent strain (49.6%), followed by G1P[8] (20.3%) and G12P[8] (14.3%). Other genotypes detected throughout the three-year period were G4P[8] (3.8%), G2P[4] (1.5%), and G3P[8] (0.8%) (Figure 1). Mixed infections caused by G1 + G3P[8] (four cases), G1 + G9P[8] (three cases), G3 + G9P[8] (two cases), and G9 + G12P[8] (one case) were detected. Among the 133 rotavirus strains, 131 were genotype P[8] (97.7%; 95% CI: 93.5–99.5) and only 2 were genotype P[4] (1.5%; 95% CI: 0.2–5.3). No strains of genotype P[6] were detected.

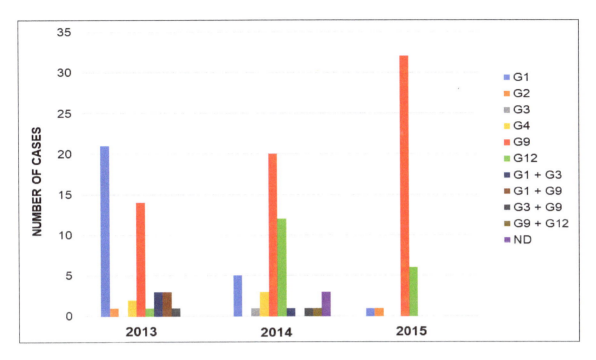

**Figure 1.** Temporal distribution of rotavirus G genotypes during the three-year study period. Regarding P genotypes, 98% of the strains were P[8] genotype with an overall dominance of G9P[8]. Abbreviations: ND, not determined.

*3.3. Secretor (FUT2) Status*

Rotavirus preferentially infected secretor (98.5%) (95% CI: 94.7–99.8) and Lewis b positive children 92.5% (95% CI: 86.6–96.3) (Table 1). Among the rotavirus-infected secretor individuals, the distribution of homozygous and heterozygous alleles for the *FUT2* gene was 38% and 61%, respectively. In the control group, 70% were secretors and 30% non-secretors (Table 1).

**Table 1.** Distribution of histo-blood group antigens (HBGAs) in rotavirus-infected children ($n = 133$), in the control group ($n = 50$), and in blood donors ($n = 283,399$).

| | Patients ($n = 133$) (%) | | Controls [a] ($n = 50$) (%) | | $p$ Value [b] | Odds Ratio [c] 95% CI | | Donors ($n = 283,399$) (%) | | $p$ Value [b] |
|---|---|---|---|---|---|---|---|---|---|---|
| **Blood Group** | | | | | | | | | | |
| O | 50 | (37.6) | 15 | (36.6) | 0.365 | * | | 146,454 | (51.7) | 0.003 |
| A | 64 | (48.1) | 17 | (41.5) | | 0.89 | (0.4–2) | 110,273 | (38.9) | |
| B | 10 | (7.5) | 7 | (17.1) | | 2.31 | (0.7–7.2) | 19,054 | (6.7) | |
| AB | 9 | (6.8) | 2 | (4.9) | | 0.78 | (0.1–3.6) | 7618 | (2.7) | |
| **Secretor (FUT2)** | | | | | | | | | | |
| Secretor | 131 | (98.5) | 35 | (70) | 0.000 | * | | NA | | – |
| Non-secretor | 2 | (1.5) | 15 | (30) | | 25 | (6.7–100) | NA | | |
| **Lewis (FUT3)** | | | | | | | | | | |
| Negative | 8 | (6) | 3 | (6) | 1.000 | * | | 31,090 | (11) | 0.091 |
| Positive | 125 | (94) | 47 | (94) | | 0.97 | (0.26–4.84) | 252,309 | (89) | |
| **Lewis A** | | | | | | | | | | |
| Negative | 73 | (54.9) | 15 | (30) | 0.005 | * | | 225,219 | (79.5) | 0.000 |
| Positive | 60 | (45.1) | 35 | (70) | | 2.81 | (1.42–5.78) | 56,180 | (20.5) | |
| **Lewis B** | | | | | | | | | | |
| Negative | 10 | (7.5) | 18 | (36) | 0.000 | * | | 88,784 | (31.3) | 0.000 |
| Positive | 123 | (92.5) | 32 | (64) | | 0.15 | (0.06–0.35) | 194,615 | (68.7) | |

Table 1. Cont.

| | Patients (n = 133) (%) | | Controls [a] (n = 50) (%) | | p Value [b] | Odds Ratio [c] 95% CI | | Donors (n = 283,399) (%) | | p Value [b] |
|---|---|---|---|---|---|---|---|---|---|---|
| **Lewis A/B** | | | | | | | | | | |
| Le a− b− | 8 | (6) | 3 | (6) | | * | | 31,090 | (11) | |
| Le a− b+ | 65 | (48.9) | 12 | (24) | 0.000 | 0.49 | (0.1–2.6) | 194,129 | (68.5) | 0.000 |
| Le a+ b− | 2 | (1.5) | 15 | (30) | | 16.47 | (2.6–169.7) | 57,694 | (20.3) | |
| Le a+ b+ | 58 | (43.6) | 20 | (40) | | 0.9 | (0.2–4.6) | 486 | (0.2) | |

Abbreviations: CI, confidence interval; Le, Lewis; NA, not available; [a] ABO blood group phenotype was determined in 41 children in the control group; [b] $X^2$ test with two-tailed significance. When $n < 5$, the Fisher exact test with two-tailed significance was used; [c] unadjusted odds ratio; * reference category for the odds ratio estimation.

### 3.4. Lewis and ABO Phenotypes

Among the 133 children with rotavirus infection, the phenotypic HBGA distribution was Le$^{a−b−}$ (6.0%), Le$^{a−b+}$ (48.9%), Le$^{a+b−}$ (1.5%), and Le$^{a+b+}$ (43.6%), with 98.5% being secretors (H type 1 positive) and 1.5% non-secretors (Table 1). Distribution of Lewis phenotypes, secretor status, and ABO blood groups in the control group is also shown in Table 1. In our study, children with Lewis b positive phenotype (Le$^{a−b+}$ and Le$^{a+b+}$) (92.5%) were more commonly infected with rotaviruses than those with phenotype Lewis b negative ($p < 0.05$). By contrast, in the control group only 64% individuals were Lewis b positive (Table 1). The percentage of infected children with Lewis a positive phenotype was 45.1% (95% CI: 36.5–54.0), which was lower than the control group (70%; 95% CI: 55.4–82.1) ($p < 0.05$).

The distribution of the ABO blood group phenotypes among rotavirus-infected children was not homogenous, as 37.6% were group O, 48.1% group A, 7.5% group B, and 6.8% group AB (Table 1). This pattern of ABO blood group distribution was similar in the control group (Table 1) and the differences found were not statistically significant ($p = 0.365$).

### 3.5. Association between HBGAs and Rotavirus Genotypes

The rotavirus genotypes most frequently isolated in our study, G1P[8], G9P[8], and G12P[8], infected more patients with blood groups A and O. However, when we compared the distribution of ABO blood groups in patients to the control group, the difference observed was not statistically significant ($p = 0.365$). When compared with blood donors, group A and AB individuals were at a higher risk of being among gastroenteritis patients than group O individuals ($p = 0.003$) (Table 1).

G1P[8] and G9P[8] genotypes infected mainly blood group A patients (51.8% and 45.4%, respectively), while the G12P[8] genotype was more frequently isolated in group O patients (47.4%) (Table 2). No significant differences were found in the ABO group antigens among children infected with different G genotypes ($p = 0.826$). All rotavirus genotypes more frequently infected *FUT2* heterozygous individuals, except G12P[8] genotype, which was slightly more prevalent (57.9%) among *FUT2* homozygous individuals (Table 2).

Table 2. Association between ABO blood group, secretor status (secretor, heterozygous/homozygous, non-secretor), and Lewis phenotypes with the infecting G/P rotavirus genotypes.

| | G1P[8] (n = 27) (%) | | G2P[4] (n = 2) (%) | | G3P[8] (n = 1) (%) | | G4P[8] (n = 5) (%) | | G9P[8] (n = 66) (%) | | G12P[8] (n = 19) (%) | | p Value [a] |
|---|---|---|---|---|---|---|---|---|---|---|---|---|---|
| **Blood Group** | | | | | | | | | | | | | |
| O | 10 | (37) | 0 | (0) | 0 | (0) | 2 | (40) | 24 | (36.4) | 9 | (47.4) | |
| A | 14 | (51.8) | 2 | (100) | 1 | (100) | 3 | (60) | 30 | (45.4) | 7 | (36.8) | 0.826 |
| B | 2 | (7.4) | 0 | (0) | 0 | (0) | 0 | (0) | 7 | (10.6) | 1 | (5.3) | |
| AB | 1 | (3.7) | 0 | (0) | 0 | (0) | 0 | (0) | 5 | (7.6) | 2 | (10.5) | |

Table 2. Cont.

|  | G1P[8] (n = 27) | (%) | G2P[4] (n = 2) | (%) | G3P[8] (n = 1) | (%) | G4P[8] (n = 5) | (%) | G9P[8] (n = 66) | (%) | G12P[8] (n = 19) | (%) | p Value [a] |
|---|---|---|---|---|---|---|---|---|---|---|---|---|---|
| **Secretor** | | | | | | | | | | | | | |
| Heterozygous | 16 | (59.3) | 2 | (100) | 1 | (100) | 3 | (60) | 44 | (66.7) | 8 | (42.1) | |
| Homozygous | 10 | (37) | 0 | (0) | 0 | (0) | 2 | (40) | 22 | (33.3) | 11 | (57.9) | 0.265 |
| Non-secretor | 1 | (3.7) | 0 | (0) | 0 | (0) | 0 | (0) | 0 | (0) | 0 | (0) | |
| **Lewis A / B** | | | | | | | | | | | | | |
| Le a– b– | 4 | (50) | 0 | (0) | 0 | (0) | 0 | (0) | 2 | (25) | 1 | (12.5) | |
| Le a– b+ | 15 | (23.1) | 1 | (1.5) | 0 | (0) | 3 | (4.6) | 30 | (46.1) | 11 | (16.9) | 0.146 |
| Le a+ b– | 1 | (50) | 0 | (0) | 0 | (0) | 0 | (0) | 0 | (0) | 0 | (0) | |
| Le a+ b+ | 7 | (12.1) | 1 | (1.7) | 1 | (1.7) | 2 | (3.4) | 34 | (58.6) | 7 | (12.1) | |

[a] $X^2$ test with two-tailed significance. When $n < 5$, the Fisher exact test with two-tailed significance was used.

Regarding the patients' Lewis phenotype no statistically significant differences were found in the distribution of rotavirus G genotypes ($p = 0.146$) (Table 2).

## 4. Discussion

Several studies have related rotavirus susceptibility to human histo-blood group antigens (HBGAs), namely to the secretor status associated with the presence of at least one functional *FUT2* (fucosyltransferase-2) allele, and with Lewis antigens (Le$^a$ and Le$^b$), which depend on the *FUT3* gene [17,26,27]. These antigens are oligosaccharide compounds made of N-acetyl-glucosamine, galactose, and fucose. The molecular bases for binding the VP8* domain from P[8] VP4 spike protein to its cellular receptor, the secretor H type 1 antigen (Fuc-α1,2-Gal-β1,3-GlcNAc; H1), and to its precursor lacto-N-biose (Gal-β1,3-GlcNAc; LNB) have recently been determined [28,29]. Capacity to synthesize secretor H type 1 antigen at the mucosae, determined by the presence of one or two functional copies of the fucosyltransferase *FUT2* gene (secretor status), has been clearly linked to infectivity in other enteric viruses such as the noroviruses [16,26]. However, some controversy existed about the contribution of H1 antigen to rotavirus infection. Epidemiological data has only recently evidenced lower incidence of rotavirus symptomatic infections in non-secretor individuals unable to produce H1 [7], as is also reported in this study.

Several interactions between rotavirus and HBGAs have been described. The recombinant protein VP8* of the genotypes P[4], P[6], and P[8], which belong to the P[II] genogroup, recognize H type 1 antigen. It was previously reported that besides the H type 1 antigen, genotypes P[4] and P[8] could also interact with the Lewis b antigen [7]. However, recent structural data obtained with other members of the P[II] genogroup (genotypes P[4], P[6], P[19]) indicate that the recognition of the VP8* from this genogroup occurs via the type 1 precursor, the lacto-N-biose (LNB, Gal β1-3 GlcNac), which interacts within the GlcNac where fucose is added by the FUT3 enzyme [28,29]. These recent discoveries are in contradiction with previous data reported by Huang and collaborators [7]. In addition, the genotypes P[9], P[14], and P[25] of the P[III] genogroup, which infect humans, bind specifically to antigen A [30], and genotype P[11] of the P[IV] genogroup, which infects infants, binds to the type 2 precursor [31].

The fact that P[4], P[6], and P[8] rotaviruses recognize the secretor H antigen seems to be related to the higher prevalence of these genotypes worldwide. The secretor antigen is present in 80% of the population of North America and Europe [12]. Genotypes P[4] and P[8] are the most frequently found in human infections worldwide, with a higher prevalence of genotype [P8] [32]. However, the P[6] genotype is more prevalent in Africa, Asia, and in non-African newborns [33–35]. Some studies have shown a predominance of secretor Lewis-negative individuals in African, Latin American, and Asian countries, in contrast to North America and Europe, where secretor Lewis-positive individuals predominate [23,26,36]. As in North America and the rest of Europe, most of the Spanish population has a Lewis-positive secretor phenotype (FUT2+), which has been related to infection by genotypes

P[4] and P[8], but not by genotype P[6]. This would explain why almost 98% of the rotaviruses detected in this study were P[8] genotypes but none were P[6] genotype. However, in surveys conducted in Burkina Faso, where the majority of the population is Lewis negative, a majority presence of P[6] genotype infections is observed [8]. These Burkina Faso results were interpreted to mean that Lewis b antigen could be a requisite for infection with rotavirus genotypes P[4] and P[8] [8]. Nevertheless, as previously mentioned, this interpretation is not consistent with new, recently reported structural data [28,29]. Something similar happens with non-African neonates; although they are genetically Lewis b positive, expression of these antigens on the surface of erythrocytes can be delayed for the first two months of life, during which time they are Lewis negative [37]. However, it is important to note that these studies were performed in red blood cells, which may not reflect the presence of Lewis antigens on enterocytes and/or in secretions of the intestinal tract. In addition, very little is known about HBGA expression and evolution during development or with concomitant infections in small children. Seven patients in our study got rotavirus infection within the first three months of life, all of them secretor Lewis b positive. The fact that these children express the Lewis b antigen in their mucosae at such a young age has not been observed in other studies [37]. It has been reported that the delay in expression of certain Lewis antigens during the first months of life, despite having an active *FUT3* gene, reinforces the idea that the Lewis antigen might indeed have a preventative effect against rotavirus infection and be part of the age-related restriction factors found in this viral infection.

The G9P[8] genotype proved the most prevalent in our geographical area during the study period with secretor phenotype (FUT2+), as described in other studies carried out in France and Vietnam [36,38]. In our study, the presence of Lewis b antigen in patients (92.5%) was higher than described for the general population of our geographical area, where 69% of individuals are Lewis b positive, estimated from a total of 283,399 individuals (according to unpublished data from the Transfusion Centre of the Autonomous Region of Valencia, Spain). By contrast, 6% of patients were Lewis negative (identical to the 6% described in the control group), but they were nevertheless infected with a P[8] genotype, which contrasts with the results by Nordgren et al. (2014) [8]. This raises the possibility of the secretor H type 1 antigen, rather than the Lewis antigens, being the relevant factor for rotavirus P[8] genotype infection. However, these data must be reinforced by further analyses of P genotypes other than P[8]. It has also been recently reported that the Lewis a phenotype is a restriction factor for RotaTeq and Rotarix vaccine uptake in Nicaraguan children [20]. Moreover, it must be taken into account that aside from HBGA expression, intestinal microbiota composition may play a significant role in susceptibility to rotavirus infections [39].

It was suggested that certain rotavirus P genotypes may be prone to infect blood group A individuals [31] and supporting this we found that group A and AB individuals were more commonly found among patients than group O individuals. As expected, we found a lower infection rate among previously vaccinated than unvaccinated patients [40], and observed no differences in the G genotypes of the infecting rotavirus strains and the brand of vaccine administered (Rotarix or RotaTeq).

Interestingly, it has recently been reported that HBGA-binding specificities of human rotaviruses are associated with the disease, but not with in vitro infection [41]. In this regard, further research is needed to clarify how HBGAs determine rotavirus infection and disease in the human host.

## 5. Conclusions

Our results confirm that genetic background leading to different HBGA expression is linked to susceptibility to group A rotavirus symptomatic infection. Rotavirus P[8] infection is manifestly more frequent in secretor (FUT2+) than in non-secretor individuals, although no significant differences between rotavirus G genotypes were found.

**Author Contributions:** R.P.-O. and J.B. designed and supervised the study. R.P.-O., C.S.-B., N.C.-V., and J.B. collected samples and data. R.P.-O., C.S.-B., S.V.-V., J.R.-D., and J.B. performed the laboratory analyses and interpreted the results. R.P.-O. and J.B. prepared the initial manuscript draft. All authors have read and approved the final version.

**Acknowledgments:** We are grateful to Emma Castro Izaguirre for supplying blood donor data and to José Bermúdez for performing statistical analyses.

## References

1. Tate, J.E.; Burton, A.H.; Boschi-Pinto, C.; Steele, A.D.; Duque, J.; Parashar, U.D. WHO-coordinated Global Rotavirus Surveillance Network. 2008 estimate of worldwide rotavirus-associated mortality in children younger than 5 years before the introduction of universal rotavirus vaccination programmes: A systematic review and meta-analysis. *Lancet Infect. Dis.* **2012**, *12*, 136–141. [CrossRef]
2. WHO. Meeting of the Strategic Advisory Group of Experts on immunization, October 2009–Conclusions and recommendations. *Biologicals.* **2010**, *38*, 170–177. [CrossRef] [PubMed]
3. Armah, G.E.; Sow, S.O.; Breiman, R.F.; Dallas, M.J.; Tapia, M.D.; Feikin, D.R.; Binka, F.N.; Steele, A.D.; Laserson, K.F.; Anasah, N.A.; et al. Efficacy of pentavalent rotavirus vaccine against severe rotavirus gastroenteritis in infants in developing countries in sub-Saharan Africa: A randomised, double-blind, placebo-controlled trial. *Lancet* **2010**, *376*, 606–614. [PubMed]
4. Madhi, S.A.; Cunliffe, N.A.; Steele, D.; Witte, D.; Kirsten, M.; Louw, C.; Ngwira, B.; Victor, J.C.; Gillard, P.H.; Cheuvart, B.B.; et al. Effect of human rotavirus vaccine on severe diarrhea in African infants. *N. Engl. J. Med.* **2010**, *362*, 289–298. [PubMed]
5. Harris, V.C.; Armah, G.; Fuentes, S.; Korpela, K.E.; Parashar, U.; Victor, J.C.; Tate, J.; de Weerth, C.; Giaquinto, C.; Wiersinga, W.J.; et al. Significant correlation between the infant gut microbiome and rotavirus vaccine response in rural Ghana. *J. Infect. Dis.* **2017**, *215*, 34–41. [CrossRef]
6. Harris, V.C.; Haak, B.W.; Handley, S.A.; Jiang, B.; Velasquez, D.E.; Hykes, B.L., Jr.; Droit, L.; Berbers, G.A.N.; Kemper, E.M.; van Leeuwen, E.M.M.; et al. Effect of antibiotic-mediated microbiome modulation on rotavirus vaccine immunogenicity: A human, randomized-control proof-of-concept trial. *Cell Host Microbe* **2018**, *24*, 197–207. [CrossRef] [PubMed]
7. Huang, P.; Xia, M.; Tan, M.; Zhong, W.; Wei, C.; Wang, L.; Morrow, A.; Jiang, X. Spike protein VP8* of human rotavirus recognizes histo-blood group antigens in a type-specific manner. *J. Virol.* **2012**, *86*, 4833–4843. [CrossRef]
8. Nordgren, J.; Sharma, S.; Bucardo, F.; Nasir, W.; Günaydin, G.; Ouermi, D.; Nitiema, L.W.; Becker-Dreps, S.; Simpore, J.; Hammarstrom, L.; et al. Both lewis and secretor status mediate susceptibility to rotavirus infections in a rotavirus genotype-dependent manner. *Clin. Infect. Dis.* **2014**, *59*, 1567–1573. [CrossRef]
9. Jiang, X.; Liu, Y.; Tan, M. Histo-blood group antigens as receptors for rotavirus, new understanding on rotavirus epidemiology and vaccine strategy. *Emerg. Microbes Infect.* **2017**, *6*, e22. [CrossRef] [PubMed]
10. Henry, S.; Jovall, P.Å.; Ghardashkhani, S.; Elmgren, A.; Martinsson, T.; Larson, G.; Samuelsson, B. Structural and immunochemical identification of Le(a), Le(b), H type 1, and related glycolipids in small intestinal mucosa of a group O Le(a-b-) nonsecretor. *Glycoconj J.* **1997**, *14*, 209–223. [CrossRef]
11. Marionneau, S.; Cailleau-Thomas, A.; Rocher, J.; Le Moullac-Vaidye, B.; Ruvoën, N.; Clément, M.; Le Pendu, J. ABH and Lewis histo-blood group antigens, a model for the meaning of oligosaccharide diversity in the face of a changing world. *Biochimie* **2001**, *83*, 565–573.
12. Le Pendu, J. Histo-blood group antigen and human milk oligosaccharides: Genetic polymorphism and risk of infectious diseases. *Adv. Exp. Med. Biol.* **2004**, *554*, 135–143.
13. Böhm, R.; Fleming, F.E.; Maggioni, A.; Dang, V.T.; Holloway, G.; Coulson, B.S.; von Itzstein, M.; Haselhorst, T. Revisiting the role of histo-blood group antigens in rotavirus host-cell invasion. *Nat. Commun.* **2015**, *6*, 5907. [CrossRef] [PubMed]
14. Payne, D.C.; Currier, R.L.; Staat, M.A.; Sahni, L.C.; Selvarangan, R.; Halasa, N.B.; Englund, J.A.; Weinberg, G.A.; Boom, J.A.; Szilagyi, P.G.; et al. Epidemiologic association between FUT2 secretor status and severe rotavirus gastroenteritis in children in the United States. *JAMA Pediatr.* **2015**, *169*, 1040–1045. [CrossRef] [PubMed]
15. Zhang, X.-F.; Long, Y.; Tan, M.; Zhang, T.; Huang, Q.; Jiang, X.; Tan, W.-F.; Li, J.-D.; Hu, G.-F.; Tang, S.; et al. P[8] and P[4] Rotavirus infection associated with secretor phenotypes among children in South China. *Sci. Rep.* **2016**, *6*, 34591. [PubMed]
16. Lindesmith, L.; Moe, C.; Marionneau, S.; Ruvoen, N.; Jiang, X.; Lindblad, L.; Stewart, P.; LePendu, J.; Baric, R. Human susceptibility and resistance to Norwalk virus infection. *Nat. Med.* **2003**, *9*, 548–553. [PubMed]

17. Hutson, A.M.; Atmar, R.L.; Graham, D.Y.; Estes, M.K. Norwalk virus infection and disease is associated with ABO histo-blood group type. *J. Infect. Dis.* **2002**, *185*, 1335–1337. [CrossRef]
18. Todd, S.; Page, N.A.A.; Duncan Steele, A.; Peenze, I.; Cunliffe, N.A. Rotavirus Strain Types Circulating in Africa: Review of Studies Published during 1997–2006. *J. Infect. Dis.* **2010**, *202*, S34–S42. [CrossRef]
19. Nordgren, J.; Nitiema, L.W.; Sharma, S.; Ouermi, D.; Traore, A.S.; Simpore, J.; Svensson, L. Emergence of unusual G6P[6] rotaviruses in children, Burkina Faso, 2009–2010. *Emerg. Infect Dis.* **2012**, *18*, 589–597. [CrossRef]
20. Bucardo, F.; Nordgren, J.; Reyes, Y.; Gonzalez, F.; Sharma, S.; Svensson, L. The Lewis A phenotype is a restriction factor for Rotateq and Rotarix vaccine-take in Nicaraguan children. *Sci. Rep.* **2018**, *8*, 1502. [CrossRef]
21. Ayouni, S.; Sdiri-Loulizi, K.; de Rougemont, A.; Estienney, M.; Ambert-Balay, K.; Aho, S.; Hamami, S.; Aouni, M.; Neji-Guediche, M.; Pothier, P.; et al. Rotavirus P[8] Infections in Persons with Secretor and Nonsecretor Phenotypes, Tunisia. *Emerg. Infect. Dis.* **2015**, *21*, 2055–2058. [CrossRef]
22. Iturriza-Gómara, M.; Dallman, T.; Bányai, K.; Böttiger, B.; Buesa, J.; Diedrich, S.; Fiore, L.; Johansen, K.; Koopmans, M.; Korsun, N.; et al. Rotavirus genotypes co-circulating in Europe between 2006 and 2009 as determined by EuroRotaNet, a pan-European collaborative strain surveillance network. *Epidemiol. Infect.* **2011**, *139*, 895–909. [CrossRef]
23. Nordgren, J.; Nitiema, L.W.; Ouermi, D.; Simpore, J.; Svensson, L. Host genetic factors affect susceptibility to norovirus infections in Burkina Faso. *PLoS ONE* **2013**, *8*, e69557. [CrossRef]
24. Serpa, J.; Mendes, N.; Reis, C.A.; Santos Silva, L.F.; Almeida, R.; Le Pendu, J.; David, L. Two new FUT2 (fucosyltransferase 2 gene) missense polymorphisms, 739G→A and 839T→C, are partly responsible for non-secretor status in a Caucasian population from Northern Portugal. *Biochem. J.* **2004**, *383*, 469–474. [CrossRef]
25. Marionneau, S.; Ruvoën, N.; Le Moullac-Vaidye, B.; Clement, M.; Cailleau-Thomas, A.; Ruiz-Palacios, G.; Huang, P.; Jiang, X.; Le Pendu, J. Norwalk Virus binds to histo-blood group antigens present on gastroduodenal epithelial cells of secretor individuals. *Gastroenterology* **2002**, *122*, 1967–1977.
26. Carlsson, B.; Kindberg, E.; Buesa, J.; Rydell, G.E.; Lidón, M.F.; Montava, R.; Abu Mallouh, R.; Grahn, A.; Rodriguez-Diaz, J.; Bellido, J.; et al. The G428A nonsense mutation in FUT2 provides strong but not absolute protection against symptomatic GII.4 norovirus infection. *PLoS ONE* **2009**, *4*, e5593.
27. Tan, M.; Jiang, X. Histo-blood group antigens: A common niche for norovirus and rotavirus. *Expert Rev. Mol. Med.* **2014**, *16*, e5. [CrossRef]
28. Liu, Y.; Ramelot, T.A.; Huang, P.; Liu, Y.; Li, Z.; Feizi, T.; Zhong, W.; Wu, F.T.; Tan, M.; Kennedy, M.A.; et al. Glycan specificity of P[19] rotavirus and comparison with those of related P genotypes. *J. Virol.* **2016**, *90*, 9983–9996. [CrossRef]
29. Hu, L.; Sankaran, B.; Laucirica, D.R.; Patil, K.; Salmen, W.; Ferreon, A.C.M.; Tsoi, P.S.; Lasanajak, Y.; Smith, D.F.; Ramani, S.; et al. Glycan recognition in globally dominant human rotaviruses. *Nat. Commun.* **2018**, *9*, 2631.
30. Hu, L.; Crawford, S.E.; Czako, R.; Cortes-Penfield, N.W.; Smith, D.F.; Le Pendu, J.; Estes, M.K.; Prasad, B.V. Cell attachment protein VP8* of a human rotavirus specifically interacts with A-type histo-blood group antigen. *Nature* **2012**, *485*, 256–259. [CrossRef]
31. Liu, Y.; Huang, P.; Jiang, B.; Tan, M.; Morrow, A.L.; Jiang, X. Poly-LacNAc as an age-specific ligand for rotavirus P[11] in neonates and infants. *PLoS ONE* **2013**, *8*, e78113. [CrossRef]
32. Santos, N.; Hoshino, Y. Global distribution of rotavirus serotypes/genotypes and its implication for the development and implementation of an effective rotavirus vaccine. *Rev. Med. Virol.* **2005**, *15*, 29–56.
33. Das, S.; Varghese, V.; Chaudhuri, S.; Barman, P.; Kojima, K.; Dutta, P.; Bhattacharya, S.K.; Krishnan, T.; Kobayashi, N.; Naik, T.N. Genetic variability of human rotavirus strains isolated from eastern and northern India. *J. Med. Virol.* **2004**, *72*, 156–161. [CrossRef]
34. Shim, J.O.; Son, D.W.; Shim, S.-Y.; Ryoo, E.; Kim, W.; Jung, Y.-C. Clinical characteristics and genotypes of rotaviruses in a neonatal intensive care unit. *Pediatr. Neonatol.* **2012**, *53*, 18–23.
35. Waggie, Z.; Hawkridge, A.; Hussey, G.D. Review of rotavirus studies in Africa: 1976–2006. *J. Infect. Dis.* **2010**, *202*, S23–S33.
36. Van Trang, N.; Vu, H.T.; Le, N.T.; Huang, P.; Jiang, X.; Anh, D.D. Association between norovirus and rotavirus infection and histo-blood group antigen types in Vietnamese children. *J. Clin. Microbiol.* **2014**, *52*, 1366–1374.

37. Ameno, S.; Kimura, H.; Ameno, K.; Zhang, X.; Kinoshita, H.; Kubota, T.; Ijiri, I. Lewis and Secretor gene effects on Lewis antigen and postnatal development of Lewis blood type. *Biol. Neonatol.* **2001**, *79*, 91–96. [CrossRef]
38. Imbert-Marcille, B.M.; Barbé, L.; Dupé, M.; Le Moullac-Vaidye, B.; Besse, B.; Peltier, C.; Ruvoen-Clouet, N.; Le Pendu, J. A FUT2 gene common polymorphism determines resistance to rotavirus a of the P[8] genotype. *J. Infect. Dis.* **2014**, *209*, 1227–1230.
39. Rodríguez-Díaz, J.; García-Mantrana, I.; Vila-Vicent, S.; Gozalbo-Rovira, R.; Buesa, J.; Monedero, V.; Collado, M.C. Relevance of secretor status genotype and microbiota composition in susceptibility to rotavirus and norovirus infections in humans. *Sci. Rep.* **2017**, *7*, 45559. [CrossRef]
40. Pérez-Ortín, R.; Santiso-Bellón, C.; Vila-Vicent, S.; Carmona-Vicente, N.; Rodríguez-Díaz, J.; Buesa, J. Rotavirus symptomatic infection among vaccinated children in Valencia, Spain. *BMC Infect. Dis.* submitted.
41. Barbé, L.; Le Moullac-Vaidye, B.; Echasserieau, K.; Bernardeau, K.; Carton, T.; Bovin, N.; Nordgren, J.; Svensson, L.; Ruvoen-Clouet, N.; Le Pendu, J. Histo-blood group antigen-binding specificities of human rotaviruses are associated with gastroenteritis but not with in vitro infection. *Sci. Rep.* **2018**, *8*, 12961. [CrossRef] [PubMed]

# Epidemiological Trends of Five Common Diarrhea-Associated Enteric Viruses Pre- and Post-Rotavirus Vaccine Introduction in Coastal Kenya

Arnold W. Lambisia [1,2,*,†], Sylvia Onchaga [1,†], Nickson Murunga [1], Clement S. Lewa [1], Steven Ger Nyanjom [2] and Charles N. Agoti [1,3]

1. Kenya Medical Research Institute (KEMRI)-Wellcome Trust Research Programme, Centre for Geographic Medicine Research-Coast, Kilifi 230-80108, Kenya; onchagasylvia@gmail.com (S.O.); nmurunga@kemri-wellcome.org (N.M.); clewa@kemri-wellcome.org (C.S.L.); cnyaigoti@kemri-wellcome.org (C.N.A.)
2. Department of Biochemistry, Jomo Kenyatta University of Agriculture and Technology, Juja 62000-00200, Kenya; snyanjom@jkuat.ac.ke
3. School of Health and Human Sciences, Pwani University, Kilifi 195-80108, Kenya
* Correspondence: ALambisia@kemri-wellcome.org;
† Joint First Authors.

**Abstract:** Using real-time RT-PCR, we screened stool samples from children aged <5 years presenting with diarrhea and admitted to Kilifi County Hospital, coastal Kenya, pre- (2003 and 2013) and post-rotavirus vaccine introduction (2016 and 2019) for five viruses, namely rotavirus group A (RVA), norovirus GII, adenovirus, astrovirus and sapovirus. Of the 984 samples analyzed, at least one virus was detected in 401 (40.8%) patients. Post rotavirus vaccine introduction, the prevalence of RVA decreased (23.3% vs. 13.8%, $p < 0.001$) while that of norovirus GII increased (6.6% vs. 10.9%, $p = 0.023$). The prevalence of adenovirus, astrovirus and sapovirus remained statistically unchanged between the two periods: 9.9% vs. 14.2%, 2.4% vs. 3.2 %, 4.6% vs. 2.6%, ($p = 0.053$, 0.585 and 0.133), respectively. The median age of diarrhea cases was higher post vaccine introduction (12.5 months, interquartile range (IQR): 7.9–21 vs. 11.2 months pre-introduction, IQR: 6.8–16.5, $p < 0.001$). In this setting, RVA and adenovirus cases peaked in the dry months while norovirus GII and sapovirus peaked in the rainy season. Astrovirus did not display clear seasonality. In conclusion, following rotavirus vaccine introduction, we found a significant reduction in the prevalence of RVA in coastal Kenya but an increase in norovirus GII prevalence in hospitalized children.

**Keywords:** viral diarrhea; real-time PCR; rotavirus vaccination; Kenya

## 1. Introduction

In the year 2016 alone, approximately 300,000 children aged <5 years succumbed to diarrhea in sub-Saharan Africa [1]. Viral pathogens including rotavirus group A (RVA), adenovirus (type 40/41), astrovirus, norovirus (genogroup GI and GII) and sapovirus are among the top causative agents of severe diarrhea globally [2,3]. Understanding their epidemiological patterns such as prevalence, incidence, seasonality, clinical severity and infection age distribution in local settings is essential for designing and prioritizing interventions. Historically, RVA has been the single most important cause of severe childhood diarrhea, responsible for ~38% (95% CI: 4.8–73.4%) of hospital cases (<5 years) pre-vaccine introduction [4]. However, RVA prevalence has been rapidly declining since 2009 and was approximately 23% (95% CI: 0.7–57.7%) in 2016, in settings where the rotavirus vaccine was in use [4]. Due to the shared ecological niche and the apparent decline of all-cause gastroenteritis-associated hospital admissions, it has been hypothesized that rotavirus vaccination has likely impacted the epidemiology of the other enteric viruses [5]. However, there are contradicting reports on the specific impact of rotavirus vaccination on the prevalence of the individual enteric viruses—for example, norovirus [6,7]. This has not been adequately examined in African populations where diarrhea burden is highest. Kenya began rotavirus vaccination in July 2014 using the monovalent Rotarix® (RV1), derived from G1P[8] strain, administered at 6 and 10 weeks of life. RV1 vaccine coverage in Kenya has increased over time since 2014 but is varied by age group, number of doses and geographic region in Kenya [8]. Within Kilifi County, coastal Kenya, coverage in 2017 in <1-year-olds was 73% (at least one dose) vs. 65% (complete two doses), while in <12–24 month-olds, it was 86% (at least one dose) vs. 84% (complete two doses) [9].

The KEMRI/Wellcome Trust Research Programme (KWTRP) has been running surveillance of RVA since 2002 in children admitted to the Kilifi County Hospital (KCH). The current study screened archived diarrheal samples from KCH, spanning both the pre- and post-rotavirus vaccine introduction periods in Kenya for RVA, astrovirus, adenovirus (all serotypes), sapovirus and norovirus (only GII) using real-time reverse-transcription polymerase chain reaction (RT-PCR) approach. We update on the prevalence of these viral diarrheal agents and their seasonal patterns pre and post introduction of the rotavirus vaccination program in Kenya.

## 2. Results

*2.1. Study Population Characteristics*

Out of 2156 children aged <5 years who presented with diarrhea at KCH during the four selected years (2003, 2013, 2016 and 2019), 1397 (64.8%) provided a stool sample; see Table 1. Overall, the demographic characteristics of the eligible children sampled, and eligible children not sampled, differed in age strata distribution ($p = 0.001$) and discharge outcome ($p < 0.001$); see Table 1. The main reasons for failure to sample eligible children were as follows: death ($n = 21$, 2.8%), discharge or transfer before sample collection ($n = 296$, 40.0%), consent refusal ($n = 315$, 41.5%) or other ($n = 127$, 16.7%). Among the sampled cases, 984 (70.4%) had a specimen available and tested by real-time RT-PCR for the five enteric viruses, and these were included in subsequent analysis. The median age of the sampled participants was significantly higher for the post-vaccine introduction period compared to pre-vaccine introduction period ($p < 0.001$); see Table 2.

**Table 1.** Characteristics of children under 5 years of age admitted to Kilifi County Hospital (KCH), coastal Kenya, with diarrhea symptoms that were sampled versus those who were not sampled in the study.

| Characteristics | All Subjects | Sampled (%) | Not Sampled (%) | *p*-Value |
|---|---|---|---|---|
| Total Admissions | 2156 | 1397 (64.8) | 759 (35.2) | |
| **Admissions Per Year** | | | | |
| 2003 | 1007 (46.7) | 587 (42.0) | 420 (55.3) | |
| 2013 | 332 (15.4) | 254 (18.2) | 78 (10.3) | |
| 2016 | 334 (15.5) | 257 (18.4) | 77 (10.1) | |
| 2019 | 483 (22.4) | 299 (21.4) | 184 (24.2) | |
| **Gender** | | | | 0.838 |
| Male | 1262 (58.5) | 815 (58.3) | 447 (58.9) | |
| Female | 894 (41.5) | 582 (41.7) | 312 (41.1) | |
| **Age** | | | | |
| Median (IQR) | 12.4 (7.7–20.5) | 11.7 (7.4–19.7) | 13.8 (8.5–22.1) | <0.001 |
| Mean (SD) | 15.7 (11.4) | 15.0 (11.1) | 16.9 (12.0) | <0.001 |
| **Age Group** | | | | 0.001 |
| 0–11 Months | 1045 (48.4) | 718 (51.4) | 326 (43.0) | |
| 12–23 Months | 716 (33.2) | 444 (31.8) | 272 (35.8) | |
| 24–59 Months | 396 (18.4) | 235 (16.8) | 161 (21.2) | |

Table 1. Cont.

| Characteristics | All Subjects | Sampled (%) | Not Sampled (%) | p-Value |
|---|---|---|---|---|
| Discharge Outcome ($n = 2153$) [#] | | | | <0.001 |
| Alive | 1918 (88.9) | 1306 (93.5) | 612 (80.5) | |
| Dead | 235 (10.9) | 89 (6.4) | 146 (19.3) | |

SD means standard deviation; IQR means interquartile range. Not sampled: sample was not collected due to lack of consent, time-up, death and others. [#] Discharge outcome data for three subjects were missing.

Table 2. Characteristics of children under 5 years of age admitted to KCH, coastal Kenya, with diarrhea symptoms and tested pre-vaccine introduction versus those tested post-vaccine introduction.

| Characteristics | Total | Pre-Vaccine Introduction (%) | Post-Vaccine Introduction (%) | p-Value |
|---|---|---|---|---|
| Number of Samples Tested | 984 | 454 (46.1) | 530 (53.9) | |
| Samples Tested (Year) | | | | |
| 2003 | 223 | 223 | - | |
| 2013 | 231 | 231 | - | |
| 2016 | 239 | - | 239 | |
| 2019 | 291 | - | 291 | |
| Gender | | | | 0.847 |
| Male | 570 (57.9) | 261 (57.5) | 309 (58.3) | |
| Female | 414 (42.1) | 193 (42.5) | 221 (41.7) | |
| Age | | | | |
| Mean (SD) | 15 (11.2) | 13.4 (9.9) | 16.3 (12) | <0.001 |
| Median (IQR) | 11.7 (7.3–19.3) | 11.2 (6.8–16.5) | 12.5 (7.9–21) | <0.001 |
| Age group | | | | 0.003 |
| 0–11 Months | 505 (51.3) | 252 (55.5) | 253 (47.7) | |
| 12–23 Months | 323 (32.8) | 148 (32.6) | 175 (33.0) | |
| 24–59 Months | 156 (15.9) | 54 (11.9) | 102 (19.3) | |
| Disease Severity in RVA Cases = $n$ (139) | | | | |
| Mild | 12 (8.6) | 7 (10.6) | 5 (6.8) | 0.441 |
| Moderate | 50 (36.0) | 26 (39.4) | 24 (32.9) | |
| Severe | 77 (55.4) | 33 (50) | 44 (60.3) | |
| Discharge Outcome = $n$ (982) [#] | | | | 0.556 |
| Alive | 925 (94.2) | 425 (93.6) | 500 (94.7) | |
| Dead | 57 (5.8) | 29 (6.4) | 28 (5.3) | |

SD means standard deviation; IQR means interquartile range; RVA means rotavirus group A. Values given are the counts and percentages are provided in brackets. [#] Discharge outcome for two subjects was missing. Disease Severity Was Calculated Using the Vesikari Clinical Severity Scoring System Manual [10].

## 2.2. Overall Virus Detection

Of the 984 samples analyzed, at least one of the viruses was detected in 401 samples (40.8%) at the real-time RT-PCR cycle threshold (Ct) value of <35.0. The lower the Ct value, the higher the virus titer in the sample. The detection frequency differed significantly for adenovirus ($p = 0.001$) and sapovirus ($p < 0.001$) pre- and post-rotavirus vaccine introduction when the Ct cut-off value was gradually lowered (<30, <35, <40), unlike for RVA, astrovirus and norovirus GII; see Figure 1. All our subsequent analyses were undertaken at Ct value <35.0 Single infections were detected in 354 specimens (36.0%) and included RVA ($n = 149$, 42.1%), adenovirus ($n = 91$, 25.7%), norovirus GII ($n = 75$, 21.2%), sapovirus ($n = 20$, 5.7%) and astrovirus ($n = 18$, 5.1%).

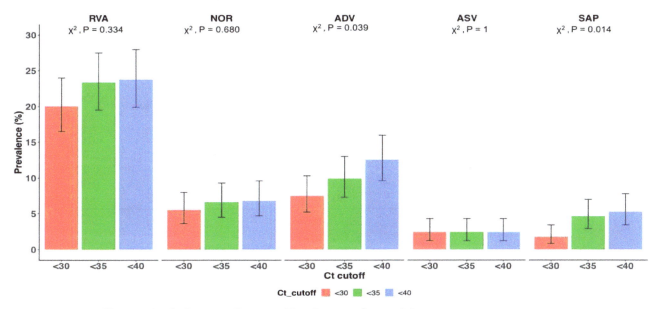
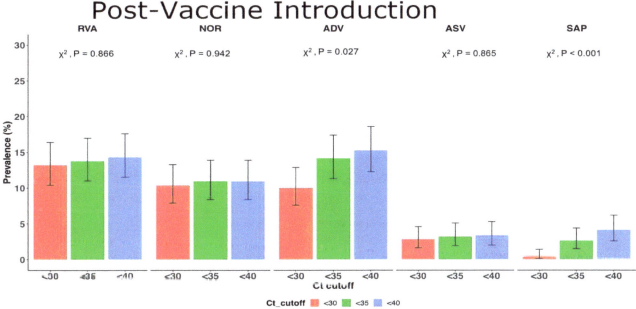

**Figure 1.** Detection frequency of RVA, adenovirus, norovirus GII, astrovirus and sapovirus at different cycle threshold (Ct) cutoffs for children under 5 years of age admitted to KCH Kenya with diarrhea symptoms. The error bars represent 95% confidence interval for the proportions. Proportions were compared using chi-square test. RVA stands for rotavirus group A, ADV stands for adenovirus, NOR stands for norovirus GII, ASV stands for astrovirus and SAP stands for sapovirus.

*2.3. Patterns Pre-Post Vaccine Introduction*

RVA showed a significant decrease (23.3% vs. 13.8%, $p < 0.001$) in prevalence while norovirus GII showed a significant increase (6.6% vs. 10.9%, $p = 0.02$) post-vaccine introduction compared to pre-vaccine introduction; see Table 3. There were no significant changes in the prevalence of astrovirus ($p = 0.585$), adenovirus ($p = 0.053$) and sapovirus ($p = 0.133$) pre- and post-RVA vaccine introduction (chi-squared ($\chi^2$) test); see Table 3. Notably, norovirus GII had a gradual increase in prevalence across the four years, from 6.7% (95% CI: 3.8–10.9%) to 12.4% (95% CI: 8.8–16.7%); see Figure 2. RVA was the most commonly detected virus across all years, except in year 2019, in which adenovirus had the highest prevalence; see Figure 2.

**Table 3.** Comparison of the prevalence of viral detection in children under 5 years of age admitted to KCH Kenya with diarrhea symptoms pre- and post-rotavirus vaccine introduction.

| Viruses Detected | Total | Pre-Vaccine Introduction (%) | Post-Vaccine Introduction (%) | *p*-Value |
|---|---|---|---|---|
| Samples Tested | 984 | 454 (46.1) | 530 (53.9) | |
| Rotavirus Group A | 179 (18.2) | 106 (23.3) | 73 (13.8) | <0.001 |
| Adenovirus | 120 (12.2) | 45 (9.9) | 75 (14.2) | 0.053 |
| Norovirus GII | 88 (8.9) | 30 (6.6) | 58 (10.9) | 0.023 |
| Astrovirus | 28 (2.8) | 11 (2.4) | 17 (3.2) | 0.585 |
| Sapovirus | 35 (3.6) | 21 (4.6) | 14 (2.6) | 0.133 |

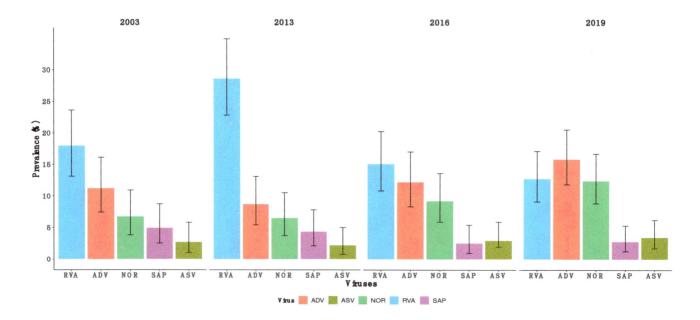

**Figure 2.** Prevalence of RVA, adenovirus, norovirus GII, astrovirus and sapovirus in 2003, 2013, 2016 and 2019 in children under 5 years of age admitted to KCH Kenya with diarrhea symptoms. The error bars represent 95% confidence interval for the proportions. Proportions were compared using chi-square test. Abbreviations used for viruses as in Figure 1.

Notably, RVA and sapovirus cases in the post-vaccine introduction period had statistically significant lower and higher median Ct values, respectively, compared to the pre-vaccine period (Wilcoxon, *p* value < 0.001); see Figure 3. This was not observed for the other three screened viruses pre- and post-rotavirus vaccine introduction. The median age of the RVA positive cases was significantly higher for the post-vaccine introduction period (14.0 months) compared to the pre-vaccine introduction period (10.4 months) (Wilcoxon, $p < 0.001$). A similar shift was not observed for the other viruses; see Figure 4.

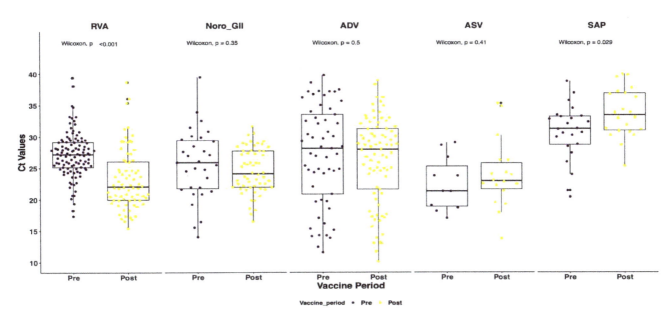

**Figure 3.** Distribution of Ct values among cases under 5 years of age admitted to KCH Kenya with diarrhea symptoms pre- and post-vaccine introduction. RVA stands for rotavirus group A, ADV stands for adenovirus, NOR GII stands for norovirus GII, ASV stands for astrovirus and SAP stands for sapovirus.

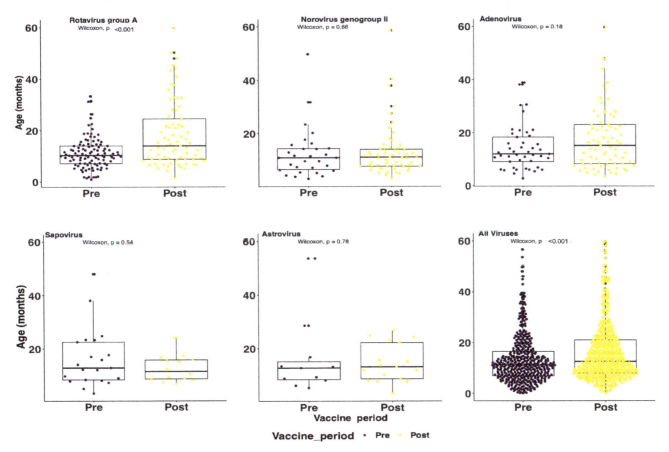

**Figure 4.** Distribution of age in months among cases under 5 years of age admitted to KCH Kenya with diarrhea symptoms pre- and post-vaccine introduction.

## 2.4. Virus Coinfections (i.e., Two or More Viruses in a Single Specimen)

These were detected in 47 specimens (4.8%). In 583 specimens (59.2%), none of the targeted viruses was detected. The prevalence of coinfections pre-vaccine was 4.4% (95% CI: 2.7–6.7%), while in the post-vaccine introduction period, this value was 5.7% (95% CI: 3.9–8.0%), $p = 0.454$. RVA and astrovirus were the most common coinfections in the pre-vaccine introduction period ($n = 6$), while in the post-vaccine introduction period, it was RVA and adenovirus ($n = 15$); see Table 4.

**Table 4.** Coinfections pre- and post-rotavirus vaccine introduction. RVA stands for rotavirus group A, ADV stands for adenovirus, NOR GII stands for norovirus GII, ASV stands for astrovirus and SAP stands for sapovirus.

| PATHOGEN COINFECTION | PRE-VACCINE INTRODUCTION | POST-VACCINE INTRODUCTION |
|---|---|---|
| RVA & NOR GII | 1 | 2 |
| RVA & ADV | 2 | 15 |
| RVA & ASV | 3 | 0 |
| RVA & SAP | 6 | 1 |
| NOR GII & ADV | 3 | 4 |
| NOR GII & ASV | 0 | 1 |
| NOVGII & SAP | 2 | 1 |
| ADV & ASV | 1 | 3 |
| ADV & SAP | 1 | 1 |
| ASV & SAP | 1 | 2 |

Abbreviations used for viruses as in Figure 3.

## 2.5. Circulating RVA Genotypes Pre- and Post-Vaccine Introduction

G1P[8] was the predominant RVA genotype pre vaccine introduction. However, in the post-vaccine introduction period, the predominant genotypes were G2P[4] (2016) and G3P[8] (2019); see Table 5.

**Table 5.** Frequency of RVA genotypes detected in coastal Kenya pre- (2003 and 2013) and post- (2016 and 2019) vaccine introduction.

| Year | 2003 | | 2013 | | 2016 | | 2019 | |
|---|---|---|---|---|---|---|---|---|
| | No. of Cases | % | No. of Cases | % | No. of Cases | % | No. of Cases | % |
| RVA Positive | 40 | | 66 | | 36 | | 37 | |
| Genotyped | 2 | 5.0 | 48 | 72.7 | 34 | 94.4 | 36 | 97.3 |
| **Genotypes** | | | | | | | | |
| G1P[8] | 1 | 50.0 | 43 | 89.6 | 5 | 14.7 | 1 | 2.8 |
| G2P[4] | - | - | 2 | 4.2 | 29 | 85.3 | - | - |
| G3P[8] | - | - | 1 | 2.1 | - | - | 34 | 94.4 |
| G9P[8] | 1 | 50.0 | 1 | 2.1 | - | - | - | - |
| G10P[8] | - | - | 1 | 2.1 | - | - | - | - |
| G8P[8] | - | - | - | - | - | - | 1 | 2.8 |

## 2.6. Seasonality of the Detected Viruses

We constrained this analysis to the years 2013, 2016 and 2019, where >70% of the eligible patients had been analyzed. Pre-vaccine introduction (in 2013), for RVA, there were two peak months, in June and September. However, post-vaccine introduction (in 2016 and 2019), there was only a single peak month for RVA in September and August, respectively. For norovirus GII, cases were observed throughout the year, with peak months varying from year-to-year, in July, April and June in 2013, 2016 and 2019, respectively. Similarly, adenovirus cases appeared to occur throughout the year, with two peak months in 2013 (June and September) and one peak month in 2016 and 2019 (August for both). For sapovirus and astrovirus, we observed less than five cases monthly between January and August and no cases in the last quarter of each the three years; see Figure 5.

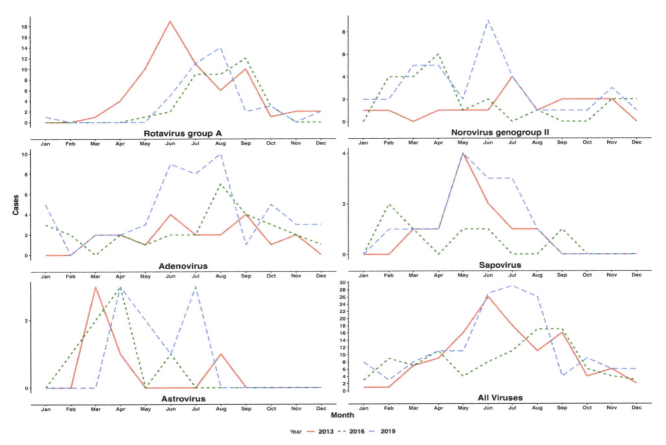

**Figure 5.** The frequency of detection of RVA, adenovirus, norovirus GII, astrovirus and sapovirus by month in children under 5 years of age admitted to KCH Kenya with diarrhea in 2013, 2016 and 2019.

*2.7. Primer/Probe Mismatches with Contemporary Sequences*

Nucleotide mismatches were observed in either or both the primers and probes and the viral target sequences for all the viruses except for norovirus GII; see Figure 6. The RVA forward primer had a G-A and A-G mismatches at positions 12 and 15, respectively. Adenovirus had two mismatches in the forward primer (C-G and G-A), three mismatches in the probe (C-T, C-T and T-C) and two mismatches in the reverse primer (T-C and C-T), and none of them were within five bases of the 3' end. Mismatches within the sapovirus primer/probe binding sites were pronounced in sapovirus genogroup V and included six mismatches in the forward primer, three mismatches in the probe and two mismatches in the reverse primer. Some of the mismatches were within five bases of the 3' end (forward primer: C-G, probe: T-C, reverse primer: A-C and T-C). Astrovirus primers and probe did not have pronounced mismatches present in all the sequences—rather, they had mismatches in individual sequences; see Figure 6.

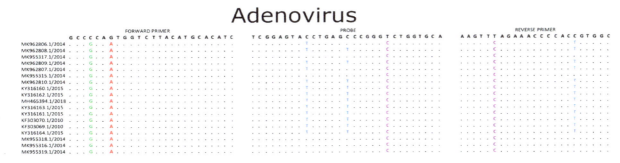

**Figure 6.** *Cont.*

Figure 6. The primers and probes target sites for RVA, adenovirus and norovirus GII, sapovirus and astrovirus were aligned using MAFFT v.7.31313 and the alignments were trimmed to the region of the primer and probe target sites. Nucleotide differences between the expected primer and probe target sites and the viral sequences were identified and highlighted. Dots indicate identity with primer or probe sequences.

## 3. Discussion

We observed a significant decrease in the prevalence of RVA in the post-vaccine introduction period in KCH, concurring with findings of a recent multi-site study in Kenya that reported RVA vaccine effectiveness of ~64% (95% CI: 35–80%) and a reduction in rotavirus-associated hospital admissions two years post-vaccine introduction of ~80% (95% CI: 46–93%) [9,11]. Note that Kenya rotavirus vaccine coverage was considered medium in 2018 (70–79%) [12]. Our pre- and post-vaccine introduction analysis observed a significant increase in the prevalence of norovirus GII in KCH post-rotavirus vaccine introduction, as similarly observed in the United States, Nicaragua and Bolivia following RVA vaccine introduction [13–15]. It is unclear if this has been driven by an established biological interaction between these two viruses or that this reflects natural norovirus GII fluctuation in prevalence across multiple years.

The shift in the predominant genotypes pre- and post-vaccine introduction from G1P[8] to G2P[4] in 2016 and G3P[8] in 2019 in our setting has also been described elsewhere, e.g., in Belgium, Madagascar and Ethiopia [16–18]. G3P[8] was the predominant genotype in this setting in 2018 [19] and it continued being the dominant genotype in 2019. Although these dominant post-vaccine genotypes are either partially or fully heterotypic to the Rotarix G1P[8] strain, in their surface exposed immunodominant proteins, there is not enough evidence yet to directly attribute their increased incidence to vaccine introduction [20]. Additional analysis will help to bring better understanding on the reason behind their dominance.

Despite RV vaccine introduction in Kilifi, Kenya, no significant difference was observed in the discharge outcome for all causes of diarrhea pre- and post-rotavirus vaccine introduction. We suggest two explanations for this. Firstly, the majority of the children who were eligible to be in this study and died did not have a sample collected to determine their RVA and other enteric pathogens' status. Secondly, inpatient mortality of children treated for diarrhea in Kilifi County Hospital has been previously found to be predicted by a positive HIV test, bacteremia and poor nutritional status [21]. This may have not changed pre- or post-introduction of rotavirus vaccination.

RVA Ct values were decreased in post-vaccine samples compared to pre-vaccination years. This was despite RVA disease severity remaining unchanged between the two periods. Different extraction methods were used to process the samples between 2003, 2013 and 2016, 2019. However, according to Liu et al., the difference in the extraction methods for enteric pathogen studies is not significant, except for norovirus GII, which showed a higher Ct value with kits targeting RNA purification alone compared to those targeting total nucleic acid (TNA) (difference within 1 Ct value). Different extraction kits were used in this study because raw stool samples from 2003 to 2016 were already destroyed following a directive by the WHO in 2016 that was part of the larger global polio eradication effort.

It has been previously noted the introduction to rotavirus vaccines may result in the shift of diarrhea disease burden to slightly older age groups [20]. Our study found a significant increase in the median age of diarrhea cases post-vaccine introduction (12.5 months) compared 11.2 months pre-introduction. This in part may be explained by the higher immunity at both individual and population levels against rotavirus that wanes as children grow older.

On local seasonality patterns, in each year, a peak month(s) of occurrence was observed for RVA, norovirus GII, sapovirus and adenovirus but not astrovirus. The Kilifi area has a tropical climate with two rainy seasons; the main rains usually peak in May (up to July) while the short rains usually peak in November (can run from October to December). RVA and adenovirus appeared to peak in the dry months while norovirus GII and sapovirus peaked in the rainy season. Similar patterns in the seasonality of RVA, adenovirus, norovirus GII and sapovirus have been observed elsewhere [22–25]. The seasonality of astrovirus is not well described.

The performance of qPCR assays can be impacted by mismatches within the last five bases at the 3' end of primers and probe or/and the number of mismatches being more than five in the primers and probe [26,27]. The mismatches observed in the primer and probe binding sites of adenovirus, astrovirus and sapovirus may have impaired the real-time PCR function by blocking the amplification or increasing the quantification cycles. Consequently, this may have impacted the estimated frequency of detection of these viruses. Unlike for RVA, the magnitude of the mismatches in qPCR function could have been shown better using recent local sequences of the other viruses.

This study had limitations: firstly, we did not analyze healthy children in the community to inform on the background prevalence of the five viruses in our study population. Secondly, the adenovirus assay was not specific to type 40/41 alone; thus, some of the adenoviruses detected may not be associated with diarrhea. Thirdly, a significant number of eligible cases were not sampled, including those who died before sampling. This potentially biased prevalence of the screened pathogens in the study population. Fourthly, extracting TNA from samples after many years of storage could lead to lower Ct values due to deterioration. Finally, the seasonality of examined pathogens will be best described if we examine more years.

In conclusion, we found a significant decline in the prevalence of rotavirus in hospitalized children in coastal Kenya after rotavirus vaccine introduction. This finding reinforces evidence of the continued benefit of rotavirus vaccination in this setting. Concomitantly, there has been a surge in norovirus GII prevalence, but the factors driving this increase are unclear and will require future investigation. The observation that the screened viruses peak at different times of the year also would benefit further investigation in order to understand drivers of their transmission and inform the design of effective intervention measures.

## 4. Materials and Methods

### 4.1. Study Site and Population

This study was undertaken at KCH, a referral hospital serving the Kilifi County population, which is majorly a rural population. We utilized stool specimens collected during routine surveillance of rotavirus in children with diarrhea as one of their illness symptoms, aged below five years and admitted to KCH [9,11]. Diarrhea was defined as observation of three or more loose stools in the preceding 24-h period. In this study, we selected two pre-vaccine years (2003 and 2013) and two post-vaccine years (2016 and 2019) for analysis. A stool specimen was collected from children who met the diarrhea case-definition following parental or guardian consent. The study protocol was approved by the Scientific and Ethics Review Unit (SSC#2861 and SERU#CGMRC/113/3624) based at KEMRI, Nairobi, Kenya.

### 4.2. Laboratory Methods

Irrespective of their previously determined rotavirus status, TNA were extracted from 0.2 g of 2003 and 2013 specimens (or 200 µL if liquid) using the cador Pathogen 96 QIAcube HT Kit (Qiagen, Manchester, UK). For 2016 and 2019 specimens, TNA were extracted using QIAamp Fast DNA Stool Mini kit (Qiagen, Manchester, UK) as per the manufacturer's instructions. Fecal specimens from the post-vaccine period (0.2 mg or 200 µL) were subjected to bead beating prior to TNA extraction and collected in a 200 µL of elution buffer [28].

The TNA extracts were screened for the five viruses by a two-step real-time RT-PCR assay [29]. First, cDNA was synthesized in a total volume of 20 µL using random hexamers and 5µL of TNA using the Omniscript Reverse Transcriptase kit (Qiagen, Manchester, UK), as per the manufacturer's instructions. Two µL of the cDNA was henceforth used for real-time RT-PCR in a total volume of 20 µL using the QuantiFast RT-PCR Kit (Qiagen, Manchester, UK) and run on the ABI 7500 Real-Time PCR System (Applied Biosystems, Foster City, CA, USA). Primers and probes were adopted from previously published work [30]. The presence of nucleotide mismatches in the primer and probe binding sites was investigated by aligning the primers/probes to genomic sequences deposited in GenBank from 2010 to 2019, using MAFFT v.7.313 [31]. The adenovirus probe/primer pair used in this study detected adenovirus serotypes beyond type 40/41. We used three Ct cut-off values (<40.0, <35.0

and <30.0) to define positive samples. Samples that were positive for RVA in 2003, 2013, 2016 and 2019 were processed for RVA genotyping using VP4 and VP7 RT-PCR, followed by either dideoxy sanger sequencing, as described elsewhere [19], or next-generation sequencing on the Illumina Miseq platform [32].

*4.3. Statistical Analysis*

All statistical analyses were performed using R version 3.6.1 [33]. Prevalence was defined as the proportion of these viruses in a hospital-admitted diarrhea patient population during the study period in Kilifi, Kenya. Means and medians of continuous variables were compared using a Kruskal Wallis and Wilcoxon rank-sum test, respectively. Binary data were summarized using proportions and comparisons between groups made using $\chi^2$ statistics. A $p$ value of <0.05 was considered statistically significant. Diarrhea severity in RVA positive cases pre- (year 2013) and post- (years 2016 and 2019) was assessed using the Vesikari Clinical Severity Scoring System Manual [10], with a modification in the treatment parameter. If the participant was given oral rehydration therapy or intravenous fluid therapy, they received a score of one or two, respectively.

**Author Contributions:** Conceptualization, A.W.L. and C.N.A.; methodology, A.W.L. and C.N.A.; formal analysis, A.W.L., N.M. and C.N.A.; investigation, A.W.L., S.O., C.S.L. and C.N.A.; resources, D.J.N. and C.N.A.; data curation, A.W.L. and N.M.; writing—original draft preparation, A.W.L.; writing—review and editing, A.W.L., S.O., N.M., C.S.L., S.G.N. and C.N.A.; visualization, A.W.L. supervision, S.G.N. and C.N.A., project administration, C.N.A.; funding acquisition, C.N.A. All authors have read and agreed to the published version of the manuscript.

**Acknowledgments:** We thank all the study participants for their contribution of study samples, their parents/guardians, members of the viral epidemiology and control research group (http://virec-group.org/) and colleagues at the KEMRI Wellcome Trust Research Programme for their useful discussions during the preparation of the manuscript. We are grateful to James Nokes of KEMRI-Wellcome Trust for his comments and suggestions on the presentation of this work This paper is published with the permission of the Director of KEMRI.

## References

1. Troeger, C.; Blacker, B.F.; Khalil, I.A.; Rao, P.C.; Cao, S.; Zimsen, S.R.; Albertson, S.B.; Stanaway, J.D.; Deshpande, A.; Abebe, Z.; et al. Estimates of the global, regional, and national morbidity, mortality, and aetiologies of diarrhoea in 195 countries: A systematic analysis for the Global Burden of Disease Study 2016. *Lancet Infect. Dis.* **2018**, *18*, 1211–1228. [CrossRef]
2. Platts-Mills, J.A.; Liu, J.; Rogawski, E.T.; Kabir, F.; Lertsethtakarn, P.; Siguas, M.; Khan, S.S.; Praharaj, I.; Murei, A.; Nshama, R.; et al. Use of quantitative molecular diagnostic methods to assess the aetiology, burden, and clinical characteristics of diarrhoea in children in low-resource settings: A reanalysis of the MAL-ED cohort study. *Lancet Glob. Health* **2018**, *6*, e1309–e1318. [CrossRef]
3. Liu, J.; Platts-Mills, J.A.; Juma, J.; Kabir, F.; Nkeze, J.; Okoi, C.; Operario, D.J.; Uddin, J.; Ahmed, S.; Alonso, P.L.; et al. Use of quantitative molecular diagnostic methods to identify causes of diarrhoea in children: A reanalysis of the GEMS case-control study. *Lancet* **2016**. [CrossRef]
4. Aliabadi, N.; Antoni, S.; Mwenda, J.M.; Weldegebriel, G.; Biey, J.N.M.; Cheikh, D.; Fahmy, K.; Teleb, N.; Ashmony, H.A.; Ahmed, H.; et al. Global impact of rotavirus vaccine introduction on rotavirus hospitalisations among children under 5 years of age, 2008–2016: Findings from the Global Rotavirus Surveillance Network. *Lancet Glob. Health* **2019**, *7*, e893–e903. [CrossRef]
5. Yu, W.J.; Chen, S.Y.; Tsai, C.N.; Chao, H.C.; Kong, M.S.; Chang, Y.J.; Chiu, C.H. Long-term impact of suboptimal rotavirus vaccines on acute gastroenteritis in hospitalized children in Northern Taiwan. *J. Formos. Med. Assoc.* **2018**, *117*, 720–726. [CrossRef] [PubMed]
6. Muhsen, K.; Kassem, E.; Rubenstein, U.; Goren, S.; Ephros, M.; Shulman, L.M.; Cohen, D. No evidence of an increase in the incidence of norovirus gastroenteritis hospitalizations in young children after the introduction of universal rotavirus immunization in Israel. *Hum. Vaccines Immunother.* **2019** *15*, 1284–1293. [CrossRef]
7. Halasa, N.; Piya, B.; Stewart, L.S.; Rahman, H.; Payne, D.C.; Woron, A.; Thomas, L.; Constantine-Renna, L.; Garman, K.; McHenry, R.; et al. The Changing Landscape of Pediatric Viral Enteropathogens in the Post-Rotavirus Vaccine Era. *Clin. Infect. Dis.* **2020**, *53*, 1689–1699. [CrossRef]

8. Wandera, E.A.; Mohammad, S.; Ouko, J.O.; Yatitch, J.; Taniguchi, K.; Ichinose, Y. Variation in rotavirus vaccine coverage by sub-counties in Kenya. *Trop. Med. Health* **2017**. [CrossRef]
9. Otieno, G.P.; Bottomley, C.; Khagayi, S.; Adetifa, I.; Ngama, M.; Omore, R.; Ogwel, B.; Owor, B.E.; Bigogo, G.; Ochieng, J.B.; et al. Impact of the Introduction of Rotavirus Vaccine on Hospital Admissions for Diarrhea Among Children in Kenya: A Controlled Interrupted Time-Series Analysis. *Clin. Infect. Dis.* **2019**, 1–8. [CrossRef]
10. Lewis, K. Vesikari Clinical Severity Scoring System Manual. Path. 2011, pp. 1–50. Available online: https://www.path.org/publications/files/VAD_vesikari_scoring_manual.pdf (accessed on 22 July 2020).
11. Khagayi, S.; Omore, R.; Otieno, G.P.; Ogwel, B.; Ochieng, J.B.; Juma, J.; Apondi, E.; Bigogo, G.; Onyango, C.; Ngama, M.; et al. Effectiveness of monovalent rotavirus vaccine against hospitalization with acute rotavirus gastroenteritis in Kenyan children. *Clin. Infect. Dis.* **2020**, *70*, 2298–2305. [CrossRef]
12. VIEW-hub, International Vaccine Access Center (IVAC), Johns Hopkins Bloomberg School of Public Health. Available online: https://view-hub.org/map/?set=wuenic-coverage&group=vaccine-coverage&category=rv (accessed on 31 July 2020).
13. Bucardo, F.; Reyes, Y.; Svensson, L.; Nordgren, J. Predominance of norovirus and sapovirus in nicaragua after implementation of universal rotavirus vaccination. *PLoS ONE* **2014**, *9*, e98201. [CrossRef] [PubMed]
14. McAtee, C.L.; Webman, R.; Gilman, R.H.; Mejia, C.; Bern, C.; Apaza, S.; Espetia, S.; Pajuelo, M.; Saito, M.; Challappa, R.; et al. Burden of norovirus and rotavirus in children after rotavirus vaccine introduction, Cochabamba, Bolivia. *Am. Trop. Med. Hyg.* **2016**. [CrossRef] [PubMed]
15. Payne, D.C.; Vinjé, J.; Szilagyi, P.G.; Edwards, K.M.; Staat, M.A.; Weinberg, G.A.; Hall, C.B.; Chappell, J.; Bernstein, D.I.; Curns, A.T.; et al. Norovirus and medically attended gastroenteritis in US children. *N. Engl. J. Med.* **2013**. [CrossRef] [PubMed]
16. Gelaw, A.; Pietsch, C.; Liebert, U.G. Molecular epidemiology of rotaviruses in Northwest Ethiopia after national vaccine introduction. *Infect. Genet. Evol.* **2018**. [CrossRef] [PubMed]
17. Rahajamanana, V.L.; Raboba, J.L.; Rakotozanany, A.; Razafindraibe, N.J.; Andriatahirintsoa, E.J.P.R.; Razafindrakoto, A.C.; Mioramalala, S.A.; Razaiarimanga, C.; Weldegebriel, G.G.; Burnett, E.; et al. Impact of rotavirus vaccine on all-cause diarrhea and rotavirus hospitalizations in Madagascar. *Vaccine* **2018**. [CrossRef] [PubMed]
18. Zeller, M.; Rahman, M.; Heylen, E.; De Coster, S.; De Vos, S.; Arijs, I.; Novo, L.; Verstappen, N.; Van Ranst, M.; Matthijnssens, J. Rotavirus incidence and genotype distribution before and after national rotavirus vaccine introduction in Belgium. *Vaccine* **2010**. [CrossRef]
19. Mwanga, M.J.; Owor, B.E.; Ochieng, J.B.; Ngama, M.H.; Ogwel, B.; Onyango, C.; Juma, J.; Njeru, R.; Gicheru, E.; Otieno, G.P.; et al. Rotavirus group A genotype circulation patterns across Kenya before and after nationwide vaccine introduction, 2010–2018. *BMC Infect. Dis.* **2020**, *20*, 504. [CrossRef]
20. Pitzer, V.E.; Bilcke, J.; Heylen, E.; Crawford, F.W.; Callens, M.; De Smet, F.; Van Ranst, M.; Zeller, M.; Matthijnssens, J. Did Large-Scale Vaccination Drive Changes in the Circulating Rotavirus Population in Belgium? *Sci. Rep.* **2015**, *5*, 1–14. [CrossRef]
21. Talbert, A.; Ngari, M.; Bauni, E.; Mwangome, M.; Mturi, N.; Otiende, M.; Maitland, K.; Walson, J.; Berkley, J.A. Mortality after inpatient treatment for diarrhea in children: A cohort study. *BMC Med.* **2019**. [CrossRef]
22. Ahmed, S.M.; Lopman, B.A.; Levy, K. A Systematic Review and Meta-Analysis of the Global Seasonality of Norovirus. *PLoS ONE* **2013**, *8*, e75922. [CrossRef]
23. Dey, S.K.; Phathammavong, O.; Nguyen, T.D.; Thongprachum, A.; Chan-It, W.; Okitsu, S.; Mizuguchi, M.; Ushijima, H. Seasonal pattern and genotype distribution of sapovirus infection in Japan, 2003–2009. *Epidemiol. Infect.* **2012**, *140*, 74–77. [CrossRef] [PubMed]
24. Omore, R.; Tate, J.E.; O'Reilly, C.E.; Ayers, T.; Williamson, J.; Moke, F.; Schilling, K.A.; Awuor, A.O.; Jaron, P.; Ochieng, J.B.; et al. Epidemiology, seasonality and factors associated with rotavirus infection among children with moderate-to-severe diarrhea in rural western Kenya, 2008–2012: The Global Enteric Multicenter Study (GEMS). *PLoS ONE* **2016**, *11*, e0160060. [CrossRef] [PubMed]
25. Vetter, M.R.; Staggemeier, R.; Vecchia, A.D.; Henzel, A.; Rigotto, C.; Spilki, F.R. Seasonal variation on the presence of adenoviruses in stools from non-diarrheic patients. *Braz. J. Microbiol.* **2015**, *46*, 749–752. [CrossRef] [PubMed]
26. Stadhouders, R.; Pas, S.D.; Anber, J.; Voermans, J.; Mes, T.H.; Schutten, M. The effect of primer-template

mismatches on the detection and quantification of nucleic acids using the 5' nuclease assay. *Mol. Diagn.* **2010**, *12*, 109–117. [CrossRef]
27. Lefever, S.; Pattyn, F.; Hellemans, J.; Vandesompele, J. Single-nucleotide polymorphisms and other mismatches reduce performance of quantitative PCR assays. *Clin. Chem.* **2013**, *59*, 1470–1480. [CrossRef]
28. Liu, J.; Gratz, J.; Amour, C.; Nshama, R.; Walongo, T.; Maro, A.; Mduma, E.; Platts-Mills, J.; Boisen, N.; Nataro, J.; et al. Optimization of quantitative PCR methods for enteropathogen detection. *PLoS ONE* **2016**, *11*, e0158199. [CrossRef]
29. Bennett, S.; Gunson, R.N. The development of a multiplex real-time RT-PCR for the detection of adenovirus, astrovirus, rotavirus and sapovirus from stool samples. *Virol. Methods* **2017**, *242*, 30–34. [CrossRef]
30. Van Maarseveen, N.M.; Wessels, E.; de Brouwer, C.S.; Vossen, A.C.; Claas, E.C. Diagnosis of viral gastroenteritis by simultaneous detection of Adenovirus group F, Astrovirus, Rotavirus group A, Norovirus genogroups I and II, and Sapovirus in two internally controlled multiplex real-time PCR assays. *Clin. Virol.* **2010**. [CrossRef]
31. Katoh, K.; Standley, D.M. MAFFT multiple sequence alignment software version 7: Improvements in performance and usability. *Mol. Biol. Evol.* **2013**. [CrossRef]
32. Magagula, N.B.; Esona, M.D.; Nyaga, M.M.; Stucker, K.M.; Halpin, R.A.; Stockwell, T.B.; Seheri, M.L.; Steele, A.D.; Wentworth, D.E.; Mphahlele, M.J. Whole genome analyses of G1P[8] rotavirus strains from vaccinated and non-vaccinated South African children presenting with diarrhea. *Med. Virol.* **2015**, *87*, 79–101. [CrossRef]
33. R Core Team. *R: A Language and Environment for Statistical Computing*; R Foundation for Statistical Computing: Vienna, Austria, 2019. Available online: https://www.R-project.org/ (accessed on 22 October 2019).

# Phylogenetic Analyses of Rotavirus A from Cattle in Uruguay Reveal the Circulation of Common and Uncommon Genotypes and Suggest Interspecies Transmission

Matías Castells [1,2,*], Rubén Darío Caffarena [2,3], María Laura Casaux [2], Carlos Schild [2], Samuel Miño [4], Felipe Castells [5], Daniel Castells [6], Matías Victoria [1], Franklin Riet-Correa [2], Federico Giannitti [2], Viviana Parreño [4] and Rodney Colina [1,*]

[1] Laboratorio de Virología Molecular, CENUR Litoral Norte, Centro Universitario de Salto, Universidad de la República, Rivera 1350, Salto 50000, Uruguay; matvicmon@yahoo.com

[2] Instituto Nacional de Investigación Agropecuaria (INIA), Plataforma de Investigación en Salud Animal, Estación Experimental la Estanzuela, Ruta 50 km 11, Colonia 70000, Uruguay; rdcaffarena@gmail.com (R.D.C.); mlcasaux@gmail.com (M.L.C.); schild.co@gmail.com (C.S.); frcorrea@inia.org.uy (F.R.-C.); fgiannitti@inia.org.uy (F.G.)

[3] Facultad de Veterinaria, Universidad de la República, Alberto Lasplaces 1620, Montevideo 11600, Uruguay

[4] Sección de Virus Gastroentéricos, Instituto de Virología, CICVyA, INTA Castelar, Buenos Aires 1686, Argentina; mino.samuel@inta.gob.ar (S.M.); vivipar3015@gmail.com (V.P.)

[5] Doctor en Veterinaria en Ejercicio Libre, Asociado al Laboratorio de Virología Molecular, CENUR Litoral Norte, Centro Universitario de Salto, Universidad de la República, Rivera 1350, Salto 50000, Uruguay; felicastells@gmail.com

[6] Centro de Investigación y Experimentación Dr. Alejandro Gallinal, Secretariado Uruguayo de la Lana, Ruta 7 km 140, Cerro Colorado, Florida 94000, Uruguay; castells@adinet.com.uy

* Correspondence: matiascastellsbauer@gmail.com (M.C.); rodneycolina1@gmail.com (R.C.);

**Abstract:** Uruguay is one of the main exporters of beef and dairy products, and cattle production is one of the main economic sectors in this country. Rotavirus A (RVA) is the main pathogen associated with neonatal calf diarrhea (NCD), a syndrome that leads to significant economic losses to the livestock industry. The aims of this study are to determine the frequency of RVA infections, and to analyze the genetic diversity of RVA strains in calves in Uruguay. A total of 833 samples from dairy and beef calves were analyzed through RT-qPCR and sequencing. RVA was detected in 57.0% of the samples. The frequency of detection was significantly higher in dairy (59.5%) than beef (28.4%) calves ($p < 0.001$), while it did not differ significantly among calves born in herds that were vaccinated (64.0%) or not vaccinated (66.7%) against NCD. The frequency of RVA detection and the viral load were significantly higher in samples from diarrheic (72.1%, 7.99 $\log_{10}$ genome copies/mL of feces) than non-diarrheic (59.9%, 7.35 $\log_{10}$ genome copies/mL of feces) calves ($p < 0.005$ and $p = 0.007$, respectively). The observed G-types (VP7) were G6 (77.6%), G10 (20.7%), and G24 (1.7%), while the P-types were P[5] (28.4%), P[11] (70.7%), and P[33] (0.9%). The G-type and P-type combinations were G6P[11] (40.4%), G6P[5] (38.6%), G10P[11] (19.3%), and the uncommon genotype G24P[33] (1.8%). VP6 and NSP1-5 genotyping were performed to better characterize some strains. The phylogenetic analyses suggested interspecies transmission, including transmission between animals and humans.

**Keywords:** rotavirus; bovine; genotypes; interspecies transmission; diarrhea

## 1. Introduction

Neonatal calf diarrhea (NCD) is a syndrome of worldwide distribution and the major cause of mortality of dairy calves before weaning [1]. NCD has a negative impact on animal welfare and leads to significant economic losses to the livestock industry [2–5].

Rotavirus A (RVA) is the main pathogen associated with NCD [6,7]. RVA (species *Rotavirus A*; genus *Rotavirus*; subfamily *Sedoreovirinae*; family *Reoviridae*) is a nonenveloped virus with a triple-layered capsid and a genome composed of 11 segments of double-stranded RNA [8]. RVA is widespread in dairy farms in Uruguay, and viable viral particles have been detected in sources of drinking water used for calves [9], suggesting water contamination and waterborne transmission.

Rotaviruses are classified by a binary system of G and P types for VP7 and VP4, respectively, determined by sequence analyses. In 2008, a complete genome classification system, named genotype constellation, assigning a specific genotype to each of the 11 genome segments was developed [10]. The VP7-VP4-VP6-VP1-VP2-VP3-NSP1-NSP2-NSP3-NSP4-NSP5/6 genes of rotavirus strains are classified using the abbreviations Gx-P[x]-Ix-Rx-Cx-Mx-Ax-Nx-Tx-Ex-Hx (where x is the genotype number), respectively.

Recently, since the inclusion of gene segments other than VP7 and VP4 in molecular analyses, gene reassortment has been described as a common event in RVA, sometimes between virus strains originated from different hosts, suggesting interspecies transmission [10–13].

Surveys describing the epidemiology of RVA in cattle in South America are mainly restricted to Brazil and Argentina; no published data about RVA epidemiology in Uruguayan calves are available. However, other viruses such as bovine coronavirus and bovine astrovirus have been detected in Uruguay [14,15].

Uruguay is one of the main exporters of beef [16] and dairy products [17]. Furthermore, cattle production is one of the main economic sectors in this country, with almost 12 million head of cattle accounting for 33% of the total exports [18]. The aims of this study are to determine the frequency of RVA infections and to analyze the genetic diversity of the RVA strains detected in Uruguayan calves.

## 2. Results

### 2.1. Detection Frequency of RVA in Uruguayan Calves

Rotavirus A was detected in 57.0% (475/833) of the analyzed samples. The frequency of detection was significantly higher in dairy (59.5%, 456/766) than beef (28.4%, 19/67) calves (OR: 3.72, 95% CI: 2.14–6.44; $p < 0.000001$; Figure 1a). The frequency of RVA detection in live calves was higher (58.0%, 444/766) than in deceased calves (46.3%, 31/67), although this difference was not statistically significant ($p = 0.06$; Figure 1b). The frequency of detection in dairy calves born in herds that vaccinated (64.0%, 144/225) or did not vaccinate dams (66.7%, 164/246) against NCD did not differ significantly ($p = 0.5$; Figure 1c). The frequency of RVA detection was significantly higher in samples from diarrheic (72.1%, 173/240) than non-diarrheic (59.9%, 163/272) dairy calves (OR: 1.73, 95% CI: 1.19–2.50; $p < 0.005$; Figure 1d). No seasonal distribution was observed in RVA detection (data not shown).

Rotavirus A was detected in 58.8% (87/148), 70.6% (142/201), 68.2% (75/110), and 52.9% (18/34) of dairy calves in the first, second, third, and fourth weeks of life, respectively (Table 1). Statistically significant differences were observed between the second and the first weeks of age (OR: 1.69, 95% CI: 1.08–2.64; $p = 0.02$), and between the second and the fourth weeks of age (OR: 2.14, 95% CI: 1.02–4.48; $p = 0.04$). The mean age in days of RVA-positive dairy calves was significantly lower in diarrheic than nondiarrheic calves ($p = 0.02$; Table 1).

The RVA viral load was significantly higher in diarrheic than nondiarrheic dairy calves ($p = 0.007$; Table 1), ranging between $1.14 \times 10^4$ and $7.36 \times 10^{12}$ genome copies/milliliter (gc/mL) of feces. In all four age groups, the frequency of RVA detection was higher in diarrheic than nondiarrheic dairy calves: 69.0% (40/58) vs. 52.2% (47/90) in the first week, 72.1% (98/136) vs. 67.7% (44/65) in the second week, 68.8% (22/32) vs. 67.9% (53/78) in the third week, and 85.7% (6/7) vs. 44.4% (12/27) in the fourth week of age. A statistically significant difference was observed only within the first week (OR: 2.03, 95% CI: 1.01–4.07; $p = 0.04$).

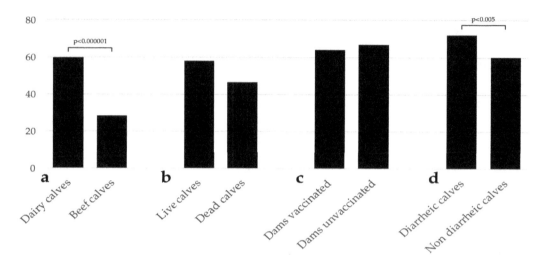

**Figure 1.** Frequency of Rotavirus A (RVA) detection in calves. (**a**) Frequency of RVA detection in dairy vs. beef calves; (**b**) frequency of RVA detection in live vs. deceased calves; (**c**) frequency of RVA detection in calves from vaccinated [a] vs. unvaccinated dairy herds; (**d**) frequency of RVA detection in diarrheic vs. non diarrheic dairy calves. Comparisons with statistically significant differences are indicated. [a] Most of the vaccines against neonatal calf diarrhea available in Uruguay include two RVA strains.

**Table 1.** Frequency of RVA detection and viral load in feces of diarrheic and nondiarrheic calves.

|  | Mean Age [a] | Viral Load [b] | Calves Age | | | |
|---|---|---|---|---|---|---|
|  |  |  | First Week | Second Week | Third Week | Fourth Week |
| Diarrheic | 11.9 [1] | 7.99 [2] | 69.0 [3] | 72.1 | 68.8 | 85.7 |
| Non-diarrheic | 13.5 [1] | 7.35 [2] | 52.2 [3] | 67.7 | 67.9 | 44.4 |
| Total | 12.7 | 7.67 | 58.8 [4] | 70.6 [4,5] | 68.2 | 52.9 [5] |

[a] Mean age in days of RVA-positive calves. [b] Mean RVA viral load expressed as log10 of RVA genome copies per milliliter of feces. Equal numbers in superscript refer to values with statistically significant differences ($p < 0.05$).

## 2.2. VP7 and VP4 Genotyping

We obtained 58 and 116 sequences for VP7 and VP4, respectively. The detected G-types (VP7) were G6 (77.6%, 45/58), G10 (20.7%, 12/58), and G24 (1.7%, 1/58), while the P-types (VP4) were P[5] (28.4%, 33/116), P[11] (70.7%, 82/116), and P[33] (0.9%, 1/116). The following G- and P-type combinations were obtained for 57 strains: G6P[11] (40.4%, 23/57), G6P[5] (38.6%, 22/57), G10P[11] (19.3%, 11/57), and G24P[33] (1.8%, 1/57). Furthermore, 60 strains had undetermined G- or P-type: GXP[11] (80.0%, 48/60), GXP[5] (18.3%, 11/60), and G10P[X] (1.7%, 1/60).

## 2.3. VP6 and NSP1-5 Genotyping

Ten samples, including representative VP7 and VP4 genotype combinations observed, were selected for VP6 and NSP1-5 gene characterization: 2 G6P[5], 2 G6P[11], 2 G10P[11], 2 GXP[11], 1 G10P[X], and 1 G24P[33] (Table 2). All the strains were I2 (VP6), N2 (NSP2), and E12 (NSP4). Nine were H3 and one could not be determined HX (NSP5). Five strains were A3, four were A13, and one could not be determined AX (NSP1). Eight strains were T6, one was T9, and one could not be determined TX (NSP3).

Table 2. Genotype constellation of 10 RVA strains from Uruguayan calves.

| Strain | VP7 | VP4 | VP6 | NSP1 | NSP2 | NSP3 | NSP4 | NSP5 |
|---|---|---|---|---|---|---|---|---|
| RVA/Cow-wt/URY/LVMS781/2015/G6P[5] | G6 | P[5] | I2 | AX | N2 | T6 | E12 | H3 |
| RVA/Cow-wt/URY/LVMS1788/2016/GxP[11] | GX | P[11] | I2 | A3 | N2 | T6 | E12 | H3 |
| RVA/Cow-wt/URY/LVMS1812/2016/G6P[5] | G6 | P[5] | I2 | A3 | N2 | T6 | E12 | H3 |
| RVA/Cow-wt/URY/LVMS1837/2016/G10P[11] | G10 | P[11] | I2 | A13 | N2 | TX | E12 | H3 |
| RVA/Cow-wt/URY/LVMS2625/2016/G10P[11] | G10 | P[11] | I2 | A13 | N2 | T6 | E12 | H3 |
| RVA/Cow-wt/URY/LVMS3024/2016/G24P[33] | G24 | P[33] | I2 | A13 | N2 | T9 | E12 | H3 |
| RVA/Cow-wt/URY/LVMS3027/2016/G6P[11] | G6 | P[11] | I2 | A3 | N2 | T6 | E12 | H3 |
| RVA/Cow-wt/URY/LVMS3031/2016/G6P[11] | G6 | P[11] | I2 | A3 | N2 | T6 | E12 | H3 |
| RVA/Cow-wt/URY/LVMS3053/2016/G10P[x] | G10 | P[X] | I2 | A13 | N2 | T6 | E12 | HX |
| RVA/Cow-wt/URY/LVMS3206/2016/GxP[11] | GX | P[11] | I2 | A3 | N2 | T6 | E12 | H3 |

Uncommon genotypes are shadowed in grey.

## 2.4. Phylogenetic Analyses

The phylogenetic analyses showed an intricate genetic scenario. The analyses of the VP7 gene showed that G6 and G10 Uruguayan strains clustered in two and one different lineages, respectively, with sequences obtained from cattle. Specifically, the G6P[5] Uruguayan strains clustered in one lineage (split into two sublineages) with Argentinian strains, and the G6P[11] Uruguayan strains clustered separately in a lineage with Slovenian strains (Figure 2). The G10 Uruguayan strains clustered in a lineage (split into two sublineages) with Argentinian strains (Figure 3). Brazilian G6 and G10 strains clustered separately with Uruguayan and Argentinian G6 and G10 strains.

The phylogenetic analyses of the VP4 gene showed that P[5] Uruguayan strains clustered in a lineage with Argentinian G6P[5] strains obtained from cattle, and Brazilian P[5] strains clustered separate (Figure 4). The P[11] Uruguayan strains clustered in three lineages with sequences obtained from cattle, two of the lineages were comprised of G6 and G10 Argentinian strains (and one of these lineages is split into two sublineages), and the other lineage comprised of G6P[11] Brazilian strains, although P[11] Uruguayan strains were distinct to the majority of the Brazilian P[11] strains (Figure 5).

In the phylogenetic tree of the NSP1 gene, we observed that Uruguayan strains clustered in three different genetic lineages of the genotype A3: one jointly with human strains from Paraguay and Brazil, another with Italian and Belgian human strains, and another with a goat strain from Argentina and, in one genetic lineage of the genotype A13, with an Argentinian strain from a cow (Figure S1).

The phylogenetic analysis of the NSP2 gene showed that the Uruguayan strains were clustered in two separate lineages: one with Argentinian strains from cow and goat, and the other with strains from guanaco and vicuña from Argentina and strains from humans from Australia (Figure S2).

On the other hand, the phylogenetic analysis of the NSP3 gene showed that the T6 Uruguayan strains were clustered in three sublineages within one lineage: one together with strains distributed worldwide (including vaccine strains), one with Argentinian (vicuña and guanaco), Japanese (cow), Slovenian (human), and Paraguayan (human) strains, and the third with a goat strain from Argentina and a human strain from Belgium. The T9 strain clustered with the other four T9 strains detected so far (from Japan and the USA; Figure S3).

For the NSP4 gene, we observed that besides the Uruguayan strains obtained in our study, only sequences from South America were available. The phylogenetic analysis showed that Uruguayan strains clustered in four different lineages together with strains from several host species (cows, guanacos, horses, goats, and humans), all from this subcontinent (Figure S4).

The phylogenetic analysis of the NSP5 gene showed that the Uruguayan strains were clustered in three sublineages within one lineage: one together with strains distributed worldwide in several host species), other with an Argentinian strain from a cow and a Paraguayan strain obtained from a human, and another with a strain from a guanaco from Argentina, a strain from a yak from China, and a strain from a human from Hungary (Figure S5).

Lastly, the phylogenetic analysis of the VP6 gene showed that the Uruguayan strains were clustered in three lineages: one conformed only with Uruguayan strains, another lineage with an Argentinian strain from a cow, and another lineage with South American strains from various hosts (human, llama, sheep, and goat), Japanese strains from human and cow, and a roe deer Slovenian strain (Figure S6).

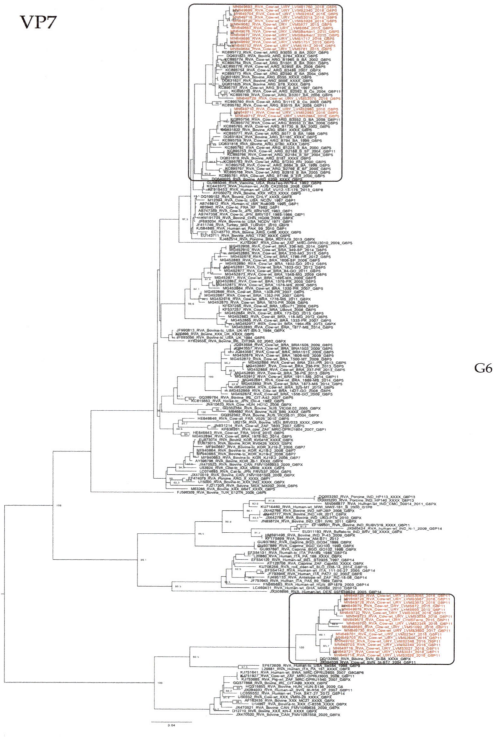

**Figure 2.** Maximum likelihood tree of the G6 genotype of the VP7 gene. The best nucleotide substitution model (TIM2 + I + G) and the maximum likelihood tree were obtained with W-IQ-TREE. Uruguayan strains are shown in red. Shimodaira–Hasegawa-approximate likelihood-ratio test (SH-aLRT) values ≥ 80 are shown.

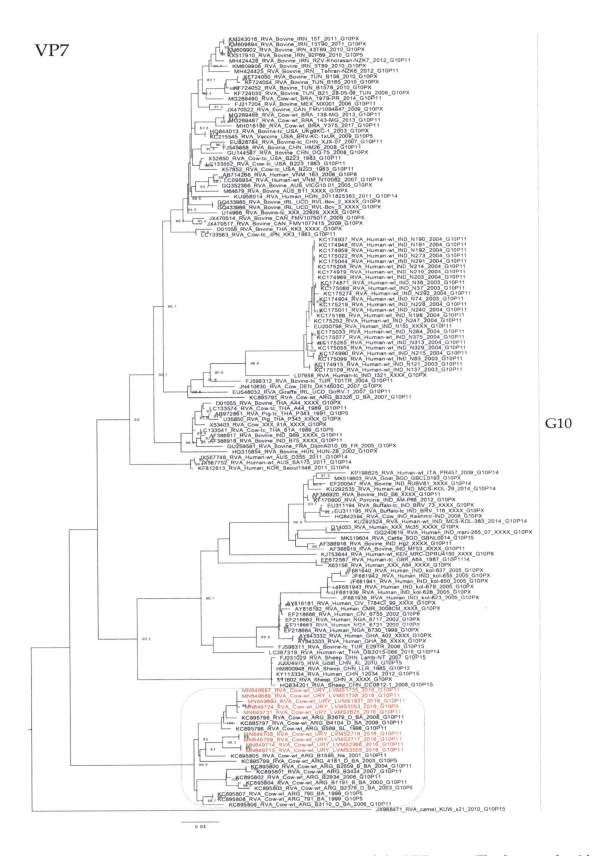

**Figure 3.** Maximum likelihood tree of the G10 genotype of the VP7 gene. The best nucleotide substitution model (TPM3 + G) and the maximum likelihood tree were obtained with W-IQ-TREE. Uruguayan strains are shown in red. SH-aLRT values ≥ 80 are shown.

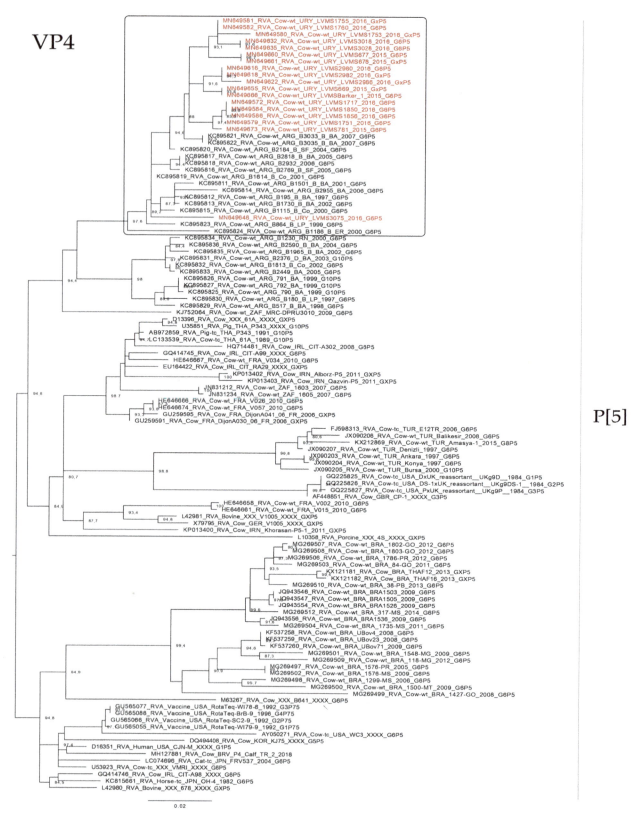

**Figure 4.** Maximum likelihood tree of the P[5] genotype of the VP4 gene. The best nucleotide substitution model (TIM + G) and the maximum likelihood tree were obtained with W-IQ-TREE. Uruguayan strains are shown in red. SH-aLRT values ≥ 80 are shown.

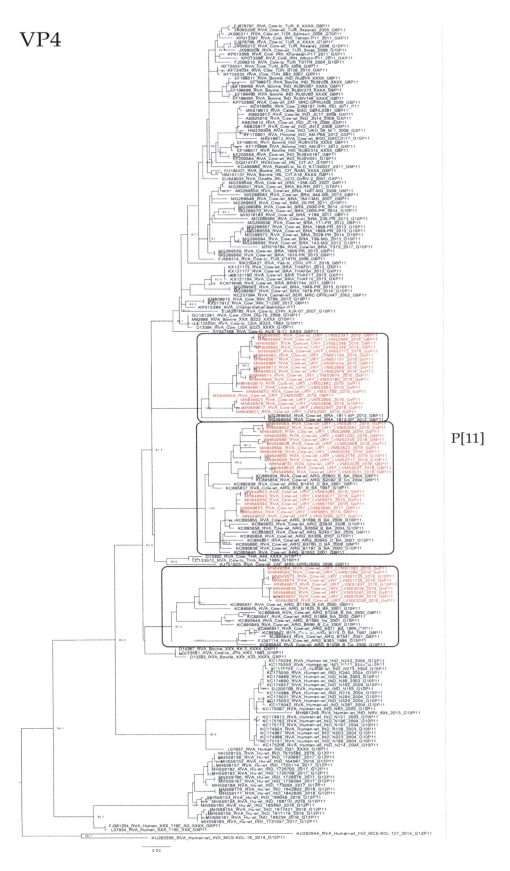

**Figure 5.** Maximum likelihood tree of the P[11] genotype of the VP4 gene. The best nucleotide substitution model (TPM3u + G) and the maximum likelihood tree were obtained with W-IQ-TREE. Uruguayan strains are shown in red. SH-aLRT values ≥ 80 are shown.

## 3. Discussion

Rotavirus A was detected in feces and intestinal contents collected from dairy and beef calves with a frequency of 57%, which was higher than reports from Argentina and Brazil (17–42%) [19–22], and other geographic regions (20–49%) [7,23–25]. On the other hand, in Australia, the frequency of RVA detection was 80%, which is higher than the detected in our study [6]. Interestingly, most of the mentioned studies were conducted by assays different than RT-qPCR, except the one conducted in Australia. It is well documented that the RT-qPCR for RVA detection has a higher sensitivity than other assays, reducing the risk of false-negatives (i.e., ELISA, electron microscopy, PAGE, immunochromatography, and conventional PCR) [6,26–28], which could explain the higher frequency observed in Uruguay when compared with neighboring countries while reducing the risk of false-positive results, also given its higher specificity. Furthermore, the use of RT-qPCR, which is known to detect very few genomic copies, allows pathogen detection in clinical and subclinical calves. In addition, in many field situations, the time of onset of diarrhea is not known, so the peak of pathogen shedding may have already passed, or the infection could be just settling down by the time of sampling [29]. The limit of detection in our study ($10^4$ gc/mL of feces) and the higher RVA viral load in diarrheic than nondiarrheic calves are in agreement with the stated by Torres-Medina et al. [29]. On the other hand, we also observed high viral loads in some nondiarrheic calves.

Infection with RVA has long been associated with diarrhea [29–31], as observed in our study, where RVA detection was more frequent in diarrheic than in nondiarrheic calves, independently of their age (up to 4 weeks). Concerning the calves' age, we observed that the proportion of calves shedding RVA was higher in the second and third weeks of age, as observed in Brazil [19,32] and elsewhere [33]. In addition, the mean age of RVA-positive calves in our study is similar to the age reported previously [31], and we observed that diarrheic calves positive for RVA were younger than nondiarrheic calves, indicating that calves are exposed to this pathogen early after birth.

Although the sampling between beef and dairy farms was unequal, our results indicate that the circulation of RVA was higher in dairy than beef calves. This contrasts with the reported results in neighboring countries, where RVA was more frequently detected in beef than dairy calves [19,20] or in a similar frequency [21]. Our results also contrast with those observed in a study conducted in Australia [6].

A common practice used to prevent NCD is the vaccination of pregnant cows/heifers during the last stage of pregnancy to protect the calves by the transference of passive maternal antibodies through colostrum intake. Most available vaccines in the Uruguayan market include bovine rotavirus A strains (most of them include two strains, G6 and G10, as detailed by the manufacturers). In this study, we observed a similar frequency of RVA detection in calves from vaccinated and unvaccinated herds. Failure in the protection against RVA infection by the vaccine was reported in studies conducted in Argentina and Brazil [34–37]; although vaccines are not effective in preventing RVA infection, they significantly reduce morbidity, the severity of diarrhea, and mortality related to RVA [38].

In this study, we determined the RVA genotypes circulating in calves in Uruguay. Overall, the VP7 and VP4 genotypes observed in this country are the most prevalent in cattle worldwide [39], although, unexpectedly, we detected a G24P[33] strain, which thus far had only been reported from an asymptomatic cow and her calf in Japan [11]. The G24P[33] strain detected in Uruguay was obtained from a 10-day-old asymptomatic dairy calf sampled in August 2016.

Regarding the VP6 and NSP1-5 genotyping, the Uruguayan strains, including the G24P[33], showed a relatively conserved genotype constellation I2-A3/A13-N2-T6/T9-E12-H3, corresponding to VP6 and NSP1-5 genotypes, respectively. These genotypes are commonly found in cattle, with the exception of T9 [40]. The T9 genotype has been sporadically detected in two cows from Japan [11], in a child from Japan [41], and in a child from the USA [42]. This genotype has been associated with atypical VP7 and VP4 genotypes (G21P[29], G24P[33], G8P[14], and G24P[14]). In this study, we observed the T9 genotype associated with G24P[33]. Indepth analysis of the RVA/Cow-wt/URY/LVMS3024/2016/G24P[33] strain revealed almost the same genotype constellation as the RVA/Cow-wt/JPN/Dai-10/2007/G24P[33] strain from Japan, with the unusual G24, P[33], and T9 genotypes. The only difference was observed in the NSP4 gene that was E12 in the Uruguayan strain and E2 in the Japanese. It is interesting to note that all the Uruguayan strains were E12, a genotype widely detected in cattle [12], guanacos [12], horses [43,44], goats [45], and children [46,47] in South America. This reinforces the notion that the E12 genotype may be restricted to South America, as previously postulated [44].

The rare G24P[33] strain detected in our study represented a challenge. The G24, P[33], and T9 genotypes observed in this strain provides information for a possible introduction of the virus from Japan to Uruguay, or vice versa. The expansion of the Wagyu beef industry beyond Japan [48] could have influenced the dispersion of some RVA strains through live cattle exports. On the other hand, the E12 genotype in the Uruguayan G24P[33] strain and E2 genotype in the Japanese G24P[33] strain represented a probable gene reassortment, which is a more plausible scenario than the emergence of two independent strains with the same rare genotype constellation except for NSP4. Further studies should be conducted to determine the evolution and possible emergence of these rare genotypes.

In the phylogenetic analyses of all the genes, it can be observed that Uruguayan strains clustered mainly with South American strains. The only gene that did not show any South American-specific lineage was NSP3, in which the Uruguayan strains clustered mainly with Argentinian strains, but also with strains from other continents. These data, together with the identification of the E12 genotype in all the Uruguayan sequences, suggest a South American origin of RVA lineages [44]. Furthermore, the phylogenetic analyses showed an intricate pattern of diversity, with evidence of gene reassortments, interspecies transmission, local dispersion of some strains, and circulation of strains that are most prevalent in cattle worldwide.

The analyses of VP7 and VP4 showed a conserved pattern with all the Uruguayan strains clustering, with strains detected only in cattle and mainly from Argentina, indicating a probable host species and geographic linkage. Due to the shortage of G24 and P[33] sequences in the database (2 and 1, respectively), no phylogenetic analyses were performed for these genotypes. In the VP7 and VP4 phylogenetic analysis, the majority of strains characterized in this study clustered closely with strains detected in Argentinian cattle. The exceptions were one G6 lineage that clustered with European strains isolated from cattle, and one in P[11] sublineage that clustered with Brazilian strains isolated from cattle. There is a clear phylogenetic relationship between the strains detected in the cattle in Uruguay and Argentina, whereas Brazilian strains were, in general, phylogenetically distant from the Uruguayan strains. In addition, Uruguayan strains clustered together among themselves, suggesting that limited introductions of RVA into the country have occurred, but the strains were widely dispersed in the cattle. A possible explanation for the genetic similarity between the Uruguayan and Argentinian strains and their divergence to the Brazilian strains could be explained, in part, by the breed of cattle. In Uruguay and Argentina, most of the cattle breeds are *Bos taurus*, while in Brazil, there are mostly *Bos indicus* or *Bos indicus* x *Bos taurus* crosses. Although it has not been studied in cattle, different human subpopulations appeared to have different susceptibility infection and clinical disease, and this susceptibility is dependent on the rotavirus genotype, and in some cases, it also depends on different rotavirus strains of the same genotype [49].

Based on the phylogenetic analyses, we observed evidence of gene reassortment and interspecies transmission events. Regarding the former event, in addition to the previously mentioned gene reassortment of the G24P[33] strain, strong evidence was observed in the strains RVA/Cow-wt/URY/LVMS1812/2016/G6P[5] and RVA/Cow-wt/URY/LVMS3206/2016/GxP[11] because both strains clustered together in all the genes, except in VP4 (which showed different genotypes, (P[5] and P[11], respectively), indicating that a possible gene reassortment event may have occurred. Another piece of evidence was observed in the RVA/Cow-wt/URY/LVMS1788/2016/GxP[11] strain because it clustered together with other Uruguayan strains in most of the genes, except in NSP1 and NSP3 genes, which clustered alone in different genetic lineages, also suggesting a gene reassortment event. Furthermore, the strain RVA/Cow-wt/URY/LVMS1837/2016/G10P[11] clustered together with RVA/Cow-wt/URY/LVMS2625/2016/G10P[11] and RVA/Cow-wt/URY/LVMS3053/2016/G10P[x] in most of the genes, but clustered separately in distant genetic lineages in NSP2 and NSP5; this was probably due to gene reassortment. On the other hand, an interesting observation was that, in general, G6 strains tended to cluster together in most of the genes, and the same was observed for the G10 strains, with the exceptions aforementioned.

Regarding interspecies transmission, we observed that in the analyses of VP7 and VP4, all the Uruguayan strains clustered with other bovine strains, so these gene segments seem to be more host-specific than the other genes. On the other hand, and based on the phylogenetic analyses, we observed evidence suggesting interspecies transmission because the bovine strains detected in Uruguay closely clustered with strains detected in other host species. We observed that bovine Uruguayan strains A13 (NSP1 gene) clustered together with strains isolated from humans and a goat, possibly indicating events of interspecies transmission. Two lineages showed a close relationship between Uruguayan bovine strains and human strains (from South America and Europe); these human strains were reported to be Artiodactyl-like and a product of interspecies transmission [10,47,50], as well as the goat strain of a third lineage [45], which is in accordance with our results. In the NSP2-5 and VP6 genes, we observed that the Uruguayan bovine strains clustered in some lineages with strains isolated from other host species (human, goat, guanaco, vicuna, roe deer, llama, and sheep), mainly from South America, that were proposed to be originated by interspecies transmission [12,45,47,51], again in accordance with our results. Another piece of evidence supporting this event was observed in the NSP4; all the RVA strains detected in South America were E12, independent of the host species where they were isolated (horse, cow, guanaco, human, goat), suggesting interspecies transmission and fixation of this genotype in South America [44]. The interspecies transmission of RVA is widely documented [10–13], and our results support this event. In South America, it is common to raise different livestock species on the same farm in close contact with humans [45], which increases the possibility of interspecies transmission. Our results support that interspecies transmission is a common event in South America, including the possibility of zoonotic transmission [45,51,52].

Lastly, our study had some limitations. In Uruguay, dairy farming is concentrated in the southwest region and calves are raised under intensive production systems that facilitated the collection of the samples, while beef calves are mostly bred in extensive production systems and dispersed throughout the country, which hindered the access to samples. This resulted in an overrepresentation of dairy (92%) versus beef (8%) samples in our study. Another limitation was that we had no spiked control to determine if there was inhibition of the qPCR, which may lead to false-negatives. Regarding coinfections, the methodology used has the limitation that sequences obtained from a single animal would have only represented the predominant strain and/or sequences with multiple traces that were not included in the study. It is important to mention that, from our analyses, we could not determine the route nor the time in which the gene reassortment and the interspecies transmission events took place.

## 4. Materials and Methods

### 4.1. Samples

Fecal samples of 766 live calves and intestinal contents from 67 naturally-deceased calves were collected from 833 different calves from dairy and beef herds in Uruguay between 2015 and 2018. Sampled herds were distributed in 10 of the 19 regions of the country (Figure 6), and throughout the year, including samples collected in the four climate seasons. In addition, 766 samples were from dairy calves, and 67 from beef calves. We compared the frequency of the RVA infection between groups only for dairy calves. A total of 240 dairy calves had diarrhea at the time of sampling, while 272 were nondiarrheic dairy calves (this information was unavailable for 321 calves). The distribution by age in the first, second, third, and fourth weeks of life was 148, 201, 110, and 34 dairy calves, respectively (the age was unavailable for 340 calves). A total of 225 calves were from dairy herds vaccinated against NCD and 246 calves were from nonvaccinated dairy herds (herd vaccination history was unavailable for 362 calves).

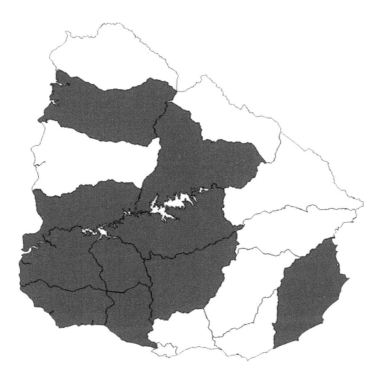

**Figure 6.** Map of Uruguay, the regions from which samples were collected shown in grey.

### 4.2. Sample Suspension, RNA Extraction, Reverse Transcription, Detection and Quantification of RVA

Samples were diluted 1:10 (*v*:*v*) in phosphate-buffered saline solution, centrifuged at 3000× *g* for 20 min at 4 °C, and supernatants were collected and stored at −80 °C. Viral RNA was extracted using a QIAamp® cador® Pathogen Mini Kit (Qiagen®, Hilden, Germany), following the manufacturer's instructions. Reverse transcription (RT) was carried out with RevertAid® Reverse Transcriptase (Thermo Fisher Scientific®, Waltham, MA, USA) and random hexamers primers (Qiagen®), following the manufacturer's instructions. All RNAs and cDNAs were stored at −80 °C until further viral analyses. Screening and quantification of the samples for RVA identification were carried out through a quantitative polymerase chain reaction (qPCR) targeted to the NSP3 gene, as described elsewhere [9]. Briefly, 12.5 µL of SensiFAST™ Probe No-ROX Kit (Bioline®, London, UK), 5.0 µL of nuclease-free water, 1.0 µL of 10 µM forward primer, 1.0 µL of 10 µM reverse primer, 0.5 µL of 10 µM probe, and 5 µL of cDNA were mixed in 0.2-mL PCR tubes. All samples were analyzed in duplicate. In order to validate the complete process, an RVA-positive (G6P[5] strain) and an RVA-negative fecal sample were used as positive and negative controls, respectively.

### 4.3. Rotavirus A Genotyping

Quantitative-PCR positive samples were subsequently subjected to amplification of VP7 and VP4 (VP8*). Briefly, 12.5 µL of MangoMix™ (Bioline®), 5 µL of cDNA, 5.5 µL of nuclease-free water, 1 µL of dimethyl sulfoxide, 0.5 µL of 20 µM forward primer and 0.5 µL of 20 µM reverse primer were mixed in 0.2-mL PCR tubes. Forward and reverse primers for VP7 and VP4 (VP8*) amplification are described elsewhere [20,53]. In addition, 10 samples, including representative VP7 and VP4 genotype combinations observed in this study, were selected for VP6 and NSP1-5 gene characterization. Primers and cycling conditions were used, as described elsewhere [10], and PCR reagents were used, as described above. Genotyping was performed using the web-based genotyping tool RotaC v2.0 [54].

### 4.4. PCR Product Purification, Sequencing, and GenBank Accession Numbers

PCR products were visualized in 1–2% agarose gels and positive samples were purified using PureLink™ Quick Gel Extraction and PCR Purification Combo Kit (Invitrogen®, Carlsbad, CA, USA), according to the manufacturer's instructions. Both cDNA strands were sequenced by Macrogen Inc. (Seoul, Korea). Sequences were deposited in GenBank with accession numbers: MN649559—MN649674 (VP4), MN649675—MN649732 (VP7), MN649733—MN649742 (VP6), MN649743—MN649751 (NSP1), MN649752—MN649761 (NSP2), MN649762—MN649770 (NSP3), MN649771—MN649780 (NSP4), and MN649781—MN649789 (NSP5).

*4.5. Phylogenetic Analysis*

All the available sequences corresponding to the genotypes observed in the RVA strains detected in this study, previously determined with RotaC, were downloaded from the Virus Variation Resource (http://www.ncbi.nlm.nih.gov/genome/viruses/variation/) [55]. A dataset was created for each genotype, and multiple sequence alignments were obtained using Clustal W implemented in MEGA 7 software [56]. The final alignment of each gene comprised all the worldwide sequences that covered the length of the sequences obtained in this study. The length of the sequences and the nucleotide position, involved in the phylogenetic analysis of each gene, are detailed in Table 3. The nucleotide substitution models that best fit each dataset (Table 3) and the maximum likelihood trees were obtained using W-IQ-TREE (available at http://iqtree.cibiv.univie.ac.at) [57]. The branches support was estimated with the Shimodaira–Hasegawa-approximate likelihood-ratio test (SH-aLRT) [58]. Trees were visualized in FigTree (http://tree.bio.ed.ac.uk/software/figtree/).

**Table 3.** Information about the final alignments obtained for the phylogenetic analyses.

| | NSP1 | NSP2 | NSP3 | NSP4 | NSP5 | VP4 (P[5]) | VP4 (P[11]) | VP6 | VP7 (G6) | VP7 (G10) |
|---|---|---|---|---|---|---|---|---|---|---|
| Sequences lenght * | 1005 | 954 | 917 | 528 | 597 | 645 | 654 | 1143 | 852 | 837 |
| Genomic position * | 165–1169 | Complete ORF | 47–963 | Complete ORF | Complete ORF | 130–774 | 124–795 | Complete ORF | 121–972 | 73–909 |
| Best nucleotide substitution model | TIM + I + G | TIM + G | TIM3 + G | HKY + G | TN + I + G | TIM + G | TPM3u + G | TIM + I + G | TIM2 + I + G | TPM3 + G |

* Reference strain: WC3.

*4.6. Statistical Analyses*

Data were organized and graphics were generated using Microsoft® Office Excel. Categorical data were evaluated with RStudio v1.0.136 software through Pearson's chi-squared tests. Odds ratios (OR) and 95% confidence intervals (CI) were calculated with jamovi software (available at https://www.jamovi.org/). Viral load values (genome copies/milliliter of feces) were log10 transformed. For the viral load and mean age analyses, the Shapiro–Wilk test was performed, rejecting the normality of the data, so the Mann–Whitney U test was performed with the same software. For all tests, differences were considered statistically significant if the obtained $p$-value was < 0.05.

## 5. Conclusions

Rotavirus A is widespread in cattle in Uruguay and is associated with diarrhea in calves, with a peak of viral shedding at 2–3 weeks of age, and higher viral shedding in diarrheic versus non-diarrheic calves. Even though the main genotypes observed in this country are the most prevalent worldwide, a rare strain was detected with a G24-P[33]-I2-A13-N2-T9-E12-H3 genotype constellation. The E12 genotype detected in all strains, regardless of the VP7 and VP4 genotypes, appears to be a South American geographic marker. An intricate genetic scenario was evidenced, with gene reassortment and interspecies transmission events, including transmission between animals and humans.

**Supplementary Materials:**
Figure S1: Maximum likelihood tree of the NSP1 gene. The best nucleotide substitution model (TIM + I + G) and the maximum likelihood tree were obtained with W-IQ-TREE. Uruguayan strains are shown in different colors. SH-aLRT values ≥ 80 are shown. Figure S2: Maximum likelihood tree of the NSP2 gene. The best nucleotide substitution model (TIM + G) and the maximum likelihood tree were obtained with W-IQ-TREE. Uruguayan strains are shown in different colors. SH-aLRT values ≥ 80 are shown. Figure S3: Maximum likelihood tree of the NSP3 gene. The best nucleotide substitution model (TIM3 + G) and the maximum likelihood tree were obtained with W-IQ-TREE. Uruguayan strains are shown in different colors. SH-aLRT values ≥ 80 are shown.

Figure S4: Maximum likelihood tree of the NSP4 gene. The best nucleotide substitution model (HKY + G) and the maximum likelihood tree were obtained with W-IQ-TREE. Uruguayan strains are shown in different colors. SH-aLRT values ≥ 80 are shown. Figure S5: Maximum likelihood tree of the NSP5 gene. The best nucleotide substitution model (TN + I + G) and the maximum likelihood tree were obtained with W-IQ-TREE. Uruguayan strains are shown in different colors. SH-aLRT values ≥ 80 are shown. Figure S6: Maximum likelihood tree of the VP6 gene. The best nucleotide substitution model (TIM + I + G) and the maximum likelihood tree were obtained with W-IQ-TREE. Uruguayan strains are shown in different colors. SH-aLRT values ≥ 80 are shown.

**Author Contributions:** Conceptualization, M.C. and R.C.; methodology, M.C., R.D.C., M.L.C., C.S., S.M., F.C. and D.C.; resources, M.C., F.R.-C., F.G., V.P. and R.C.; writing—original draft preparation, M.C.; writing—review and editing, M.C., R.D.C., M.L.C., S.M., F.C., D.C., M.V., F.R.-C., F.G., V.P. and R.C.; funding acquisition, M.C., F.R.-C. and R.C. All authors have read and agreed to the published version of the manuscript.

**Acknowledgments:** M.C. acknowledges support from the "Agencia Nacional de Investigación e Innovación" (ANII) through a PhD scholarship, and "Comisión Sectorial de Investigación Científica" (CSIC) and ANII for mobility fellowships.

## References

1. Urie, N.J.; Lombard, J.E.; Shivley, C.B.; Kopral, C.A.; Adams, A.E.; Earleywine, T.J.; Olson, J.D.; Garry, F.B. Preweaned heifer management on US dairy operations: Part V. Factors associated with morbidity and mortality in preweaned dairy heifer calves. *J. Dairy Sci.* **2018**, *101*, 9229–9244. [CrossRef]
2. Waltner-Toews, D.; Martin, S.W.; Meek, A.H. The effect of early calfhood health status on survivorship and age at first calving. *Can. J. Vet. Res.* **1986**, *50*, 314–317. [PubMed]
3. Donovan, G.A.; Dohoo, I.R.; Montgomery, D.M.; Bennett, F.L. Calf and disease factors affecting growth in female Holstein calves in Florida, USA. *Prev. Vet. Med.* **1998**, *33*, 1–10. [CrossRef]
4. Østerås, O.; Solbu, H.; Refsdal, A.O.; Roalkvam, T.; Filseth, O.; Minsaas, A. Results and evaluation of thirty years of health recordings in the Norwegian dairy cattle population. *J. Dairy Sci.* **2007**, *90*, 4483–4497. [CrossRef]
5. Windeyer, M.C.; Leslie, K.E.; Godden, S.M.; Hodgins, D.C.; Lissemore, K.D.; LeBlanc, S.J. Factors associated with morbidity, mortality, and growth of dairy heifer calves up to 3 months of age. *Prev. Vet. Med.* **2014**, *113*, 231–240. [CrossRef] [PubMed]
6. Izzo, M.M.; Kirkland, P.D.; Mohler, V.L.; Perkins, N.R.; Gunn, A.A.; House, J.K. Prevalence of major enteric pathogens in Australian dairy calves with diarrhoea. *Aust. Vet. J.* **2011**, *89*, 167–173. [CrossRef]
7. Al Mawly, J.; Grinberg, A.; Prattley, D.; Moffat, J.; French, N. Prevalence of endemic enteropathogens of calves in New Zealand dairy farms. *N. Z. Vet. J.* **2015**, *63*, 147–152. [CrossRef]
8. Estes, M.; Greenberg, H. Rotaviruses. In *Fields Virology*, 6th ed.; Knipe, D.M., Howley, P.M., Cohen, J.I., Griffin, D.E., Lamb, R.A., Martin, M.A., Racaniello, V.R., Roizman, B., Eds.; Wolters Kluwer Business/Lippincott Williams and Wilkins: Philadelphia, PA, USA, 2013.
9. Castells, M.; Schild, C.; Cattarena, D.; Bok, M.; Giannitti, F.; Armendano, J.; Riet-Correa, F.; Victoria, M.; Parreño, V.; Colina, R. Prevalence and viability of group A rotavirus in dairy farm water sources. *J. Appl. Microbiol.* **2018**, *124*, 922–929. [CrossRef]
10. Matthijnssens, J.; Ciarlet, M.; Heiman, E.; Arijs, I.; Delbeke, T.; McDonald, S.M.; Palombo, E.A.; Iturriza-Gómara, M.; Maes, P.; Patton, J.T.; et al. Full genome-based classification of rotaviruses reveals a common origin between human Wa-Like and porcine rotavirus strains and human DS-1-like and bovine rotavirus strains. *J. Virol.* **2008**, *82*, 3204–3219. [CrossRef]
11. Abe, M.; Ito, N.; Masatani, T.; Nakagawa, K.; Yamaoka, S.; Kanamaru, Y.; Suzuki, H.; Shibano, K.; Arashi, Y.; Sugiyama, M. Whole genome characterization of new bovine rotavirus G21P[29] and G24P[33] strains provides evidence for interspecies transmission. *J. Gen. Virol.* **2011**, *92*, 952–960. [CrossRef]
12. Matthijnssens, J.; Potgieter, C.A.; Ciarlet, M.; Parreño, V.; Martella, V.; Bányai, K.; Garaicoechea, L.; Palombo, E.A.; Novo, L.; Zeller, M.; et al. Are human P[14] rotavirus strains the result of interspecies transmissions from sheep or other ungulates that belong to the mammalian order Artiodactyla? *J. Virol.* **2009**, *83*, 2917–2929. [CrossRef] [PubMed]
13. Matthijnssens, J.; Rahman, M.; Martella, V.; Xuelei, Y.; De Vos, S.; De Leener, K.; Ciarlet, M.; Buonavoglia, C.; Van Ranst, M. Full genomic analysis of human rotavirus strain B4106 and lapine rotavirus strain 30/96 provides evidence for interspecies transmission. *J. Virol.* **2006**, *80*, 3801–3810. [CrossRef]

14. Castells, M.; Giannitti, F.; Caffarena, R.D.; Casaux, M.L.; Schild, C.; Castells, D.; Riet-Correa, F.; Victoria, M.; Parreño, V.; Colina, R. Bovine coronavirus in Uruguay: Genetic diversity, risk factors and transboundary introductions from neighboring countries. *Arch. Virol.* **2019**, *164*, 2715–2724. [CrossRef] [PubMed]
15. Castells, M.; Bertoni, E.; Caffarena, R.D.; Casaux, M.L.; Schild, C.; Victoria, M.; Riet-Correa, F.; Giannitti, F.; Parreño, V.; Colina, R. Bovine astrovirus surveillance in Uruguay reveals high detection rate of a novel *Mamastrovirus* species. *Viruses* **2019**, *12*, 32. [CrossRef] [PubMed]
16. Food and Agriculture Organization of the United Nations. *Meat Market Review*; FAO: Rome, Italy, 2018.
17. International Dairy Federation. The World Dairy Situation 2013. In *Bulletin of the International Dairy Federation 470/2013*; International Dairy Federation: Schaerbeek, Belgium, 2013.
18. DIEA. Anuario Estadístico Agropecuario. 2018. Available online: https://descargas.mgap.gub.uy/DIEA/Anuarios/Anuario2018/Anuario_2018.pdf (accessed on 19 March 2020).
19. Alfieri, A.A.; Parazzi, M.E.; Takiuchi, E.; Médici, K.C.; Alfieri, A.F. Frequency of group A rotavirus in diarrhoeic calves in Brazilian cattle herds, 1998–2002. *Trop. Anim. Health Prod.* **2006**, *38*, 521–526. [CrossRef] [PubMed]
20. Garaicoechea, L.; Bok, K.; Jones, L.R.; Combessies, G.; Odeón, A.; Fernandez, F.; Parreño, V. Molecular characterization of bovine rotavirus circulating in beef and dairy herds in Argentina during a 10-year period (1994–2003). *Vet. Microbiol.* **2006**, *118*, 1–11. [CrossRef] [PubMed]
21. Badaracco, A.; Garaicoechea, L.; Rodríguez, D.; Uriarte, E.L.; Odeón, A.; Bilbao, G.; Galarza, R.; Abdala, A.; Fernandez, F.; Parreño, V. Bovine rotavirus strains circulating in beef and dairy herds in Argentina from 2004 to 2010. *Vet. Microbiol.* **2012**, *158*, 394–399. [CrossRef]
22. Da Silva Medeiros, T.N.; Lorenzetti, E.; Alfieri, A.F.; Alfieri, A.A. G and P genotype profiles of rotavirus A field strains circulating in beef and dairy cattle herds in Brazil, 2006–2015. *Comp. Immunol. Microbiol. Infect. Dis.* **2019**, *64*, 90–98. [CrossRef]
23. Madadgar, O.; Nazaktabar, A.; Keivanfar, H.; Zahraei Salehi, T.; Lotfollah Zadeh, S. Genotyping and determining the distribution of prevalent G and P types of group A bovine rotaviruses between 2010 and 2012 in Iran. *Vet. Microbiol.* **2015**, *179*, 190–196. [CrossRef]
24. Pourasgari, F.; Kaplon, J.; Karimi-Naghlani, S.; Fremy, C.; Otarod, V.; Ambert-Balay, K.; Mirjalili, A.; Pothier, P. The molecular epidemiology of bovine rotaviruses circulating in Iran: A two-year study. *Arch. Virol.* **2016**, *161*, 3483–3494. [CrossRef] [PubMed]
25. Mohamed, F.F.; Mansour, S.M.G.; El-Araby, I.E.; Mor, S.K.; Goyal, S.M. Molecular detection of enteric viruses from diarrheic calves in Egypt. *Arch. Virol.* **2017**, *162*, 129–137. [CrossRef] [PubMed]
26. Pang, X.L.; Lee, B.; Boroumand, N.; Leblanc, B.; Preiksaitis, J.K.; Yu Ip, C.C. Increased detection of rotavirus using a real time reverse transcription-polymerase chain reaction (RT-PCR) assay in stool specimens from children with diarrhea. *J. Med. Virol.* **2004**, *72*, 496–501. [CrossRef] [PubMed]
27. Gutiérrez-Aguirre, I.; Steyer, A.; Boben, J.; Gruden, K.; Poljsak-Prijatelj, M.; Ravnikar, M. Sensitive detection of multiple rotavirus genotypes with a single reverse transcription-real-time quantitative PCR assay. *J. Clin. Microbiol.* **2008**, *46*, 2547–2554. [CrossRef] [PubMed]
28. De La Cruz Hernández, S.I.; Anaya Molina, Y.; Gómez Santiago, F.; Terán Vega, H.L.; Monroy Leyva, E.; Méndez Pérez, H.; García Lozano, H. Real-time RT-PCR, a necessary tool to support the diagnosis and surveillance of rotavirus in Mexico. *Diagn. Microbiol. Infect. Dis.* **2018**, *90*, 272–276. [CrossRef]
29. Torres-Medina, A.; Schlafer, D.H.; Mebus, C.A. Rotaviral and coronaviral diarrhea. *Vet. Clin. N. Am. Food Anim. Pract.* **1985**, *1*, 471–493. [CrossRef]
30. Foster, D.M.; Smith, G.W. Pathophysiology of diarrhea in calves. *Vet. Clin. N. Am. Food Anim. Pract.* **2009**, *25*, 13–36. [CrossRef] [PubMed]
31. Blanchard, P.C. Diagnostics of dairy and beef cattle diarrhea. *Vet. Clin. N. Am. Food Anim. Pract.* **2012**, *28*, 443–464. [CrossRef]
32. Coura, F.M.; Freitas, M.D.; Ribeiro, J.; de Leme, R.A.; de Souza, C.; Alfieri, A.A.; Facury Filho, E.J.; de Carvalho, A.Ú.; Silva, M.X.; Lage, A.P.; et al. Longitudinal study of Salmonella spp., diarrheagenic Escherichia coli, Rotavirus, and Coronavirus isolated from healthy and diarrheic calves in a Brazilian dairy herd. *Trop. Anim. Health Prod.* **2015**, *47*, 3–11. [CrossRef]
33. Saif, L.J.; Smith, K.L. Enteric viral infections of calves and passive immunity. *J. Dairy Sci.* **1985**, *68*, 206–228. [CrossRef]
34. Badaracco, A.; Garaicoechea, L.; Matthijnssens, J.; Louge Uriarte, E.; Odeón, A.; Bilbao, G.; Fernandez, F.;

Parra, G.I.; Parreño, V. Phylogenetic analyses of typical bovine rotavirus genotypes G6, G10, P[5] and P[11] circulating in Argentinean beef and dairy herds. *Infect. Genet. Evol.* **2013**, *18*, 18–30. [CrossRef] [PubMed]

35. Barreiros, M.A.; Alfieri, A.F.; Médici, K.C.; Leite, J.P.; Alfieri, A.A. G and P genotypes of group A rotavirus from diarrhoeic calves born to cows vaccinated against the NCDV (P[1], G6) rotavirus strain. *J. Vet. Med. B Infect. Dis. Vet. Public Health* **2004**, *51*, 104–109. [CrossRef]

36. Da Silva Medeiros, T.N.; Lorenzetti, E.; Alfieri, A.F.; Alfieri, A.A. Phylogenetic analysis of a G6P[5] bovine rotavirus strain isolated in a neonatal diarrhea outbreak in a beef cattle herd vaccinated with G6P[1] and G10P[11] genotypes. *Arch. Virol.* **2015**, *160*, 447–451. [CrossRef] [PubMed]

37. Rocha, T.G.; Silva, F.D.; Gregori, F.; Alfieri, A.A.; Buzinaro, M.D.; Fagliari, J.J. Longitudinal study of bovine rotavirus group A in newborn calves from vaccinated and unvaccinated dairy herds. *Trop. Anim. Health Prod.* **2017**, *49*, 783–790. [CrossRef] [PubMed]

38. Parreño, V.; Béjar, C.; Vagnozzi, A.; Barrandeguy, M.; Costantini, V.; Craig, M.I.; Yuan, L.; Hodgins, D.; Saif, L.; Fernández, F. Modulation by colostrum-acquired maternal antibodies of systemic and mucosal antibody responses to rotavirus in calves experimentally challenged with bovine rotavirus. *Vet. Immunol. Immunopathol.* **2004**, *100*, 7–24. [CrossRef]

39. Papp, H.; László, B.; Jakab, F.; Ganesh, B.; De Grazia, S.; Matthijnssens, J.; Ciarlet, M.; Martella, V.; Bányai, K. Review of group A rotavirus strains reported in swine and cattle. *Vet. Microbiol.* **2013**, *165*, 190–199. [CrossRef] [PubMed]

40. Komoto, S.; Pongsuwanna, Y.; Tacharoenmuang, R.; Guntapong, R.; Ide, T.; Higo-Moriguchi, K.; Tsuji, T.; Yoshikawa, T.; Taniguchi, K. Whole genomic analysis of bovine group A rotavirus strains A5-10 and A5-13 provides evidence for close evolutionary relationship with human rotaviruses. *Vet. Microbiol.* **2016**, *195*, 37–57. [CrossRef] [PubMed]

41. Okitsu, S.; Hikita, T.; Thongprachum, A.; Khamrin, P.; Takanashi, S.; Hayakawa, S.; Maneekarn, N.; Ushijima, H. Detection and molecular characterization of two rare G8P[14] and G3P[3] rotavirus strains collected from children with acute gastroenteritis in Japan. *Infect. Genet. Evol.* **2018**, *62*, 95–108. [CrossRef]

42. Ward, M.L.; Mijatovic-Rustempasic, S.; Roy, S.; Rungsrisuriyachai, K.; Boom, J.A.; Sahni, L.C.; Baker, C.J.; Rench, M.A.; Wikswo, M.E.; Payne, D.C.; et al. Molecular characterization of the first G24P[14] rotavirus strain detected in humans. *Infect. Genet. Evol.* **2016**, *43*, 338–342. [CrossRef]

43. Garaicoechea, L.; Miño, S.; Ciarlet, M.; Fernández, F.; Barrandeguy, M.; Parreño, V. Molecular characterization of equine rotaviruses circulating in Argentinean foals during a 17-year surveillance period (1992–2008). *Vet. Microbiol.* **2011**, *148*, 150–160. [CrossRef]

44. Matthijnssens, J.; Miño, S.; Papp, H.; Potgieter, C.; Novo, L.; Heylen, E.; Zeller, M.; Garaicoechea, L.; Badaracco, A.; Lengyel, G.; et al. Complete molecular genome analyses of equine rotavirus A strains from different continents reveal several novel genotypes and a largely conserved genotype constellation. *J. Gen. Virol.* **2012**, *93 Pt 4*, 866–875. [CrossRef]

45. Louge Uriarte, E.L.; Badaracco, A.; Matthijnssens, J.; Zeller, M.; Heylen, F.; Manazza, J.; Miño, S.; Van Raust, M.; Odeón, A.; Parreño, V. The first caprine rotavirus detected in Argentina displays genomic features resembling virus strains infecting members of the Bovidae and Camelidae. *Vet. Microbiol.* **2014**, *171*, 189–197. [CrossRef] [PubMed]

46. Volotão, E.M.; Soares, C.C.; Maranhão, A.G.; Rocha, L.N.; Hoshino, Y.; Santos, N. Rotavirus surveillance in the city of Rio de Janeiro-Brazil during 2000-2004: Detection of unusual strains with G8P[4] or G10P[9] specificities. *J. Med. Virol.* **2006**, *78*, 263–272. [CrossRef] [PubMed]

47. Martinez, M.; Phan, T.G.; Galeano, M.E.; Russomando, G.; Parreno, V.; Delwart, E.; Parra, G.I. Genomic characterization of a rotavirus G8P[1] detected in a child with diarrhea reveal direct animal-to-human transmission. *Infect. Genet. Evol.* **2014**, *27*, 402–407. [CrossRef]

48. Gotoh, T.; Nishimura, T.; Kuchida, K.; Mannen, H. The Japanese Wagyu beef industry: Current situation and future prospects—A review. *Asian Australas. J. Anim. Sci.* **2018**, *31*, 933–950. [CrossRef] [PubMed]

49. Sharma, S.; Hagbom, M.; Svensson, L.; Nordgren, J. The Impact of Human Genetic Polymorphisms on Rotavirus Susceptibility, Epidemiology, and Vaccine Take. *Viruses* **2020**, *12*, 324. [CrossRef] [PubMed]

50. Gómez, M.M.; Resque, H.R.; de Mello Volotao, E.; Rose, T.L.; da Silva, M.F.; Heylen, E.; Zeller, M.; Matthijnssens, J.; Leite, J.P. Distinct evolutionary origins of G12P[8] and G12P[9] group A rotavirus strains circulating in Brazil. *Infect. Genet. Evol.* **2014**, *28*, 385–388. [CrossRef]

51. Rojas, M.; Dias, H.G.; Gonçalves, J.L.S.; Manchego, A.; Rosadio, R.; Pezo, D.; Santos, N. Genetic diversity and zoonotic potential of rotavirus A strains in the southern Andean highlands, Peru. *Transbound. Emerg. Dis.* **2019**, *66*, 1718–1726. [CrossRef]
52. Matthijnssens, J.; Rahman, M.; Van Ranst, M. Two out of the 11 genes of an unusual human G6P[6] rotavirus isolate are of bovine origin. *J. Gen. Virol.* **2008**, *89*, 2630–2635. [CrossRef]
53. Gouvea, V.; Santos, N.; Timenetsky Mdo, C. VP4 typing of bovine and porcine group A rotaviruses by PCR. *J. Clin. Microbiol.* **1994**, *32*, 1333–1337. [CrossRef]
54. Maes, P.; Matthijnssens, J.; Rahman, M.; Van Ranst, M. RotaC: A web-based tool for the complete genome classification of group A rotaviruses. *BMC Microbiol.* **2009**, *9*, 238. [CrossRef]
55. Hatcher, E.L.; Zhdanov, S.A.; Bao, Y.; Blinkova, O.; Nawrocki, E.P.; Ostapchuck, Y.; Schäffer, A.A.; Brister, J.R. Virus Variation Resource—Improved response to emergent viral outbreaks. *Nucleic Acids Res.* **2017**, *45*, D482–D490. [CrossRef] [PubMed]
56. Kumar, S.; Stecher, G.; Tamura, K. MEGA7: Molecular Evolutionary Genetics Analysis Version 7.0 for Bigger Datasets. *Mol. Biol. Evol.* **2016**, *33*, 1870–1874. [CrossRef] [PubMed]
57. Trifinopoulos, J.; Nguyen, L.T.; von Haeseler, A.; Minh, B.Q. W-IQ-TREE: A fast online phylogenetic tool for maximum likelihood analysis. *Nucleic Acids Res.* **2016**, *44*, W232–W235. [CrossRef]
58. Guindon, S.; Dufayard, J.F.; Lefort, V.; Anisimova, M.; Hordijk, W.; Gascuel, O. New algorithms and methods to estimate maximum-likelihood phylogenies: Assessing the performance of PhyML 3.0. *Syst. Biol.* **2010**, *59*, 307–321. [CrossRef] [PubMed]

# Molecular Epidemiology of Rotavirus A Strains Pre- and Post-Vaccine(Rotarix®) Introduction in Mozambique, 2012–2019: Emergence of Genotypes G3P[4] and G3P[8]

Eva D. João [1,2,*], Benilde Munlela [1,3], Assucênio Chissaque [1,2], Jorfélia Chilaúle [1], Jerónimo Langa [1], Orvalho Augusto [4,5], Simone S. Boene [1,3], Elda Anapakala [1], Júlia Sambo [1,2], Esperança Guimarães [1,2], Diocreciano Bero [1], Marta Cassocera [1,2], Idalécia Cossa-Moiane [1], Jason M. Mwenda [6], Isabel Maurício [2,7], Hester G. O'Neill [8] and Nilsa de Deus [1,9]

[1] Instituto Nacional de Saúde (INS), Maputo 1008, Mozambique; benildeantnio@gmail.com (B.M.); assucenyoo@gmail.com (A.C.); Jorfeliachilaule@gmail.com (J.C.); langajeronimo@gmail.com (J.L.); simonboene@gmail.com (S.S.B.); elda.muianga07@gmail.com (E.A.); juliassiat@yahoo.com.br (J.S.); espeguima@hotmail.com (E.G.); dmbero@gmail.com (D.B.); marti.life@hotmail.com (M.C.); idaleciacossa@yahoo.com.br (I.C.-M.); ndeus1@yahoo.com (N.d.D.)
[2] Instituto de Higiene e Medicina Tropical, Universidade Nova de Lisboa, 1349-008 Lisbon, Portugal; isabel.mauricio@ihmt.unl.pt
[3] Centro de Biotecnologia, Universidade Eduardo Mondlane, Maputo 3453, Mozambique
[4] Faculdade de Medicina, Universidade Eduardo Mondlane, Maputo, P.O. Box 257, Mozambique; orvaquim@gmail.com
[5] Harris Hydraulics Laboratory, Department of Global Health, University of Washington, Seattle, WA 98195-7965, USA
[6] African Rotavirus Surveillance Network, Immunization, Vaccines and Development Program, WHO Regional Office for Africa, Brazzaville, P.O. Box 2465, Congo; mwendaj@who.int
[7] Global Health and Tropical Medicine, Instituto de Higiene e Medicina Tropical, Universidade Nova de Lisboa, 1349-008 Lisbon, Portugal
[8] Department of Microbial, Biochemical and Food Biotechnology, University of the Free State, Bloemfontein 9301, South Africa; oneillhg@ufs.ac.za
[9] Departamento de Ciências Biológicas, Universidade Eduardo Mondlane, Maputo 3453, Mozambique
* Correspondence: evadora1@hotmail.com;

**Abstract:** Group A rotavirus (RVA) remains the most important etiological agent associated with severe acute diarrhea in children. *Rotarix*® monovalent vaccine was introduced into Mozambique's Expanded Program on Immunization in September 2015. In the present study, we report the diversity and prevalence of rotavirus genotypes, pre- (2012–2015) and post-vaccine (2016–2019) introduction in Mozambique, among diarrheic children less than five years of age. Genotyping data were analyzed for five sentinel sites for the periods indicated. The primary sentinel site, Mavalane General Hospital (HGM), was analyzed for the period 2012–2019, and for all five sites (country-wide analyses), 2015–2019. During the pre-vaccine period, G9P[8] was the most predominant genotype for both HGM (28.5%) and the country-wide analysis (46.0%). However, in the post-vaccine period, G9P[8] was significantly reduced. Instead, G3P[8] was the most common genotype at HGM, while G1P[8] predominated country-wide. Genotypes G9P[4] and G9P[6] were detected for the first time, and the emergence of G3P[8] and G3P[4] genotypes were observed during the post-vaccine period. The distribution and prevalence of rotavirus genotypes were distinct in pre- and post-vaccination periods, while uncommon genotypes were also detected in the post-vaccine period. These observations support the need for continued country-wide surveillance to monitor changes in strain diversity, due to possible vaccine pressure, and consequently, the effect on vaccine effectiveness.

**Keywords:** rotavirus type A; Mozambique vaccine surveillance; G3 genotype; Rotarix

## 1. Introduction

Group A rotavirus (RVA) remains the most important etiological agent associated with severe acute diarrhea in children worldwide [1–3]. In 2016, RVA was estimated to cause more than 128,000 deaths among children younger than five years throughout the world, with more than 104,000 deaths occurring in sub-Saharan Africa [3].

RVA is a non-enveloped, double-stranded RNA virus. The segmented genome has 11 gene segments which encode six structural viral proteins (VP1, VP2, VP3, VP4, VP6, and VP7) and six non-structural viral proteins (NSP1, NSP2, NSP3, NSP4, and NSP5/6) [4–6]. The viral capsid is composed of three concentric layers which encapsulate the 11-segmented genome. The outer layer is composed of the viral spike protein, protease-sensitive VP4, and glycoprotein VP7. A dual typing system for RVA is based on the gene segments encoding VP4 (P genotypes) and VP7 (G types). The rotavirus classification-working group has identified 36 G and 51 P genotypes globally in humans and in the young of many mammalian and avian species [7–10]. Six G types (G1, G2, G3, G4, G9, G12) and 3 P types (P[8], P[4], P[6]) predominate globally [11–14], although in Africa and Asia genotypes, such as G5, G6, and G8, are also described as important [15]. The six most frequently reported G/P combinations associated with infections in humans worldwide are G1P[8], G2P[4], G3P[8], G4P[8], G9P[8], and G12P[8] [10–14,16].

In 2009, the World Health Organization (WHO) recommended the introduction of rotavirus vaccines in national immunization programs worldwide and particularly in countries with a high under-five mortality rate associated with diarrhea [17]. The WHO has coordinated the Global Network of Rotavirus surveillance (GNRS) since 2006 to support countries with evidence-based decision-making [10]. Mozambique has actively participated in WHO rotavirus surveillance since 2016. Continuous surveillance of circulating genotypes, as well as the monitoring of disease burden, is important to evaluate the effectiveness of rotavirus vaccines.

Before the introduction of rotavirus vaccines, a high rotavirus disease burden was reported in particular the southern Mozambican region. However, due to a lack of surveillance, no information was available from the center and northern regions of the country [18–20]. In the Global Enteric Multicenter Study (GEMS), which determined the burden and etiology of diarrhea in children under five years of age in four sub-Saharan African and three Asian countries, Mozambique had the highest attributable fraction (27.0%) of rotavirus-associated diarrhea among infants [20]. In Mozambique, the prevalence of rotavirus in under-five year old children from urban (Maputo City) and rural (Manhiça District) areas in 2012 and 2013 was higher than 40.0% [19]. A lower infection rate (24.0%) was, however, reported in 2011 in Gaza province, a rural area [18]. Data from the National Surveillance of Diarrhea also showed a high rotavirus infection rate of 40.2% and 38.3% in 2014 and 2015, respectively, before vaccine introduction in Mozambique [21]. The monovalent vaccine, *Rotarix®* (GlaxoSmithKline, Rixensart, Belgium), was introduced into the Expanded Program on Immunization of Mozambique in September 2015. Since then, the prevalence of rotavirus infections of 12.2% and 13.5% in 2016 and 2017, respectively, has been reported [21].

The evolution of RVA through the accumulation of point mutations, gene reassortment, recombination and interspecies transmission [5,22,23], call for rotavirus strain surveillance to elucidate the effect, if any, of rotavirus vaccine usage on the circulation of rotavirus genotypes in Mozambique. The main objective of the present study was to evaluate the distribution of rotavirus genotypes prior to (2012–2015) and following (2016–2019) rotavirus vaccine introduction in Mozambique, among diarrheic children less than five years of age.

## 2. Results

### 2.1. Comparison of Rotavirus G- and P-Types in Mozambique Pre- and Post-Vaccine Introduction

From May 2014 to December 2019, a total of 1736 diarrheal stool samples were collected in five sentinel sites as part of the National Surveillance of Diarrhea program in Mozambique. Of these stool samples, 468 tested positive for RVA by ELISA (27.0%) (Supplementary Table S1). A total of 94.0% (440/468) of these samples were genotyped, $n = 245$ from Maputo (HGM and HJM), $n = 149$ from Nampula (HCN), $n = 34$ from Quelimane (HGQ) and $n = 12$ from Beira (HCB) (Supplementary Table S2). During the pre-vaccine period (2014–2015) a total of 246 samples were genotyped and in the post-vaccine period (2016–2019) 194 samples (Supplementary Table S1). In total, 6.0% (28/468) were excluded from genotyping as an insufficient amount of sample was available.

For HGM, a total of 200 genotyped samples corresponded to the pre-vaccine period (2012–2015) and 43 to the post-vaccine period (2016–2019) (Supplementary Table S3). The samples from the pre-vaccine period also included 91 genotyped samples collected at HGM between 2012 and 2013 from a cross-sectional study [24] to extend the analyses for this particular site (Supplementary Table S3).

The analyses for HGM showed that G9 was the most prevalent G type (30.5%) in the pre-vaccine period ($n = 200$), but was significantly reduced to 9.3% during the post-vaccination period ($n = 43$). Similarly, G12 was also significantly reduced (from 18.5% to 2.3%) (Table 1). In contrast, during the pre-vaccination period, no G3 strains were detected; but during the post-vaccine period, the genotype was the most prevalent genotype (48.8%). Interestingly, a small increase in prevalence was observed for the G1 genotype, although this increase was not statistically significant (Table 1).

**Table 1.** Prevalence of G and P types at Mavalane General Hospital pre- and post-vaccine introduction in Mozambique (2012–2019).

| [1] G Type | Pre-Vaccine [5] 2012–2015 n | % | Post-Vaccine 2016–2019 n | % | OR (95% CI) | p-Value |
|---|---|---|---|---|---|---|
| G1 | 34 | **17.0** | 10 | 23.3 | 1.47 (0.59–3.44) | 0.330 |
| G12 | 37 | **18.5** | 1 | 2.3 | 0.10 (0.003–0.66) | 0.008 |
| G2 | 25 | **12.5** | 1 | 2.3 | 0.16 (0.004–1.08) | 0.054 |
| G3 | 0 | 0.0 | 21 | **48.8** | - | - |
| G8 | 6 | 3.0 | 1 | 2.3 | 0.76 (0.02–6.61) | 0.810 |
| G9 | 61 | **30.5** | 4 | 9.3 | 0.23 (0.01–0.69) | 0.004 |
| [2] Mix G | 10 | 5.0 | 1 | 2.3 | 0.45 (0.01–3.30) | 0.440 |
| [3] Gx | 27 | 13.5 | 4 | 9.3 | 0.65 (0.16–2.04) | 0.450 |
| Total | 200 | 100.0 | 43 | 100.0 | - | - |
| [1] P type | - | - | - | - | - | - |
| P[4] | 31 | 15.5 | 16 | **37.2** | 3.23 (1.44–7.04) | <0.001 |
| P[6] | 32 | 16.0 | 3 | 7.0 | 0.39 (0.07–1.36) | 0.120 |
| P[8] | 108 | **54.0** | 22 | **51.2** | 0.89 (0.43–1.83) | 0.740 |
| Mix P | 8 | 4.0 | 0 | 0.0 | - | - |
| [4] P[x] | 21 | 10.5 | 2 | 4.7 | 0.42 (0.05–0.82) | 0.230 |
| Total | 200 | 100.0 | 43 | 100.0 | - | - |

[1] It is not possible to calculate the Odds-ratio (OR) for cells with a value of 0; [2] Mix G: 2012–2015: G12G8 (2.0%), G12G9 (1.5%), G9G2 (1.5%); 2016–2019: G12G3 (2.3%); [3] x—refers to strains that were non-typeable for G; [4] x—refers to strains that were non-typeable for P; [5] Reference category: Pre-vaccine; Bold: The most prevalent genotypes per period.

P[8] was the most predominant P type in the pre-vaccine period (54.0%) (Table 1), as well as the post-vaccine period (51.2%). Only P[4] (37.2%) (Table 1) had a statistically significant increase during the post-vaccine period ($p < 0.001$). No mixed P types were detected during the post-vaccine period.

When all five sentinel sites (including HGM) were analyzed for the period of 2015–2019, a similar trend was observed for the G9 genotype. During the pre-vaccine period ($n = 213$), G9 was the most prevalent G type at 49.3%, but a significant reduction for G9 (25.3%) was reported during the post-vaccine period ($n = 194$). The emergence of G3 was also observed, becoming the most prevalent genotype, although only at 26.3% (Table 2). In contrast, a reduction in the prevalence of the G1 genotype was observed (31.5% reduced to 21.6%) for all five sentinel sites.

**Table 2.** Prevalence of G and P types at five sentinel sites in Mozambique during surveillance pre- and post-vaccine introduction (2015–2019).

| [1] G Type | [5] Pre-Vaccine 2015 | | Post-Vaccine 2016–2019 | | OR (95% CI) | *p*-Value |
|---|---|---|---|---|---|---|
| | n | % | n | % | | |
| G1 | 67 | **31.5** | 42 | **21.6** | 0.60 (0.37–0.96) | 0.030 |
| G12 | 2 | 0.9 | 2 | 1.0 | 1.18 (0.08–15.29) | 0.930 |
| G2 | 10 | 4.7 | 11 | 5.7 | 1.22 (0.46–3.28) | 0.660 |
| G3 | 0 | 0 | 51 | **26.3** | - | - |
| G8 | 0 | 0 | 3 | 1.5 | - | - |
| G9 | 105 | **49.3** | 49 | **25.3** | 0.35 (0.22–0.54) | <0.001 |
| [2] Mix G | 0 | 0 | 12 | 6.2 | - | - |
| [3] Gx | 29 | 13.6 | 24 | 12.4 | 0.90 (0.48–1.66) | 0.710 |
| Total | 213 | 100.0 | 194 | 100.0 | - | - |
| [1] P type | - | - | - | - | - | - |
| P[4] | 1 | 0.5 | 71 | **36.6** | - | - |
| P[6] | 10 | 4.7 | 37 | 19.1 | 4.78 (2.23–11.10) | <0.001 |
| P[8] | 182 | **85.4** | 76 | **39.2** | 0.10 (0.06–0.16) | <0.001 |
| [4] P[x] | 20 | 9.4 | 10 | 5.2 | 0.57 (0.23–1.32) | 0.100 |
| Total | 213 | 100.0 | 194 | 100.0 | - | - |

[1] It is not possible to calculate the Odds-ratio (OR) for cells with a value of 0; [2] Mix G—2016–2019: G12G3 (0.5%), G2G1 (0.5%), G3G1 (2.1%), G9G3 (3.1%); [3] x—refers to strains that were non-typeable for G; [4] x—Refers to strains that were non-typeable for P; [5] Reference category: Pre-vaccine; Bold: The most prevalent genotypes per period.

During the pre-vaccine period, P[8] was the most frequently detected P genotype accounting for 85.4% of all genotypes detected (Table 2). However, this high frequency was significantly reduced in the post-vaccination period to less than half (39.2%). An increase in the detection of P[6] (19.1%) and P[4] (36.6%), from almost undetectable, were recorded during this period (Table 2).

Analyses of the data recorded for samples collected at the HGM, showed a slight increase in the odds ratio for G1 type from pre-vaccine to the post-vaccine period of 1.47 times (OR = 1.47 95CI = 0.59–3.44, $p > 0.330$), but a decrease in the odds ratio for genotypes G12 of 90.0% (OR = 0.10, 95CI = 0.003–0.66, $p < 0.008$) and G9 of 77.0% (OR = 0.23, 95CI = 0.01–0.69, $p < 0.004$), respectively (Table 1). Considering all the sentinel sites, a significant decrease was observed in the odds ratio for G1 genotype from pre-vaccine to the post-vaccine period of 40.0% (OR = 0.60, 95CI = 0.37–0.96, $p < 0.030$), as well as a reduction for G9 of 65.0% (OR = 0.35, 95CI = 0.22–0.54, $p < 0.001$) (Table 2).

A reduction for genotype P[8] from pre-vaccine to the post-vaccine period was also observed at HGM (11.0%, OR= 0.89, 95CI= 0.43–1.83, $p > 0.740$, Table 1), as well as for the country-wide sentinel sites (90.0% (OR = 0.10, 95CI = 0.06 to 0.16, $p < 0.001$, Table 2). In contrast, a significant increase in the odds ratio of genotype P[4] of 3.23 times (OR = 3.23, 95CI = 1.44–7.04, $p < 0.001$) was observed at the HGM (Table 1). Analyses for all the sentinel sites showed a high prevalence for P[4] during the post-vaccine period (36.6%) compared to the pre-vaccine period (0.5%).

## 2.2. Comparison of G/P Genotype Combinations in Mozambique Pre- and Post-Vaccine Introduction

At HGM, the most predominant combinations during the pre-vaccine period were G9P[8] (28.5%), G1P[8] (17.0%), G12P[6] (13.0%) and G2P[4] (10.0%), comprising a total of 68.5% of all genotypes analyzed (Table 3). During the post-vaccine period, G1P[8] (20.9%) was still one of the predominant combinations, although G3P[8] and G3P[4] strains were detected at 25.6% and 18.6%, respectively

(Table 3). A significant reduction in G9P[8] detection was observed following vaccine introduction ($p < 0.001$). Instead, the G9 genotype was now detected in combination with P[4] and P[6] both at a frequency of 4.7% (Table 3).

Table 3. G/P type combinations prevalent at Mavalane General Hospital pre- and post-vaccine introduction in Mozambique (2012–2019).

| [1] G/P Genotype Combination | [5] Pre-Vaccine 2012–2015 | | Post-Vaccine 2016–2019 | | OR (95% CI) | $p$-Value |
|---|---|---|---|---|---|---|
| | n | % | n | % | | |
| G1P[8] | 34 | **17.0** | 9 | **20.9** | 1.29 (0.50–3.07) | 0.540 |
| G9P[8] | 57 | **28.5** | 1 | 2.3 | 0.06 (0.002–0.40) | < 0.001 |
| G12P[6] | 26 | **13.0** | 0 | 0.0 | - | - |
| G2P[4] | 20 | 10.0 | 1 | 2.3 | 0.21 (0.01–1.42) | 0.100 |
| G12P[8] | 6 | 3.0 | 0 | 0.0 | - | - |
| G3P[4] | 0 | 0.0 | 8 | **18.6** | - | - |
| G3P[8] | 0 | 0.0 | 11 | **25.6** | - | - |
| G8P[4] | 5 | 2.5 | 1 | 2.3 | 0.93 (0.02–8.61) | 0.950 |
| G9P[4] | 0 | 0.0 | 2 | 4.7 | - | - |
| G9P[6] | 0 | 0.0 | 2 | 4.7 | - | - |
| [2] Other genotypes | 5 | 2.5 | 3 | 7.0 | 2.93 (0.43–15.65) | 0.140 |
| [3] Mixed types | 13 | 6.5 | 1 | 2.3 | 0.34 (0.01–2.41) | 0.290 |
| [4] Partial G/P types | 20 | 10.0 | 2 | 4.7 | 0.44 (0.05–1.93) | 0.270 |
| Untypeables | 14 | 7.0 | 2 | 4.7 | 0.64 (0.07–3.00) | 0.570 |
| Total | 200 | 100.0 | 43 | 100.0 | - | - |

[1] It is not possible to calculate the Odds-ratio (OR) for cells with a value of 0; [2] Other genotypes: 2012–2015: G12P[4] (0.5%), G2P[6] (1.0%), G2P[8] (0.5%), G8P[8] (0.5%); 2016–2019: G1P[4] (2.3%), G3P[6] (2.3%), G12P[4] (2.3%); [3] Mixed types: 2012–2015: G12G8P[4] (1.0%), G12G8P[6] (0.5%), G12G8P[6]P[4] (0.5%), G12G9P[6] (0.5%), G12G9P[8]P[6] (1.0%), G12P[8]P[6] (1.0%), G9G2P[4] (0.5%), G9G2P[6] (0.5%), G9G2P[8] (0.5%), G9P[8]P[4] (0.5%); 2016–2019: G12G3P[4] (2.3%); [4] Partial G/P types: 2012–2015: G12P[x] (1.0%), G2P[x] (1.0%), G9P[x] (1.5%), GxP[4] (1.0%), GxP[6] (0.5%), GxP[6]P[4] (0.5%), GxP[8] (4.0%), GxP[8]P[6] (0.5%); 2016–2019: GxP[4] (2.3%), GxP[8] (2.3%); [5] Reference category: Pre-vaccine; Bold: The most prevalent genotypes per period.

The most frequent G/P combinations observed for all the sites participating in the National Surveillance of Diarrhea program during the pre-vaccine period were G9P[8] and G1P[8] at 46.0% and 31.0%, respectively. These combinations comprised a total of 77.0% of all genotypes analyzed (Table 4).

In the post-vaccine period, G1P[8] remained the most frequent G/P combination, but at a reduced frequency of 20.6%. G2P[4] (at a slightly higher frequency) and G2P[6] (similar frequency as in 2015) were, again, detected in the post-vaccine period. Similar to the analysis for HGM, G3 in combination with P[4] (14.4%) and P[8] (9.8%) were detected during the post-vaccine period, together with G9P[4] (12.4%) and G9P[6] (8.8%). Mixed infections, as determined with RT-PCR, was detected for 6.2% of the samples (Table 4).

Analyses for HGM showed an increase in the odds for G1P[8] at 1.29 times (95CI = 0.50–3.07, $p > 0.54$), but a significant decrease in the odds ratio for G9P[8] at 94.0% (OR = 0.06, 95CI = 0.002–0.40, $p < 0.001$) (Table 3).

In contrast, a significant decrease in the odds ratio for all the sentinel sites was observed for G1P[8] at 42.0% (OR = 0.58, 95CI = 0.36–0.93, $p < 0.020$) and G9P[8] at 96.0% (OR = 0.04, 95CI = 0.02–0.10, $p < 0.001$) (Table 4).

**Table 4.** G/P type combinations prevalent at five sentinel sites in Mozambique during surveillance pre- and post-vaccine introduction (2015–2019).

| [1] G/P Genotype Combination | [5] Pre-Vaccine 2015 | | Post-Vaccine 2016–2019 | | OR (95% CI) | p-Value |
|---|---|---|---|---|---|---|
| | n | % | n | % | | |
| G1P[8] | 66 | **31.0** | 40 | **20.6** | 0.58 (0.36–0.93) | 0.020 |
| G3P[4] | 0 | 0.0 | 28 | **14.4** | - | - |
| G3P[6] | 0 | 0.0 | 3 | 1.5 | - | - |
| G3P[8] | 0 | 0.0 | 19 | 9.8 | - | - |
| G8P[4] | 0 | 0.0 | 3 | 1.5 | - | - |
| G9P[4] | 0 | 0.0 | 24 | **12.4** | - | - |
| G9P[6] | 0 | 0.0 | 17 | 8.8 | - | - |
| G2P[4] | 1 | 0.5 | 3 | 1.5 | - | - |
| G2P[6] | 9 | 4.2 | 8 | 4.1 | 0.97 (0.32–2.91) | 0.959 |
| G9P[8] | 98 | **46.0** | 7 | 3.6 | 0.04 (0.02–0.10) | <0.001 |
| [2] Other genotypes | 3 | 1.4 | 4 | 2.1 | 1.47 (0.25–10.18) | 0.612 |
| [3] Mixed types | 0 | 0 | 12 | 6.2 | - | - |
| [4] Partial G/P types | 23 | 10.8 | 18 | 9.3 | 0.84 (0.41–1.70) | 0.611 |
| Untypeables | 13 | 6.1 | 8 | 4.1 | 0.66 (0.23–1.77) | 0.370 |
| Total | 213 | 100.0 | 194 | 100.0 | - | - |

[1] It is not possible to calculate the Odds-ratio (OR) for cells with a value of 0; [2] Other genotypes: 2015: G12P[8] (0.9%), G1P[6] (0.5%); 2016–2019: G12P[4] (0.5%), G12P[8] (0.5%), G1P[4] (1.0%); [3] Mixed types: 2016–2019: G12G3P[4] (0.5%),G2G1P[8] (0.5%), G3G1P[8] (2.6%),G9G3P[6] (2.6%); [4] Partial G/P types: 2015: G9P[x] (3.3%),GxP[6] (0.5%), GxP[8] (7.0%); 2016–2019: G9P[x] (1.0%),GxP[4] (4.6%), GxP[6] (1.6%), GxP[8] (2.1%); [5] Reference category: Pre-vaccine; Bold: The most prevalent genotypes per period.

*2.3. Yearly Distribution of Rotavirus Genotypes at the Mavalane General Hospital (HGM) and National Surveillance Sites*

As reported before, G12P[6] (28.6%) and G2P[4] (23.1%) were the most predominant genotype combinations at HGM during 2012–2013 [24]. In 2014 and 2015, G1P[8] and G9P[8] with 84.8% and 73.7%, respectively, were detected at the highest frequencies. In 2016, during the post-vaccine period, the most frequent genotype was G1P[8] with 66.7%. The emergence of new genotypes was observed in 2016 (G3P[4]), which increased in 2017, to the most prevalent genotype (25.0%) followed by G1P[8] (18.8%) (Table 5). In 2018, G3P[8] and G3P[4] became the most prevalent genotype combinations with 36.4% and 27.3%, respectively. Finally, in 2019, only G3P[8] were detected at the HGM. No G1P[8] strains were, therefore, detected in 2018 and 2019 (Table 5).

Since data is available for only one year for all five participating sentinel sites during the pre-vaccine period, yearly analysis for the national surveillance sites are presented from 2015–2019. The results showed that in 2015 the most frequent G/P combination was G9P[8] (46.0%), followed by G1P[8] (31.0%). In 2016, G1P[8] was detected at the highest frequency (43.6%) (Table 6). Other genotype combinations, such as G2P[6] (17.9%), G9P[6] (12.8%), G9P[4] (7.7%), and G3P[4] (2.6%), were also observed in 2016 (Table 6). These results were comparable to those from HGM.

In 2017, G1P[8], as well as G9P[4], were detected at similar frequencies (19.2%), while G3P[4] was detected at 13.5% (Table 6). In 2018 and 2019, G3P[4] and G3P[8] became the most frequently detected genotype combination with 38.7% and 60.0%, respectively (Table 6). G3 was also observed in combination with P[4] (13.5%) and P[6] (1.9%) in 2017, whereas G1P[8] genotype was not detected in 2018, although this genotype was detected at 15.0% in 2019 (Table 6). The results reported for all the sentinel sites participating in the National Surveillance of Diarrhea program is comparable to that observed for HGM for the reporting period (2015–2019), except that G1P[8] was not detected in 2019 for HGM.

**Table 5.** Prevalence of G/P type combinations at Mavalane General Hospital in Mozambique by year.

| G/P Genotype Combination | 2012 n | 2012 % | 2013 n | 2013 % | 2014 n | 2014 % | 2015 n | 2015 % | 2016 n | 2016 % | 2017 n | 2017 % | 2018 n | 2018 % | 2019 n | 2019 % |
|---|---|---|---|---|---|---|---|---|---|---|---|---|---|---|---|---|
| G1P[8] | 2 | 3.0 | 0 | 0.0 | 28 | 84.8 | 4 | 5.3 | 6 | 66.7 | 3 | 18.8 | 0 | 0.0 | 0 | 0.0 |
| G9P[8] | 1 | 1.5 | 0 | 0.0 | 0 | 0.0 | 56 | 73.7 | 0 | 0.0 | 1 | 6.3 | 0 | 0.0 | 0 | 0.0 |
| G12P[6] | 26 | 38.8 | 0 | 0.0 | 0 | 0.0 | 0 | 0.0 | 0 | 0.0 | 0 | 0 | 0 | 0.0 | 0 | 0.0 |
| G2P[4] | 5 | 7.5 | 16 | 66.7 | 0 | 0.0 | 0 | 0.0 | 0 | 0.0 | 0 | 0 | 1 | 9.1 | 0 | 0.0 |
| G12P[8] | 5 | 7.5 | 0 | 0.0 | 0 | 0.0 | 1 | 1.3 | 0 | 0.0 | 0 | 0 | 0 | 0.0 | 0 | 0.0 |
| G3P[4] | 0 | 0 | 0 | 0.0 | 0 | 0.0 | 0 | 0.0 | 1 | 11.1 | 4 | 25.0 | 3 | 27.3 | 0 | 0.0 |
| G3P[8] | 0 | 0 | 0 | 0.0 | 0 | 0.0 | 0 | 0.0 | 0 | 0.0 | 0 | 0 | 4 | 36.4 | 7 | 100.0 |
| G8P[4] | 5 | 7.5 | 0 | 0.0 | 0 | 0.0 | 0 | 0.0 | 0 | 0.0 | 0 | 0 | 1 | 9.1 | 0 | 0.0 |
| G9P[4] | 0 | 0 | 0 | 0.0 | 0 | 0.0 | 0 | 0.0 | 0 | 0.0 | 2 | 12.5 | 0 | 0.0 | 0 | 0.0 |
| G9P[6] | 0 | 0 | 0 | 0.0 | 0 | 0.0 | 0 | 0.0 | 0 | 0 | 0 | 0 | 2 | 18.2 | 0 | 0.0 |
| [1] Other genotypes | 3 | 4.5 | 0 | 0.0 | 0 | 0.0 | 2 | 2.6 | 1 | 11.1 | 2 | 12.5 | 0 | 0.0 | 0 | 0.0 |
| [2] Mixed types | 13 | 19.4 | 0 | 0.0 | 0 | 0.0 | 0 | 0.0 | 1 | 11.1 | 0 | 0 | 0 | 0.0 | 0 | 0.0 |
| [3] Partial G/P types | 5 | 7.5 | 4 | 16.7 | 4 | 12.1 | 7 | 9.2 | 0 | 0.0 | 2 | 12.5 | 0 | 0.0 | 0 | 0.0 |
| Untypeables | 2 | 3.0 | 4 | 16.7 | 1 | 3.0 | 6 | 7.9 | 0 | 0.0 | 2 | 12.5 | 0 | 0.0 | 0 | 0.0 |
| Total | 67 | 100.0 | 24 | 100.0 | 33 | 100.0 | 76 | 100.0 | 9 | 100.0 | 16 | 100.0 | 11 | 100.0 | 7 | 100.0 |

[1] Other genotypes: 2012: G12P[4] (1.5%), G2P[8] (1.5%), G8P[8] (1.5%); 2015: G2P[6] (2.6%); 2016: G12P[4] (11.1%); 2017: G1P[4] (6.3%), G3P[6] (6.3%); [2] Mixed types: 2012: G12G8P[4] (3.0%), G12G8P[6] (1.5%), G12G8P[6]P[4] (1.5%), G12G9P[6] (1.5%), G12G9P[8]P[6] (3.0%), G12P[8]P[6] (3.0%), G9G2P[4] (1.5%), G9G2P[6] (1.5%), G9G2P[8] (1.5%), G9P[8]P[4] (1.5%); 2016: G12G3P[4] (11.1%); [3] Partial G/P types: 2012: G12P[x] (3.0%), GxP[6]P[4] (1.5%), GxP[6]P[4] (1.5%), GxP[8]P[6] (1.5%); 2013: G2P[x] (8.3%), GxP[4] (8.3%); 2014: GxP[6] (3.0%), GxP[8] (9.1%); 2015: G9P[x] (4.0%), GxP[8] (5.3%); 2017: GxP[4] (6.3%), GxP[8] (6.3%); Grey: The most prevalent genotypes per year.

**Table 6.** Prevalence of G/P type combinations at five sentinel sites in Mozambique during surveillance by year.

| G/P Genotype Combination | 2015 n | 2015 % | 2016 n | 2016 % | 2017 n | 2017 % | 2018 n | 2018 % | 2019 n | 2019 % |
|---|---|---|---|---|---|---|---|---|---|---|
| G1P[8] | 66 | 31.0 | 17 | 43.6 | 20 | 19.2 | 0 | 0.0 | 3 | 15.0 |
| G3P[4] | 0 | 0.0 | 1 | 2.6 | 14 | 13.5 | 12 | 38.7 | 1 | 5.0 |
| G3P[6] | 0 | 0.0 | 0 | 0.0 | 2 | 1.9 | 1 | 3.2 | 0 | 0.0 |
| G3P[8] | 0 | 0.0 | 0 | 0.0 | 0 | 0 | 7 | 22.6 | 12 | 60.0 |
| G8P[4] | 0 | 0.0 | 0 | 0.0 | 1 | 1.0 | 2 | 6.5 | 0 | 0.0 |
| G9P[4] | 0 | 0.0 | 3 | 7.7 | 20 | 19.2 | 1 | 3.2 | 0 | 0.0 |
| G9P[6] | 0 | 0.0 | 5 | 12.8 | 9 | 8.7 | 3 | 9.7 | 0 | 0.0 |
| G2P[6] | 9 | 4.2 | 7 | 17.9 | 0 | 0 | 1 | 3.2 | 0 | 0.0 |
| G9P[8] | 98 | 46.0 | 0 | 0.0 | 6 | 5.8 | 1 | 3.2 | 0 | 0.0 |
| [1] Other genotypes | 4 | 1.9 | 3 | 7.7 | 3 | 2.9 | 1 | 3.2 | 0 | 0.0 |
| [2] Mixed types | 0 | 0.0 | 2 | 5.1 | 10 | 9.6 | 0 | 0.0 | 0 | 0.0 |
| [3] Partial G/P types | 23 | 10.8 | 0 | 0.0 | 14 | 13.5 | 2 | 6.5 | 2 | 10.0 |
| Untypeables | 13 | 6.1 | 1 | 2.6 | 5 | 4.8 | 0 | 0.0 | 2 | 10.0 |
| Total | 213 | 100.0 | 39 | 100.0 | 104 | 100.0 | 31 | 100.0 | 20 | 100.0 |

[1] Other genotypes: 2015: G12P[8] (0.9%), G1P[6] (0.5%), G2P[4] (0.5%); 2016: G12P[4] (2.6%), G2P[4] (5.1%); 2017: G12P[8] (1.0%), G1P[4] (1.9%); 2018: G2P[4] (3.2%); [2] Mixed types: 2016: G12G3P[4 (2.6%), G2G1P[8] (2.6%); 2017: G3G1P[8] (3.9%), G9G3P[6] (5.8%); [3] Partial G/P types: 2015: G9P[x] (3.3%), GxP[6] (0.5%), GxP[8] (7.0%); 2017: G9P[x] (1.9%), GxP[4] (6.7%), GxP[6] (1.9%), GxP[8] (2.9%); 2018: GxP[4] (3.2%), GxP[6] (3.2%); 2019: GxP[4] (5.0%), GxP[8] (5.0%); Grey: The most prevalent genotypes per year.

### 2.4. Geographical Distribution of Rotavirus Genotypes

A variation in rotavirus genotypes between the five sentinel sites in Mozambique was observed (Supplementary Table S4).

In the pre-vaccine period (2015), it was observed that G1P[8] occurred in all regions included in this study, with the highest frequency (78.0%) detected in the northern region, at Nampula (HCN) (Supplementary Table S4). In contrast, the G9P[8] genotype combination was mostly detected in the southern region, Maputo (HGM and HJM) at 68.8%. Other uncommon genotypes, such as G2P[6], were mostly detected at Nampula at 10.2% but were not detected in Quelimane (HGQ) or Beira (HCB) (Supplementary Table S4). Similarly, in the post-vaccine period (2016–2019), the combination G1P[8] was observed across the country. In 2016 at Maputo and Nampula, G1P[8] was the most prevalent genotype with 66.7% and 43.5%, respectively. The G1P[8] genotype was, however, also detected in Quelimane and Beira, which had small sample sizes.

In 2017 the genotype combination G3P[4] was the most prevalent (29.7%) in Maputo, while in Nampula and Quelimane G9P[4] and G9P[6] were the most prevalent at 32.7% and 35.7%, respectively. In 2018 and 2019, the G3 genotypes were predominantly detected in Maputo and Quelimane in combination with P[4] and P[8]. In Nampula and Beira, G3 was detected in combination with P[4] (Supplementary Table S4).

## 3. Discussion

Before rotavirus vaccine introduction in Mozambique, RVA surveillance studies focused in the southern region of the country [18–20]. Instituto Nacional de Saúde (INS) initiated national RVA surveillance in the southern region of Mozambique in 2014, which was expanded to other regions (center and north) in 2015. Following the country-wide introduction of *Rotarix®* in September 2015, its impact has been monitored and a substantial reduction in the prevalence of RVA infection rate to 12.2% and 13.5% in 2016 and 2017, respectively, was reported [21]. Since the country is vast, it is important to expand strain surveillance to include the entire country.

In the present analysis, rotavirus surveillance that form part of the National Surveillance of Diarrhea during 2014–2019, as well as data from a cross-section study at the HGM from 2012 and 2013, are reported [24].

During the surveillance at HGM (2012–2019), as well as country-wide sentinel sites (2015–2019), variations in the prevalence of genotypes in the pre- and post-vaccine periods were observed. Genotypes G9 and P[8] were consistently the most prevalent in the pre-vaccine period and in the post-vaccine period, genotypes G3 and P[8] were the most prevalent. However, the proportion of P[8] was reduced, and the prevalence of genotype P[4] increased. These results suggest that genotype prevalence can vary from year to year pre- or post-vaccination in Mozambique.

When comparing the most predominant G/P combinations before and after vaccine introduction at the HGM, G9P[8] was the most predominant genotype combination in the pre-vaccine period, while G1P[8] was the most prevalent genotype combination in the post-vaccine period. The country-wide surveillance also revealed a decreased odds ratio for G9P[8] after the introduction of the vaccine. However, this reduction was accompanied by the emergence of G9P[4] and G9P[6], especially in the northern part of Mozambique, after vaccine introduction. Finally, the emergence of G3P[4] and G3P[8] was also observed. These results showed that in this early phase of rotavirus strain surveillance, it is not clear whether these variations in genotype combinations between both periods were due to the rotavirus vaccine or simply natural variation in genotype frequency. Our results are consistent with previously published studies, as a number of countries from Africa, Europe and America reported a variation in the strain diversity between the two periods [16,25–30].

Countries that introduced the monovalent *Rotarix®* vaccine similar to Mozambique, reported a decline of genotype G1P[8] with a concurrent rise in other combinations in the post-vaccine period. For example, South Africa reported an increase in non-G1P[8] strains [25]. In contrast, in Malawi, the reduction of G1P[8] was not significant [27]. In Ghana, G1P[8] returned as one of the dominant strains in the fourth year post-vaccine introduction [26]. Other studies reported from England, Brazil, Belgium, Scotland, a decline in the proportion of G1P[8] with a rise in the proportion of heterotypic strains, such as G2P[4], was observed [28–31].

Additionally, Belgium reported a slightly lower vaccine effectiveness against G2P[4], and in Malawi, a lower vaccine effectiveness against G2 strains than G1 strains was reported [27].

In our analyses, HGM, with at least four years pre-vaccine data showed a slight increase of G1P[8] after vaccine introduction, although in the country-wide analyses the G1P[8] prevalence was reduced. This needs careful interpretation, due to the difference in the number of years in the pre-vaccine period, one of the limitations of this analysis.

Regarding the variation in the prevalence of some uncommon genotypes (e.g., G9P[4] G9P[6], G3P[4], G3P[6]) detected after vaccine introduction in Mozambique, it is important to mention that a number of studies in Africa [16,25,32] and Asia (India and Japan) also reported these uncommon genotypes before vaccine introduction in low frequency [33,34]. These uncommon genotypes, apart from G9P[6], were also observed in Ireland before vaccine introduction [35–37]. However, a study conducted in Ghana reported the emergence of G9P[4] at a low frequency only during the fourth rotavirus season after vaccine introduction [26].

The emergence of the genotype combinations G3P[4], detected in 2016, 2017, 2018, and G3P[8] in 2018 and 2019 was observed in Mozambique. These strains were also reported in the same period in Botswana after vaccine introduction in 2012 [38]. Botswana also reported an outbreak of G3P[8] in 2018 [39]. In addition, several countries reported G3 in combination with P[4] and P[8] during the 12th African Rotavirus Symposium 2019 [40–42]: Malawi (introduced vaccine in 2012, reported G3P[8] in 2018), South Africa (introduced vaccine in 2009, reported G3P[4] in 2015–2016), Kingdom of Eswatini (introduced vaccine in 2015, reported G3P[8] in 2018). These observations suggest that G3 strains were circulating in Southern Africa during 2015–2018, with a sharp increase in 2018. Around the world, the emergence of genotype G3P[8] and equine-like G3P[8] in 2013 in Australia and re-emergence of G3P[8] were observed in Brazil in the post-vaccine introduction [43–45]. The European Rotavirus Network (EuroRotaNet) reported 2017–2018 for the first time since inception, G3P[8] as the most prevalent strain [28].

Temporal variation of rotavirus strains was observed in Mozambique, in particular in the model site, Mavalane General Hospital (HGM), as data from a cross-sectional study that characterized rotavirus strains at the HGM from 2012 and 2013 [24], was combined with data generated at the same site as part of the National Surveillance program with its inception in 2014. As already mentioned, G12P[6] was the most predominant genotype in 2012, and in 2013, G2P[4] was the most prevalent [24]. In a similar time period, G12P[6] was also reported in the Manhiça District, while in 2011 in the Chókwè district, G12P[8] was the most prevalent genotype [18,24]. These results suggest circulation of G12 during 2011–2012 in southern Mozambique. The G12 genotype was detected at a prevalence of almost 20% in Sub-Saharan Africa during 2012–2013 [10,16]. In 2013 the G2P[4] was the predominant genotype in the Manhiça district [24] and also in South Africa in 2013 [46]. A shift in genotypes was observed in 2014 and 2015 when mostly G1P[8] and G9P[8] strains were detected.

In the post-vaccine period (2016–2019), G9P[8] was replaced by G1P[8] in 2016, while in 2017, G3P[4] was the most predominant followed by G1P[8]. In 2018 and 2019, no G1P[8] strains were detected; instead, the G3P[8] genotype was the most prevalent. The G3P[8] genotype combination is one of the most prevalent strains associated with human rotavirus infection globally [11–14]. However, G3P[4], which is considered an uncommon combination, was also detected. Studies published previously in Mozambique during the pre-vaccine period did not detect these strains. These temporal analyses clearly showed a yearly variation of rotavirus strains, complicating the assessment of vaccine introduction impact on changes in strain diversity [11–14]. These observations are further supported by data generated by the National Surveillance of Diarrhea that also showed a temporal variation of rotavirus strains and may rather represent the natural variation in rotavirus strains.

Evaluation of strains detected at the various sentinel sites between 2015–2019, showed that G1P[8] was detected at all sentinel sites, albeit at a variation in frequency. It is interesting to note that G9P[8] occurred mostly in Maputo (HGM and HJM) in the southern region of the country, while G9 in combination with P[4] and P[6] were observed mostly in the north, Nampula (HCN), and central region, Quelimane (HGQ). The occurrence of G2P[6] was mostly observed in Nampula. The emergence of G3 strains was, however, detected at all sites under surveillance suggesting that the occurrence of these strains was not location bound. Differences in the geographical distribution of genotypes within a country was previously reported [11].

Various challenges and limitations were experienced during the study. These include logistical issues, which led to a delay in the start of surveillance at some sentinel sites. The study was limited by its small sample size; therefore, it was not possible to perform in-depth temporal analyses by the site to access the genetic variability of strains. Furthermore, bias in strain diversity is possible since a low number of strains were characterized at some sentinel sites. Extended pre-vaccine genotyping data (four years) was available for only one sentinel site, whereas only one year genotyping data were available for the remainder of the sentinel sites.

Despite the circulation of diverse rotavirus strains and the emergence of some genotypes, the National Surveillance of Diarrhea reported a reduction in rotavirus prevalence during the early impact study of the rotavirus vaccine after vaccine introduction.

The whole genome characterization of rotavirus strains circulating pre- and post-vaccine introduction will be useful to evaluate any potential vaccine-induced selection of specific antigenic profiles. Moreover, with recent reports related to the emergence of double-reassortant G1P[8] on a DS-1–like genetic backbone [47–49], whole-genome characterization will be important for strains surveillance.

## 4. Materials and Methods

### 4.1. Study Population and Stool Samples Collection

RVA positive samples, as tested by Enzyme-Linked Immunosorbent Assay (ELISA), were included. Samples were obtained from children under five years of age suffering from moderate-to-severe acute and non-acute diarrhea. These samples were collected as part of an ongoing hospital-based diarrhea surveillance program, called the National Surveillance of Diarrhea (ViNaDia) that commenced in May 2014. Samples were included for this study up to December 2019. In addition, data from a cross-sectional study conducted at the Mavalane General Hospital (HGM) from January 2012 to September 2013 were also included in the analyses [24].

The National Surveillance of Diarrhea in children was led by the "Instituto Nacional de Saúde" (INS), started in May 2014 at the Mavalane General Hospital (HGM, first sentinel site) in the Maputo province (Figure 1). In March 2015, José Macamo General Hospital (HJM), also Maputo Province, and Nampula Central Hospital (HCN), in Nampula province in the northern region of the country were added. Surveillance was extended to two additional sentinel sites in June 2015: Beira Central Hospital (HCB) in Sofala Province and Quelimane General Hospital (HGQ) in the Zambézia province (Figure 1). Since 2016, Mozambique participates and actively report data to the WHO African Rotavirus Surveillance Network (ARSN). ARSN monitors rotavirus infection in children with severe acute watery diarrhea as part of a hospital-based sentinel-site surveillance program.

In the surveillance at HGM and HJM samples were collected and immediately transferred to the INS laboratory, while at HCB, HCN and HGQ, samples were collected and stored at −20 °C. Samples were transported on a weekly basis on dry ice to the INS laboratories located in Maputo City for testing and stored in −70 °C as previously described [21]. The cross-sectional study was conducted at the Centro de Investigação em Saúde de Manhiça (CISM). The sampling, testing procedures, clinical, socio-demographic information and characterization of rotavirus strains, as previously described [19,24].

### 4.2. Ethical Approval

The National Surveillance of Diarrhea in children protocol was reviewed and approved by the Mozambican National Committee on Bioethics for Health (CNBS) (reference N°: 348/CNBS/13; IRB00002657), as well as the rotavirus cross-sectional study (reference N°286/CNBS/10; IRB00002657).

## 4.3. Laboratory Testing

### 4.3.1. Rotavirus Detection and RNA Extraction

All samples analyzed, were tested for rotavirus using the commercial Enzyme-immuno-sorbent assay (ELISA) kit (Prospect, Oxoid Ltd., Hampshire, UK) following the manufacturer's instructions. Total RNA was extracted from ELISA-positive samples using the QIAamp Viral RNA protocol (QIAGEN, Hilden, Germany), and stored at −70 °C.

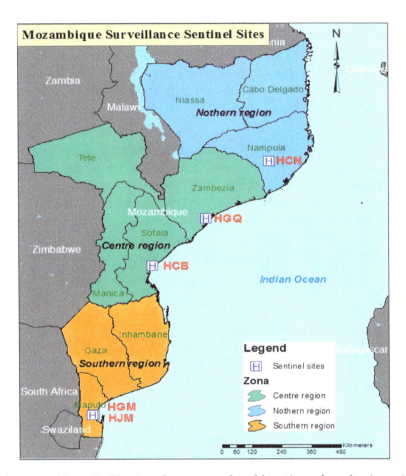

**Figure 1.** Map of Mozambique indicating the geographical location of study sites. Abbreviations for hospitals are indicated in red. HGM (Mavalane General Hospital), HJM (Jose Macamo General Hospital), HCB (Beira Central Hospital), HGQ (Quelimane General Hospital) and HCN (Nampula Central Hospital).

### 4.3.2. Reverse Transcriptase (RT) and G/P Typing PCR

Extracted RNA (8 µL) was reverse transcribed using Con2/Con3 for the partial VP4-encoding gene (VP8*, 876 bp) and sBeg9/End9 for the VP7-encoding gene. G genotypes were subsequently determined using a multiplex semi-nested PCR as described before [24]. Specific primers that identified the VP7-encoding gene with the following G genotypes: G1, aBT1; G2, aCT2; G3, aET3 or mG3; G4, aDT4; G8, aAT8; G9, aFT9, or mG9; G12, G12b; G10, mG10 in combination with the common primer RVG9 were used as described previously [50–52].

Similarly, Con3 was used in combination with specific primers that identify P genotypes: P[8], 1T-1D or 1T-1v; P[4], 2T-1; P[6], 3T-1; P[9], 4T-1, and P[10], 5T-1, P[11], mp11, P[14], P4943, as described previously [53–55]. The PCR product was analyzed using 2% agarose gel electrophoresis, stained with ethidium bromide and visualized under ultraviolet illumination.

*4.4. Data Management and Statistical Analyses*

The rotavirus vaccine, *Rotarix®*, was introduced in September 2015 in Mozambique. Therefore, the pre-vaccine period was considered to be before December 2015, due to logistical problems associated with vaccine introduction across the country.

The genotyping data from the primary sentinel site, Mavalane General Hospital (HGM), was analyzed separately from other sites because data at this site was available from 2012 and other sites from 2015.

Frequencies of identified genotypes are reported. To assess the magnitude of change in genotypes from the pre- to post-vaccine periods, unadjusted odds ratios (OR) and their 95% confidence intervals (95CI) were computed. In this analysis, the genotype was the dependent variable and time the predictor. All statistical analysis was conducted using Stata software version 15.0 (Stata Corp., College Station, TX, USA). A *p*-value of <0.05 was considered statistically significant.

## 5. Conclusions

This is the first report describing the circulation of rotavirus genotypes in three regions of Mozambique. A comparison between the pre- and post-vaccine introduction periods showed a shift in circulating genotypes following vaccine introduction. However, due to the short surveillance period, it is not clear if the observed changes were due to the introduction of the vaccine or a consequence of natural strain variation. In addition, the emergence of unusual strains, such as G3P[4] and G3P[8], was also observed, which support the need for continued country-wide surveillance to monitor changes, due to possible vaccine pressure, and consequently, the effect on vaccine effectiveness.

**Supplementary Materials:**
Table S1: Total number of stool samples collected at sentinel sites in Mozambique during surveillance between May 2014 and December 2019; Table S2: Total number of stool samples collected per sentinel sites in Mozambique during surveillance between May 2014 and December 2019; Table S3: Total number of stool samples collected at Mavalane General Hospital during a cross-sectional study (2012–2013) and the National Surveillance of Diarrhea program (2014–2019); Table S4: Distribution of rotavirus genotypes between geographical regions.

**Author Contributions:** N.d.D. and E.D.J conceptualized the main project. E.D.J., B.M., J.C., J.L., A.C., E.A., J.S., E.G., D.B., M.C., I.C.-M. and S.S.B. performed investigations. Formal analysis and methodology was done by E.D.J. and O.A. Data curation was performed by A.C., M.C. and O.A. Writing of the original draft preparation was performed by E.D.J. Review and editing was done by E.D.J., N.d.D., I.M., J.M.M. and H.G.O. Visualizations was performed by A.C. Project administration was done by J.C. Validation was done by N.d.D., H.G.O. and I.M. Supervision and funding acquisition was done by N.d.D. All authors have read and agreed to the published version of the manuscript.

**Acknowledgments:** We would like to thank the surveillance teams in Maputo, Nampula, Beira and Quelimane, as well as the parents that provided consent for the collection of stool samples and data from children. We are grateful for Centro de Investigação da Polana Caniço, INS, for providing the map illustration and to Adilson Bauhofer for assistance with data analyses.

## References

1. Troeger, C.; Khalil, I.A.; Rao, P.C.; Cao, S.; Blacker, B.F.; Ahmed, T.; Armah, G.; Bines, J.E.; Brewer, T.G.; Colombara, D.V.; et al. Rotavirus Vaccination and the Global Burden of Rotavirus Diarrhea Among Children Younger Than 5 Years. *JAMA Pediatr.* **2018**, *172*, 958–965. [CrossRef]
2. Tate, J.E.; Burton, A.H.; Boschi-Pinto, C.; Parashar, U.D. Global, Regional, and National Estimates of Rotavirus Mortality in Children <5 Years of Age, 2000–2013. *Clin. Infect. Dis.* **2016**, *62*, S96–S105. [PubMed]
3. GBD. Estimates of the global, regional, and national morbidity, mortality, and aetiologies of diarrhoea in 195 countries: A systematic analysis for the Global Burden of Disease Study 2016. *Lancet Infect. Dis.* **2018**, *18*, 1211–1228.
4. Estes, M.K.; Cohen, J. Rotavirus gene structure and function. *Microbiol. Rev.* **1989**, *53*, 410–449. [CrossRef] [PubMed]

5. Crawford, S.E.; Ramani, S.; Tate, J.E.; Parashar, U.D.; Svensson, L.; Hagbom, M.; Francco, M.A.; Greenberg, H.B.; O'Ryan, M.; Kang, G.; et al. Rotavirus infection. *Nat. Rev. Dis. Primers.* **2017**, *3*, 17083. [CrossRef]
6. Desselberger, U. Rotaviruses. *Virus Res.* **2014**, *190*, 75–96. [CrossRef]
7. Matthijnssens, J.; Ciarlet, M.; McDonald, S.M.; Attoui, H.; Banyai, K.; Brister, J.R.; Buesa, J.; Esona, M.D.; Estes, M.K.; Gentsch, J.R.; et al. Uniformity of rotavirus strain nomenclature proposed by the Rotavirus Classification Working Group (RCWG). *Arch. Virol.* **2011**, *156*, 1397–1413. [CrossRef]
8. Matthijnssens, J.; Ciarlet, M.; Heiman, E.; Arijs, I.; Delbeke, T.; McDonald, S.M.; Palombo, E.A.; Iturriza-Gómara, M.; Maes, P.; Patton, J.T.; et al. Full genome-based classification of rotaviruses reveals a common origin between human Wa-Like and porcine rotavirus strains and human DS-1-like and bovine rotavirus strains. *J. Virol.* **2008**, *82*, 3204–3219. [CrossRef]
9. Virus Classification- Laboratory of Viral Metagenomics. Available online: https://rega.kuleuven.be/cev/viralmetagenomics/virus-classification/rcwg (accessed on 20 May 2020).
10. Mwenda, J.M.; Tate, J.E.; Parashar, U.D.; Mihigo, R.; Agocs, M.; Serhan, F.; Nshimirimana, D. African rotavirus surveillance network: A brief overview. *Pediatr. Infect. Dis. J.* **2014**, *33*, S6–S8. [CrossRef]
11. Banyai, K.; Laszlo, B.; Duque, J.; Steele, A.D.; Nelson, E.A.; Gentsch, J.R.; Parashar, U.D. Systematic review of regional and temporal trends in global rotavirus strain diversity in the pre rotavirus vaccine era: Insights for understanding the impact of rotavirus vaccination programs. *Vaccine* **2012**, *30*, A122–A130. [CrossRef]
12. Gentsch, J.R.; Laird, A.R.; Bielfelt, B.; Griffin, D.D.; Banyai, K.; Ramachandran, M.; Jain, V.; Cunliffe, N.A.; Nakagomi, O.; Kirkwood, C.D.; et al. Serotype diversity and reassortment between human and animal rotavirus strains: Implications for rotavirus vaccine programs. *J. Infect. Dis.* **2005**, *192*, S146–S159. [CrossRef]
13. Leshem, E.; Lopman, B.; Glass, R.; Gentsch, J.; Banyai, K.; Parashar, U.; Patel, M. Distribution of rotavirus strains and strain-specific effectiveness of the rotavirus vaccine after its introduction: A systematic review and meta-analysis. *Lancet Infect. Dis.* **2014**, *14*, 847–856. [CrossRef]
14. Matthijnssens, J.; Bilcke, J.; Ciarlet, M.; Martella, V.; Banyai, K.; Rahman, M.; Zeller, M.; Beutels, P.; van Damme, P.; van Ranst, M. Rotavirus disease and vaccination: Impact on genotype diversity. *Fut. Microbiol.* **2009**, *4*, 1303–1316. [CrossRef]
15. Todd, S.; Page, N.A.; Duncan Steele, A.; Peenze, I.; Cunliffe, N.A. Rotavirus strain types circulating in Africa: Review of studies published during 1997–2006. *J. Infect. Dis.* **2010**, *202*, S34–S42. [CrossRef]
16. Seheri, L.M.; Magagula, N.B.; Peenze, I.; Rakau, K.; Ndadza, A.; Mwenda, J.M.; Weldegebriel, G.; Steele, A.D.; Mphahlele, M.J. Rotavirus strain diversity in Eastern and Southern African countries before and after vaccine introduction. *Vaccine* **2017**, *36*, 7222–7230. [CrossRef] [PubMed]
17. Rotavirus vaccines. WHO position paper—January 2013. *Wkly. Epidemiol. Rec.* **2013**, *88*, 49–64.
18. Langa, J.S.; Thompson, R.; Arnaldo, P.; Resque, H.R.; Rose, T.; Enosse, S.M.; Fialho, A.; Assis, R.M.S.; Silva, M.F.M.; Paulo, J.; et al. Epidemiology of Rotavirus A diarrhea in Chókwè, Southern Mozambique, from February to September, 2011. *J. Med. Virol.* **2016**, *88*, 1751–1758. [CrossRef]
19. De Deus, N.; João, E.; Cuamba, A.; Cassocera, M.; Luís, L.; Acácio, S.; Mandomando, I.; Augusto, O.; Page, N. Epidemiology of Rotavirus Infection in Children from a Rural and Urban Area, in Maputo, Southern Mozambique, before Vaccine Introduction. *J. Trop. Pediatr.* **2018**, *64*, 141–145. [CrossRef]
20. Kotloff, K.L.; Nataro, J.P.; Blackwelder, W.C.; Nasrin, D.; Farag, T.H.; Panchalingam, S.; Wu, Y.; O Sow, S.; Sur, D.; Breiman, R.F.; et al. Burden and aetiology of diarrhoeal disease in infants and young children in developing countries (the Global Enteric Multicenter Study, GEMS): A prospective, case-control study. *Lancet* **2013**, *382*, 209–222. [CrossRef]
21. De Deus, N.; Chilaule, J.J.; Cassocera, M.; Bambo, M.; Langa, J.S.; Sitoe, E.; Chissaque, A.; Anapakala, E.; Sambo, J.; Lourenço Guimarães, E.; et al. Early impact of rotavirus vaccination in children less than five years of age in Mozambique. *Vaccine* **2018**, *36*, 7205–7209. [CrossRef]
22. Matthijnssens, J.; de Grazia, S.; Piessens, J.; Heylen, E.; Zeller, M.; Giammanco, G.M.; Bányai, K.; Buonavoglia, C.; Ciarlet, M.; Martella, V.; et al. Multiple reassortment and interspecies transmission events contribute to the diversity of feline, canine and feline/canine-like human group A rotavirus strains. *Infect. Genet. Evol.* **2011**, *11*, 1396–1406. [CrossRef]
23. Matthijnssens, J.; Taraporewala, Z.F.; Yang, H.; Rao, S.; Yuan, L.; Cao, D.; Hoshino, Y.; Mertens, P.P.C.; Carner, G.R.; McNeal, M.; et al. Simian rotaviruses possess divergent gene constellations that originated from interspecies transmission and reassortment. *J. Virol.* **2009**, *84*, 2013–2026. [CrossRef] [PubMed]

24. Joao, E.D.; Strydom, A.; O'Neill, H.G.; Cuamba, A.; Cassocera, M.; Acacio, S.; Mandomando, I.; Motanyane, L.; Page, N.; de Deus, N. Rotavirus A strains obtained from children with acute gastroenteritis in Mozambique, 2012–2013: G and P genotypes and phylogenetic analysis of VP7 and partial VP4 genes. *Arch. Virol.* **2018**, *163*, 153–165. [CrossRef] [PubMed]
25. Page, N.A.; Seheri, L.M.; Groome, M.J.; Moyes, J.; Walaza, S.; Mphahlele, J.; Kahn, K.; Kapongo, C.N.; Zar, H.J.; Tempia, S.; et al. Temporal association of rotavirus vaccination and genotype circulation in South Africa: Observations from 2002 to 2014. *Vaccine* **2017**, *36*, 7231–7237. [CrossRef]
26. Lartey, B.L.; Damanka, S.; Dennis, F.E.; Enweronu-Laryea, C.C.; Addo-Yobo, E.; Ansong, D.; Kwarteng-Owusu, S.; Sagoe, K.W.; Mwenda, J.M.; Diamenu, S.K.; et al. Rotavirus strain distribution in Ghana pre- and post- rotavirus vaccine introduction. *Vaccine* **2018**, *36*, 7238–7242. [CrossRef]
27. Bar-Zeev, N.; Jere, K.C.; Bennett, A.; Pollock, L.; Tate, J.E.; Nakagomi, O.; Iturriza-Gomara, M.; Costello, A.; Mwansambo, C.; Parashar, U.D.; et al. Population Impact and Effectiveness of Monovalent Rotavirus Vaccination in Urban Malawian Children 3 Years After Vaccine Introduction: Ecological and Case-Control Analyses. *Clin. Infect. Dis.* **2016**, *62*, S213–S219. [CrossRef]
28. Hungerford, D.; Allen, D.J.; Nawaz, S.; Collins, S.; Ladhani, S.; Vivancos, R.; Iturriza-Gómara, M. Impact of rotavirus vaccination on rotavirus genotype distribution and diversity in England, September 2006 to August 2016. *Eurosurveillance* **2019**, *24*, 1700774.
29. Matthijnssens, J.; Zeller, M.; Heylen, E.; de Coster, S.; Vercauteren, J.; Braeckman, T.; van Herck, K.; Meyer, N.; Pircon, J.-Y.; Soriano-Gabarro, M.; et al. Higher proportion of G2P[4] rotaviruses in vaccinated hospitalized cases compared with unvaccinated hospitalized cases, despite high vaccine effectiveness against heterotypic G2P[4] rotaviruses. *Clin. Microbiol. Infect.* **2014**, *20*, O702–O710. [CrossRef]
30. Luchs, A.; Cilli, A.; Morillo, S.G.; de Cássia Compagnoli, C.R.; Timenetsky, M.C.S.T. Rotavirus Genotypes Circulating in Brazil, 2007-2012: Implications for the Vaccine Program. *Rev. Inst. Med. Trop.* **2015**, *57*, 305–313. [CrossRef] [PubMed]
31. Mukhopadhya, I.; Murdoch, H.; Berry, S.; Hunt, A.; Iturriza-Gomara, M.; Smith-Palmer, A.; Cameron, J.C.; Hold, G.L. Changing molecular epidemiology of rotavirus infection after introduction of monovalent rotavirus vaccination in Scotland. *Vaccine* **2016**, *35*, 156–163. [CrossRef] [PubMed]
32. Cunliffe, N.A.; Ngwira, B.M.; Dove, W.; Thindwa, B.D.; Turner, A.M.; Broadhead, R.L.; Molyneux, M.E.; Hart, A.C. Epidemiology of rotavirus infection in children in Blantyre, Malawi, 1997–2007. *J. Infect. Dis.* **2010**, *202*, S168–S174. [CrossRef] [PubMed]
33. Yamamoto, S.P.; Kaida, A.; Ono, A.; Kubo, H.; Iritani, N. Detection and characterization of a human G9P[4] rotavirus strain in Japan. *J. Med. Virol.* **2015**, *87*, 1311–1318. [CrossRef]
34. Giri, S.; Nair, N.P.; Mathew, A.; Manohar, B.; Simon, A.; Singh, T.; Suresh Kumar, S.; Mathew, M.A.; Babji, S.; Arora, R.; et al. Rotavirus gastroenteritis in Indian children < 5 years hospitalized for diarrhoea, 2012 to 2016. *BMC Public Health* **2019**, *19*, 69.
35. Cashman, O.; Collins, P.J.; Lennon, G.; Cryan, B.; Martella, V.; Fanning, S.; Staines, A.; O'Shea, H. Molecular characterization of group A rotaviruses detected in children with gastroenteritis in Ireland in 2006–2009. *Epidemiol. Infect.* **2011**, *140*, 247–259. [CrossRef]
36. Collins, P.J.; Mulherin, E.; O'Shea, H.; Cashman, O.; Lennon, G.; Pidgeon, E.; Coughlan, S.; Hall, W.; Fanning, S. Changing patterns of rotavirus strains circulating in Ireland: Re-emergence of G2P[4] and identification of novel genotypes in Ireland. *J. Med. Virol.* **2015**, *87*, 764–773. [CrossRef]
37. Lennon, G.; Reidy, N.; Cryan, B.; Fanning, S.; O'Shea, H. Changing profile of rotavirus in Ireland: Predominance of P[8] and emergence of P[6] and P[9] in mixed infections. *J. Med. Virol.* **2008**, *80*, 524–530. [CrossRef]
38. Mokomane, M.; Esona, M.D.; Bowen, M.D.; Tate, J.E.; Steenhoff, A.P.; Lechiile, K.; Gaseitsiwe, S.; Seheri, L.M.; Magagula, N.B.; Weldegebriel, G.; et al. Diversity of Rotavirus Strains Circulating in Botswana before and after introduction of the Monovalent Rotavirus Vaccine. *Vaccine* **2019**, *37*, 6324–6328. [CrossRef]
39. WHO-Botswana. Available online: https://www.afro.who.int/news/who-supports-botswana-respond-outbreak-diarrhoea-children-below-five-years-age. (accessed on 29 May 2020).
40. Rakau, K.; Gededzha, M.; Peenze, I.; Seheri, M. Rotavirus strains detected in Dr George Mukhari academic hospital and Oukasie primary healthcare, Pretoria from 2015-2016. In Proceedings of the 12th African Rotavirus Symposium, Johannesburg, South Africa, 30 July–1 August 2019.

41. Gugu, M.; Nomcebo, P.; Sindisiwe, D.; Susan, K.; Gilbert, M.; Goitom, W.; Lonkululeko, K.; Xolsile, D.; Getahun, T.; Michael, L.; et al. G3P[8] rotavirus strain causing diarrheal outbreak in the Kingdom of Eswatini, 2018. In Proceedings of the 12th African Rotavirus Symposium, Johannesburg, South Africa, 30 July–1 August 2019.
42. Mhango, C.; Chinyama, E.; Mandolo, J.; Malamba, C.; Wachepa, R.; Kanjerwa, O.; Kamng'ona, A.W.; Shawa, I.T.; Jere, K.C. Changes in rotavirus strains circulating in Malawi before vaccine introduction and six years post vaccine era. In Proceedings of the 12th African Rotavirus Symposium, Johannesburg, South Africa, 30 July–1 August 2019.
43. Carvalho-Costa, F.A.; de Assis, R.M.S.; Fialho, A.M.; Araujo, I.T.; Silva, M.F.; Gomez, M.M.; Andrade, J.S.; Rose, T.L.; Fumian, T.M.; Voloāto, E.M. The evolving epidemiology of rotavirus A infection in Brazil a decade after the introduction of universal vaccination with Rotarix(R). *BMC Pediatr.* **2019**, *19*, 42. [CrossRef]
44. Roczo-Farkas, S.; Kirkwood, C.D.; Cowley, D.; Barnes, G.L.; Bishop, R.F.; Bogdanovic-Sakran, N.; Boniface, K.; Donato, C.M.; Bines, J.E. The Impact of Rotavirus Vaccines on Genotype Diversity: A Comprehensive Analysis of 2 Decades of Australian Surveillance Data. *J. Infect. Dis.* **2018**, *218*, 546–554. [CrossRef]
45. Cowley, D.; Donato, C.M.; Roczo-Farkas, S.; Kirkwood, C.D. Emergence of a novel equine-like G3P[8] inter-genogroup reassortant rotavirus strain associated with gastroenteritis in Australian children. *J. Gen. Virol.* **2015**, *97*, 403–410. [CrossRef]
46. Page, N.; Mapuroma, F.; Seheri, M.; Kruger, T.; Peenze, I.; Walaza, S.; Cohen, C.; Groome, M.; Madhi, S. Rotavirus surveillance report, South Africa, 2013. *Commun Dis Surveill Bull.* **2014**, *12*, 130–135.
47. Jere, K.C.; Chaguza, C.; Bar-Zeev, N.; Lowe, J.; Peno, C.; Kumwenda, B.; Nakagomi, O.; Tate, J.E.; Parashar, U.D.; Heyderman, R.S.; et al. Emergence of Double- and Triple-Gene Reassortant G1P[8] Rotaviruses Possessing a DS-1-Like Backbone after Rotavirus Vaccine Introduction in Malawi. *J. Virol.* **2018**, *92*, e01246-17. [CrossRef] [PubMed]
48. Komoto, S.; Tacharoenmuang, R.; Guntapong, R.; Ide, T.; Haga, K.; Katayama, K.; Kato, T.; Ouchi, Y.; Kurahashi, H.; Tsuji, T.; et al. Emergence and Characterization of Unusual DS-1-Like G1P[8] Rotavirus Strains in Children with Diarrhea in Thailand. *PLoS ONE* **2015**, *10*, e0141739. [CrossRef] [PubMed]
49. Mwangi, P.N.; Mogotsi, M.T.; Rasebotsa, S.P.; Seheri, M.L.; Mphahlele, M.J.; Ndze, V.N.; Dennis, F.E.; Jere, K.C.; Nyaga, M.M. Uncovering the First Atypical DS-1-like G1P[8] Rotavirus Strains That Circulated during Pre-Rotavirus Vaccine Introduction Era in South Africa. *Pathogens* **2020**, *9*, 391. [CrossRef]
50. Gouvea, V.; Glass, R.I.; Woods, P.; Taniguchi, K.; Clark, H.F.; Forrester, B.; Fang, Z.Y. Polymerase chain reaction amplification and typing of rotavirus nucleic acid from stool specimens. *J. Clin. Microbiol.* **1990**, *28*, 276–282. [CrossRef]
51. Iturriza Gomara, M.; Kang, G.; Mammen, A.; Jana, A.K.; Abraham, M.; Desselberger, U.; Brown, D.; Gray, J. Characterization of G10P[11] rotaviruses causing acute gastroenteritis in neonates and infants in Vellore, India. *J. Clin. Microbiol.* **2004**, *42*, 2541–2547. [CrossRef]
52. Aladin, F.; Nawaz, S.; Iturriza-Gomara, M.; Gray, J. Identification of G8 rotavirus strains determined as G12 by rotavirus genotyping PCR: Updating the current genotyping methods. *J. Clin Virol.* **2010**, *47*, 340–344. [CrossRef]
53. Gentsch, J.R.; Glass, R.I.; Woods, P.; Gouvea, V.; Gorziglia, M.; Flores, J.; Das, B.K.; Bhan, M.K. Identification of group A rotavirus gene 4 types by polymerase chain reaction. *J. Clin. Microbiol.* **1992**, *30*, 1365–1373. [CrossRef]
54. Iturriza-Gomara, M.; Green, J.; Brown, D.W.; Desselberger, U.; Gray, J.J. Diversity within the VP4 gene of rotavirus P [8] strains: Implications for reverse transcription-PCR genotyping. *J. Clin. Microbiol.* **2000**, *38*, 898–901. [CrossRef]
55. Mphahlele, M.J.; Peenze, I.; Steele, A.D. Rotavirus strains bearing the VP4P[14] genotype recovered from South African children with diarrhoea. *Arch. Virol.* **1999**, *144*, 1027–1034. [CrossRef]

# Rotavirus A in Brazil: Molecular Epidemiology and Surveillance during 2018–2019

Meylin Bautista Gutierrez, Alexandre Madi Fialho, Adriana Gonçalves Maranhão, Fábio Correia Malta, Juliana da Silva Ribeiro de Andrade, Rosane Maria Santos de Assis, Sérgio da Silva e Mouta, Marize Pereira Miagostovich, José Paulo Gagliardi Leite and Tulio Machado Fumian *[iD]

Laboratory of Comparative and Environmental Virology, Oswaldo Cruz Institute, Oswaldo Cruz Foundation, Avenida Brasil 4365, Rio de Janeiro 21040-900, Brazil; meylin.gutierrez@ioc.fiocruz.br (M.B.G.); amfialho@ioc.fiocruz.br (A.M.F.); adriana.maranhao@ioc.fiocruz.br (A.G.M.); fabio.malta@ioc.fiocruz.br (F.C.M.); juliana@ioc.fiocruz.br (J.d.S.R.d.A.); rmsassis@ioc.fiocruz.br (R.M.S.d.A.); mouta@ioc.fiocruz.br (S.d.S.e.M.); marizepm@ioc.fiocruz.br (M.P.M.); jpgleite@ioc.fiocruz.br (J.P.G.L.)
* Correspondence: tuliomf@ioc.fiocruz.br or fumiantm@gmail.com;

**Abstract:** Rotavirus A (RVA) vaccines succeeded in lowering the burden of acute gastroenteritis (AGE) worldwide, especially preventing severe disease and mortality. In 2019, Brazil completed 13 years of RVA vaccine implementation (Rotarix™) within the National Immunization Program (NIP), and as reported elsewhere, the use of Rotarix™ in the country has reduced childhood mortality and morbidity due to AGE. Even though both marketed vaccines are widely distributed, the surveillance of RVA causing AGE and the monitoring of circulating genotypes are important tools to keep tracking the epidemiological scenario and vaccines impact. Thus, our study investigated RVA epidemiological features, viral load and G and P genotypes circulation in children and adults presenting AGE symptoms in eleven states from three out of five regions in Brazil. By using TaqMan®-based one-step RT-qPCR, we investigated a total of 1536 stool samples collected from symptomatic inpatients, emergency department visits and outpatients from January 2018 to December 2019. G and P genotypes of RVA-positive samples were genetically characterized by multiplex RT-PCR or by nearly complete fragment sequencing. We detected RVA in 12% of samples, 10.5% in 2018 and 13.7% in 2019. A marked winter/spring seasonality was observed, especially in Southern Brazil. The most affected age group was children aged >24–60 months, with a positivity rate of 18.8% ($p < 0.05$). Evaluating shedding, we found a statistically lower RVA viral load in stool samples collected from children aged up to six months compared to the other age groups ($p < 0.05$). The genotype G3P[8] was the most prevalent during the two years (83.7% in 2018 and 65.5% in 2019), and nucleotide sequencing of some strains demonstrated that they belonged to the emergent equine-like G3P[8] genotype. The dominance of an emergent genotype causing AGE reinforces the need for continuous epidemiological surveillance to assess the impact of mass RVA immunization as well as to monitor the emergence of novel genotypes.

**Keywords:** acute gastroenteritis; rotavirus A; incidence; genotyping; Brazil

## 1. Introduction

Acute gastroenteritis (AGE) remains as a major cause of mortality in children under five years old worldwide [1,2]. Among the AGE-causing pathogens, rotavirus A (RVA) is one of the leading agents, responsible for approximately 200,000 deaths per year among children <5 years old in developing countries [3–5]. Regarding severe disease, RVA accounts for around 20% and 40% of all AGE-hospitalization in countries with and without RVA vaccines implemented, respectively [6,7].

Currently, four World Health Organization (WHO)-prequalified live-attenuated oral RVA vaccines are available internationally—Rotarix™, RotaTeq™, Rotavac™, and RotaSiil™—and over 100 countries have introduced one of these vaccines into their national immunization program [8] (https://www.who.int/immunization/diseases/rotavirus/en/).

Rotaviruses belong to the *Reoviridae* family, genus *Rotavirus*. While nine rotaviruses species have been described (A–I), RVA is by far the most important species infecting humans worldwide [9,10]. The non-enveloped triple-layered viral particle has 70–75 nm in diameter with 11 segmented double-stranded RNA (dsRNA) genes, encoding for six structural (VP1-VP4, VP6, VP7) and depending on the strain, five or six non-structural proteins (NSP1-NSP5 or NSP6) [11]. Genetically, RVA is classified into G- and P-types, based on nucleotide sequence of genomic segments coding VP7 and VP4 proteins (binary classification), and currently there have been described 36 G- and 51 P-types [12]. Although many G and P combination would be possible to emerge, a few genotypes (G1P[8], G2P[4], G3P[8], G4P[8], G9P[8], and G12P[8]) have prevailed worldwide causing the majority of RVA infections in children [13–15].

Brazil has implemented the Rotarix™ vaccine in the National Immunization Program (NIP) in March 2006, which led to a significant reduction of diarrhea-associated mortality and hospitalization [16–18]. Linhares et al. [19] demonstrated the higher effectiveness of Rotarix™ among Brazilian infants aged up to 12 months and decreasing in older children. Concerning the genotype distribution in Brazil after the introduction of Rotarix™, G2P[4] was by far the most prevalent genotype detected until 2010. From 2011 onwards, a gradual decrease in the prevalence of G2P[4] was observed, being replaced by G3, G9, and G12 harboring a P[8]-type [20–23]. Nevertheless, unusual RVA genotypes have been frequently detected, such as: G3P[6], G12P[6], G8P[4], and G8P[6] and more recently the equine-like G3P[8] [17,23,24]. Similarly, recent studies from other countries have reported the detection of rare RVA genotype combination [25–28].

It has been demonstrated that the distribution of RVA genotypes over the years is characterized by natural and cyclical genotype fluctuations [20,29,30]. However, the selective pressure due to mass RVA vaccination could favor specific G and P combinations [9,31]. Therefore, the new and dynamic epidemiological scenario reinforces the need to continuously document RVA prevalence in AGE cases, molecular epidemiology and the potential emergence of unusual genotypes.

Our study investigated RVA prevalence, features and the molecular characterization of G and P genotypes among patients with AGE from three regions (Southern, Southeastern and Northeastern) in Brazil, 2018–2019. RVA was detected and quantified by quantitative RT-PCR (RT-qPCR) from diarrheic stool samples received from eleven Brazilian states, and G and P genotypes were determined by multiplex one-step RT-PCR or sequencing.

## 2. Materials and Methods

### 2.1. Stool Collection and Ethics Statements

This study included stool samples that were collected between January 2018 and December 2019 from children and adults with symptoms of AGE, characterized as ≥three liquid/semi liquid evacuations in a 24 h period. Inpatients and outpatients diarrheic stool samples were collected from eleven states from three regions of Brazil: Southern, Southeastern, and Northeastern. Samples were systematically sent together with clinical-epidemiological records to the Regional Rotavirus Reference Laboratory–Laboratory of Comparative and Environmental Virology (RRRL–LVCA). The laboratory is part of the ongoing national network for AGE surveillance and coordinated by General Coordination of Public Health Laboratories, Brazilian Ministry of Health.

This study is approved by the Ethics Committee of the Oswaldo Cruz Foundation (FIOCRUZ), number CAAE: 94144918.3.0000.5248. The surveillance is performed through a hierarchical network in which samples are provided by medical request in hospitals and health centers, monitored by the Brazilian Unified Health System (SUS). Patients' data were maintained anonymously and securely.

*2.2. Viral RNA Extraction*

Viral RNA was purified from 140 µL of clarified stool suspension (10% *w/v*) prepared with Tris-calcium buffer (pH = 7.2). Samples were subjected to an automatic nucleic acid extraction procedure using a QIAamp® Viral RNA Mini kit (QIAGEN, CA, USA) and a QIAcube® automated system (QIAGEN), according to the manufacturer's instructions. RVA RNA was eluted in 60 µL of the elution buffer AVE. The isolated RNA was immediately stored at −80 °C until the molecular analysis. In each extraction procedure, RNAse/DNAse-free water was used as negative control.

*2.3. RVA Detection and Quantification*

RVA was detected and quantified by using a TaqMan®-based quantitative one step PCR (RT-qPCR) with primers and probe targeting the conserved NSP3 segment, according to Zeng et al. (2008). Briefly, RT-qPCR reactions were performed with 5 µL of the extracted RNA in a final volume of 25 µL using the SuperScript™ III Platinum™ One-Step qRT-PCR Kit (ThermoFisher Scientific, Invitrogen Division, Carlsbad, CA, USA) in the Applied Biosystems® 7500 Real-Time PCR System (Applied Biosystems, Foster City, CA, USA). NSP3 primers and probe final concentrations used were 0.8 and 0.5 µM, respectively. The thermal cycling conditions were carried out as follows: RT step at 55 °C for 30 min, an initial denaturation step at 95 °C for 10 min and 40 cycles of PCR amplification at 95 °C for 15 s and 60 °C for 1 min. Samples that crossed the threshold line showing a characteristic sigmoid curve were regarded as positive. All runs included negative and non-template controls, and a standard curve with serial dilutions ($10^6$–$10^1$) of double-stranded DNA fragments (gBlock® Gene Fragment, Integrated DNA Technologies, Iowa, USA) containing the RVA NSP3 target region to ensure the correct interpretation of the results throughout the study. RVA viral loads were expressed as genome copies per gram (GC/g) of stool.

*2.4. Genotyping and Sequencing*

RVA-positive samples obtained by RT-qPCR were G- and P-genotyped using a one-step multiplex RT-PCR. The reactions were performed using the Qiagen One Step RT-PCR kit (Qiagen), using forward conserved primers VP7uF or VP4uF and specific reverse primers for G types G1, G2, G3, G4, G9, and G12, or P types P[4], P[6], P[8], P[9], and P[10] as recommended by the Centers for Disease Control and Prevention, USA. The G- and P-genotypes were assigned based on different amplicon sizes [base pairs (bp)] using agarose gel analysis. Sanger sequencing was also used to characterize the nucleotide (nt) sequence of specific strains, such as non-typeable samples or the equine-like G3, using consensus primers directed to the conserved regions within the VP4 and VP7 genes. The amplicons fragments of 876 bp and 881 bp for VP4 and VP7, respectively, were purified using the ExoSAP clean-up kit (ThermoFisher Scientific) and sent to the FIOCRUZ Institutional Platform for DNA sequencing (PDTIS). All primers used for RVA genotyping were based on previously studies [32–34].

*2.5. Phylogenetic Analysis*

Chromatogram analysis and consensus sequences were obtained using Geneious Prime (Biomatters Ltd., Auckland, New Zealand). RVA genotypes were confirmed in terms of closest homology sequence using Basic Local Alignment Search Tool (BLAST). Phylogenetic trees were constructed using the maximum likelihood method and the Kimura two-parameter model (2000 bootstrap replications for branch support) in MEGA X v. 10.1.7 [35], with RVA reference sequences obtained from the National Center for Biotechnology Information (NCBI) database. Nucleotide sequences obtained from clinical samples were submitted to NCBI GenBank (accession numbers: MT386419 to MT386453).

*2.6. Statistical Analysis*

Statistical analyses were performed using GraphPad Prism software v. 8.4.1 (GraphPad Software, San Diego, CA, USA). As appropriate, Mann–Whitney U test, Chi-squared or Fisher test was used to assess significant difference between RVA detection rates, years of collecting samples and age groups, as well as to compare RVA viral load according to different age groups. A *p* value < 0.05 was considered to be statistically significant.

## 3. Results

### 3.1. Rotavirus A Epidemiology

During the two-year period of this study (2018–2019), a total of 1536 stool samples were collected from symptomatic inpatients with AGE (1161 and 375 from children and adults, respectively). Overall, we detected RVA in 12% of samples (n = 185), 10.5% in 2018 and 13.7% in 2019. We observed a slight increase in RVA incidence in 2019, but without statistical significance ($p = 0.053$). Except for three months in 2018 (April, June, and December), RVA circulated year-round, with monthly detection rates varying from 1.6% to 36.7% in May 2018 and September 2019, respectively (Figure 1A). In relation to seasonal patterns, we observed higher RVA circulation during winter/spring months, especially marked in Southern region states (Figure 1B,C), whilst RVA detections were lowest in autumn months.

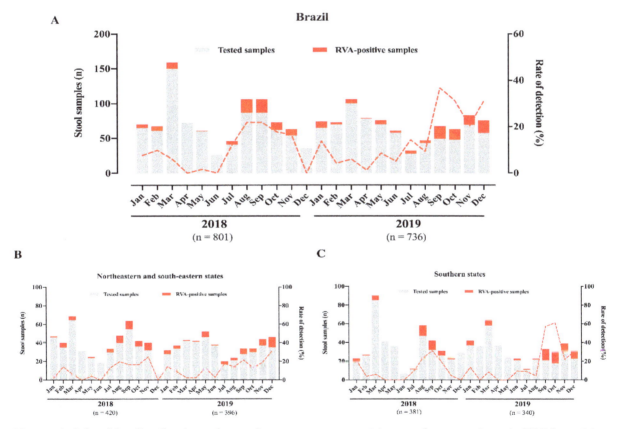

**Figure 1.** Monthly distribution of tested acute gastroenteritis samples, rotavirus A (RVA)-positive samples and RVA detection rates in Brazil (**A**), Northeastern and South-eastern states (**B**), and Southern states (**C**), during 2018–2019.

In regard to regional analysis, higher RVA prevalence was observed in the Northeast region (18.7%) compared to Southeastern and Southern regions (3.4% and 12.5%, respectively). Comparing the two year of the study, RVA detection rates were higher in 2019 for the three regions, but only with statistical significance in Southeastern region ($p = 0.022$). Table 1 shows detailed analysis by regions and states. It is interesting to note that the two states of Southern region (Santa Catarina and Rio Grande do Sul) accounted for almost half of the AGE cases and RVA-positive samples (Figure 2).

**Table 1.** Number of tested and rotavirus-positive fecal samples through laboratory-based surveillance by region and state in Brazil during 2018 and 2019.

| Region/State | No. of Fecal Samples: Positive/Tested (%) | | | p-Value (Chi-Square Test) |
|---|---|---|---|---|
| | Total | 2018 | 2019 | |
| **Southeast** | 14/381 (3.7) | 2/168 (1.2) | 12/213 (5.6) | 0.022 |
| Espírito Santo | | 1/56 | 2/101 | |
| Minas Gerais | | 1/75 | - | |
| Rio de Janeiro | | - | 10/79 | |
| **Northeast** | 81/434 (18.7) | 44/252 (17.5) | 37/182 (20.3) | 0.452 |
| Bahia | | 1/98 | 2/95 | |
| Maranhão | | 1/8 | 1/1 | |
| Paraíba | | 20/37 | - | |
| Pernambuco | | 19/68 | 30/61 | |
| Rio Grande do Norte | | - | 1/5 | |
| Sergipe | | 3/41 | 3/20 | |
| **South** | 90/720 (12.5) | 39/381 (10.2) | 51/340 (15) | 0.053 |
| Rio Grande do Sul | | 16/168 | 38/181 | |
| Santa Catarina | | 23/213 | 13/159 | |

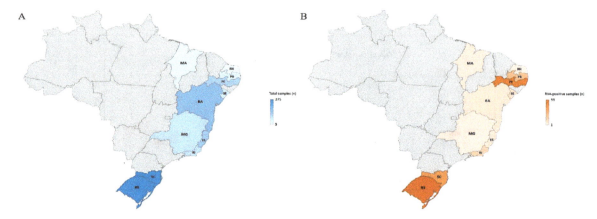

**Figure 2.** Map of Brazil highlighting the eleven states with sentinel surveillance service attended by the Rotavirus Regional Reference Laboratory, IOC, FIOCRUZ. Number of tested samples (**A**) and number of RVA-positive samples (**B**).

Most of stool samples received were from children less than five years old, representing 72.1% (1108/1536) of the AGE cases. RVA detection rate was significantly higher among children aged between 24 and 60 months (18.8%) compared to the other age groups, where detection rates varied from 9.3% to 12.1% (Table 2). We also analyzed RVA viral load (GC/g of stool) among different age groups. The median values of RVA viral loads varied from 4.2 to 6.8 $\log_{10}$ GC/g among the different age groups. RVA-positive samples showed viral load values statistically lower in AGE cases among children ≤6 months compared to older patients ($p < 0.05$) (Figure 3).

**Table 2.** Number of tested and rotavirus-positive fecal samples through laboratory-based surveillance by age group in Brazil during 2018–2019.

| Age Group (Months) | No. of Fecal Samples: Positive/Tested (%) | | | p-Value * (Chi-Square Test) |
|---|---|---|---|---|
| | 2018 | 2019 | Total | |
| 0–6 | 16/122 (13.1) | 9/101 (8.9) | 25/223 (11.2) | 0.0153 |
| >6–12 | 10/133 (7.5) | 14/116 (12) | 24/249 (9.6) | 0.0021 |
| >12–24 | 17/203 (8.3) | 18/173 (10.4) | 35/376 (9.3) | 0.0003 |
| >24–60 | 26/141 (18.4) | 23/119 (19.3) | 49/260 (18.8) | - |
| >60 | 16/202 (7.9) | 36/227 (15.8) | 52/428 (12.1) | 0.0109 |

* p-values were calculated between the age group of >24–60 and each other. All other combinations were not statistically different.

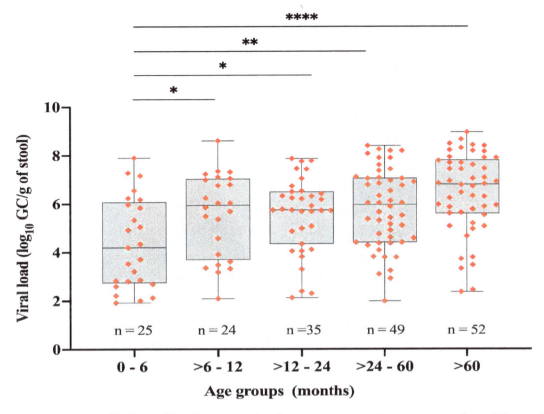

**Figure 3.** Rotavirus A (RVA) viral load expressed as $\log_{10}$ genome copies per gram of stool ($\log_{10}$ GC/g) among different age groups in Brazil, 2018–2019. Box-and-whisker plots show the first and third quartiles (equivalent to the 5th and 95th percentiles), the median (the horizontal line in the box), and range of $\log_{10}$ GC/g values. * $p \leq 0.05$; ** $p \leq 0.01$; **** $p \leq 0.0001$.

## 3.2. RVA Genotyping

A total of 186 RVA-positive samples were subjected to G and P genotyping by one-step multiplex RT-PCR. From these, 167 samples (89%) were successfully genotyped; 80 from 2018 and 87 from 2019. We characterized seven different RVA genotypes circulating during this study: G3P[8], G3P[6], G9P[8], G1P[8], G2P[6], G12P[6], and G6P[8]. G3P[8] was detected year-round and was by far, the most prevalent genotype, accounting for 83.8% (n = 67) of genotyped samples in 2018 and 65.5% (n = 57) in 2019 (Figure 4). Two other usual RVA genotypes were detected, but in lower prevalence—G1P[8] detected in one sample in 2018 and 2019, and G9P[8] detected in two and eight samples from 2018 and 2019, respectively. We also detected unusual G/P combinations, especially in 2019, as follows: G3P[6] in 6.3% of samples from 2018; G6P[8], G12P[6], and G2P[6] in 13.8%, 4.6% and 1.2% of samples from 2019 (Figure 4). G or P non-typed (NT) samples (GNTP8, GNTP6, and G3P[NT]) accounted for 5.4% of samples, and were represented mostly by samples with low RVA viral load (high Ct values).

In addition to RT-PCR genotyping, we sequenced some of the RVA-positive samples in order to get detailed information of the circulating strains and their respective lineages. We successfully obtained 22 and 21 consensus sequences of VP7 and VP4 genes, respectively. Phylogenetic analysis of the VP7 gene confirmed the characterization of Brazilian strains belonging to G3 and G6. Eighteen G3 strains from both years and from the three Brazilian regions were sequenced. From these, 94.4% (n = 17) of sequences clustered within the lineage 1, represented by equine-like G3P[8] strains. Our sequences were genetically related to previously detected equine-like G3P[8] strains from Brazil (KX469400) and other countries, such as Germany (KY000546), Slovakia (MN203563), Dominican Republic (MG652313), and Japan (LC47366). One G3 sequence clustered within lineage 3 that comprises the Wa-like G3P[8] group. The Brazilian Wa-like G3 sequence was closely related to strains from Brazil (KJ454454), Argentina (KJ583190 and KJ583201) and Hungary (JQ693568), with nt similarity varying from 98.4

to 99.8% (Figure 5A). The four G6 strains sequenced in our study, harboring a P[8]-type, clustered within lineage 1 showing moderate nt identity (97.8–98.1%) with G6P[8] strains detected in Bulgaria (KM590371 and KM590373) and with G6P[9] strains from Germany (KX880436) and Italy (KC152917). None of our G6 sequences clustered within the G6 lineage 3, that comprises human-bovine reassortant strains (Figure 5A).

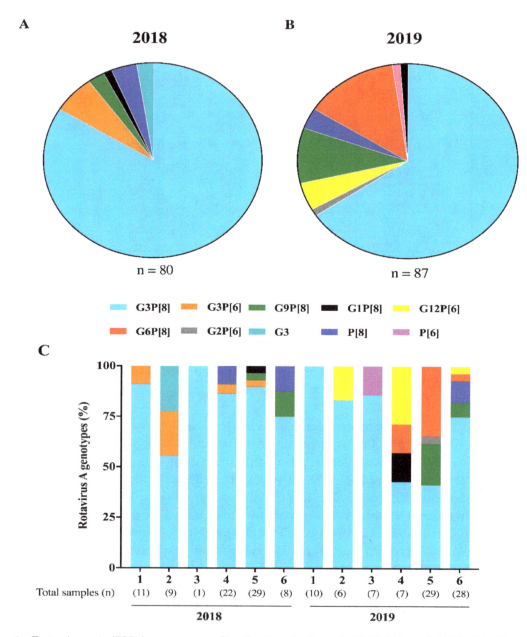

**Figure 4.** Rotavirus A (RVA) genotypes distribution in Brazil, 2018 (**A**) and 2019 (**B**). Bi-monthly genotypes circulation during the two-year of study (**C**).

Phylogenetic analysis of 21 sequences of VP4 gene, demonstrated that, except for one, all P[8] Brazilian strains harboring two different G-types (G3 and G6) grouped into lineage 3. The 20 strains were closely related (99.2–99.6% of nt similarity) to P[8]-3 Brazilian strains isolated in 2016 (KX469415 and MH569765) and strains from other countries, such as USA (MF997038), Japan (LC477395), Spain (KU550282), Australia (KU059769), and Italy (MK158257). One strain was characterized into P[6] lineage 1, and was closely related (99.5–99.7% of nt similarity) to strains detected in Argentina (KJ583199), Iraq (JX891397), and China (MG78835) (Figure 5B).

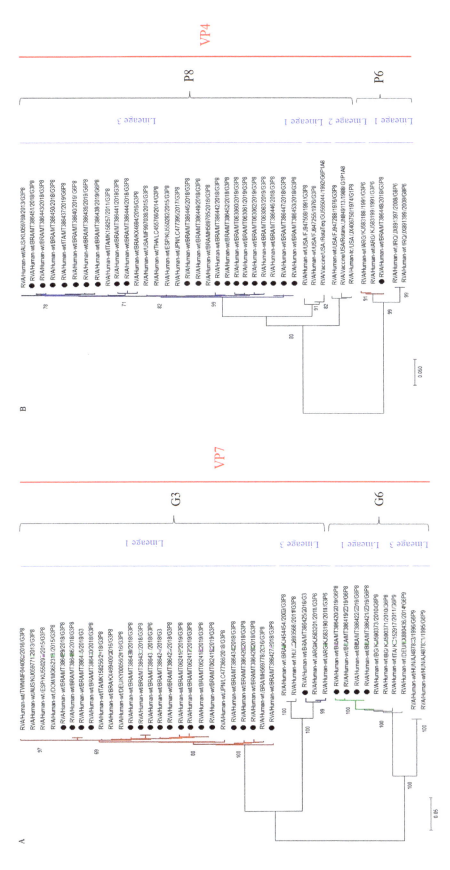

**Figure 5.** Phylogenetic analyses based on VP7 and VP4 nucleotide (nt) sequences of circulating Brazilian rotavirus strains. Strains obtained in this study are marked with a black filled circle and names contain the register number, state, and collection date (M/Y). Reference strains were downloaded from GenBank and labeled with their accession number followed by country, register number, year, and genotype. Neighbor-joining phylogenetic trees of VP4 (**A**) and VP7 (**B**) were constructed with MEGA X software and bootstrap tests (2000 replicates) based on the Kimura two-parameter model. Bootstrap values above 70% are given at branch nodes.

## 4. Discussion

In this study, we provide laboratory-based RVA national surveillance in eleven states from three regions in Brazil, during 2018–2019. We tested 1536 AGE stool samples and found an overall RVA-positivity of 12%. RVA detection rates were higher during winter/spring months and among children aged 24–60 months. By far, G3P[8] was the most frequently detected genotype, and showed a year-round circulation.

Despite the development of vaccines, RVA are still a major cause of severe AGE in infants worldwide [5]. Here, we detected RVA in 10.5% and 13.7% of samples from 2018 and 2019, respectively. In Brazil, after Rotarix™ implementation, different studies have investigated RVA circulation among AGE cases. A study from the Enteric Diseases Laboratory at Adolfo Lutz Institute, one of the three Brazilian Reference Laboratory for RVA surveillance, reported annual RVA prevalence varying from 9.9% to 25.3% during 2013–2017, with AGE samples from five states in the Midwestern and part of the Southeastern and Southern regions [24]. A previous study from our group demonstrated an overall RVA positivity of 20.8% among children up to 12 years old between 2006 and 2017, with annual detection rates varying between 5% to 35% [20]. Studies conducted at Evandro Chagas Institute, the national and regional reference center for RVA surveillance in Northern Brazil, demonstrated RVA positivity rates of 33% in samples from six states from North Brazil, 2011–2012 [23], and 24.2% in samples collected between June 2012 and June 2015 [36]. However, it is worth mentioning that both studies involved children hospitalized for severe AGE. In Argentina, RVA positivity decreased from 26.8% to 13.6% comparing the pre- and post-vaccination periods [37]. Other studies performed elsewhere have described RVA detection rates varying from 8.4% to 23.2% [38–42].

RVA seasonality has been well defined, especially for temperate climate countries, where RVA peaks during dry and cold months. In tropical areas, RVA circulates year-round without marked peaks of infections [43,44]. In Brazil, we observed a year-round RVA circulation without marked seasonality, but high detections rates of RVA was observed during winter/spring months, in agreement with other studies [42,45]. RVA highest detection rate was observed in September 2019 (36.7%) in line with findings observed over a 21-year period in Brazil [20], and also with Luchs et al. [46] that demonstrated the peak of RV incidence in September during a five-year RVA surveillance study (2007–2012) in Brazil. As a continental-size country, we analyzed separately, RVA circulation in Southern states in comparison with Southeastern and Northeastern states (Figure 1B,C). We observed more clear peaks of RVA infections in winter/spring months (June 21st to December 20th) in Southern states (Rio Grande do Sul—RS, and Santa Catarina—SC) compared to Southeastern and Northeastern Brazil. This could be explained as both RS and SC states are in a subtropical area, characterized by different climate pattern compared to the other states. A three-year study conducted in Vietnam to access RVA epidemiology in AGE cases also demonstrated varied seasonally positivity, with different RVA-detection peaks among the three regions analyzed—North, Central, and South [47]. The fact that RVA usually peaks in September in Brazil, observed here and by others [20,46], is an important information to authorities to prepare strategies to reduce AGE impacts in the health system.

Regarding RVA infections among different age groups, we observed a significantly high positivity rate among children aged >24 and 60 months compared to other age groups. This shifting in the age of children more affected by RVA illness (older children) has been observed, especially in countries that have introduced RVA mass vaccination. Our data are consistent with previous findings reported from Brazil [20] and the USA [48,49]. In contrast, countries where RVA vaccines are yet to be introduced into national immunization programs, have reported the majority of RVA positive children (~90%) within the first 2 years of life [44,47]. By analyzing RVA shedding among the age groups, we found a statistically lower viral load among children less than six months (Figure 3). We believe that this lower viral load could be mostly explained by the passive protection mediated by breast milk maternal antibodies [50], but also by the higher effectiveness and prompt immune response generated by Rotarix™ after the oral doses administered at the age of 2 and 4 months [17]. However, this second hypothesis alone could not explain the high viral load among children aged >6 and 12 months. In addition, high Ct values could indicate less severe disease [51]. In that study, authors demonstrated that the severity of diarrhea, determined by the Vesikari score, was significantly and negatively associated with Ct values of children stool samples.

Regarding RVA genotype characterization, we successfully identified G- and P-types in 89% of positive samples, by one-step multiplex RT-PCR and sequencing. By far, G3P[8] was the most prevalent genotype in both years. The phylogenetic analysis of the VP7 gene revealed that the majority of the Brazilian strains sequenced (94%) belong to the equine-like G3 genotype (G3-1). Moreover, all the P[8] strains sequenced clustered within the P[8]-3 lineage. This P[8]-3, harboring a G12-type, was the dominant strain in Brazil in 2014, detected in 75% of genotyped samples [52].

Emergent equine-like DS-1-like G3P[8] RVA strains were firstly identified in children with AGE in Australia in 2013 [53]. From 2013 onwards, the equine-like G3P[8] DS-1-like genotype has spread and become endemic worldwide [54–60]. In Brazil, the first evidence of the circulation of equine-like G3P[8] date from 2015, when Luchs et al. [24] detected the reassortant RVA strain in a touristic city of Southern Brazil, Foz do Iguaçu, that borders Argentina and Paraguay. Subsequently, these novel viruses quickly spread to other states in Brazil, being the most prevalent genotype in 2017 (66.2%). The occurrence of DS-1-like G3P[8] RVA strains was also reported in Amazon region, Northern Brazil in 2016 [60]. In the previous study from our group, we demonstrated the increase of G3P[8] from 2015, peaking in the last year of the study—2017. However, it was not investigated whether they belonged to the DS-1-like RVA group [20]. More recently, countries such as Australia, Italy and Pakistan, have demonstrated the high prevalence of the emergent equine-like G3P[8] genotype [42,45,61].

Atypical genotypes G3P[6], G6P[8], G2P[6], and G12P[6] were also detected as minor genotypes in our study. The phylogenetic analysis of the VP7 gene demonstrated that Brazilian G6-1 strains were closely related to strains circulating in Bulgaria and Italy [62,63]. The genotype G12P[6] characterized in our study has been frequently detected in Nepal, with detection rates of 46.4% in 2013 and 36% in 2014, among AGE cases in children less than five years of age [64,65]. Unexpectedly, we did not detected the former dominant G2P[4] genotype. In Brazil, after Rotarix™ implementation in March 2006, this genotype has been the most frequently detected until 2015 [66], however, the recently low prevalence of G2P[4] viruses could be explained a cyclical pattern of circulation along with the herd induced homotypic immunity and depletion of the susceptible population [20].

A major strength of our study is that we included data from eleven states, representing around 100 million inhabitants (almost half of Brazilian population). Albeit, this could be considered as a major limitation as well, since the variability in reporting and collecting AGE cases by states generates surveillance biases. Another limitation is that important RVA genes, such as VP6 and NSP4, were not characterized. Nevertheless, future studies approaching a more complete genetic characterization of G3P[8] strains, as well as unusual genotypes detected here (G3P[6] and G12P[6]) will be performed, in order to monitor RVA genotypes spread and evolution over time.

In conclusion, we found a 12% of RVA-positivity in AGE cases from Brazil, and according to global trends, the equine-like G3P[8] was the dominant genotype in 2018 and 2019. The constant shifting of RVA genotypes circulation and the potential emergence of unusual/reassortant strains reinforces the importance and the need for continuous country-based epidemiological and molecular surveillance programs.

**Author Contributions:** Conceptualization, M.B.G., M.P.M., J.P.G.L., and T.M.F.; methodology, M.B.G., A.M.F., A.G.M., F.C.M., J.d.S.R.d.A., R.M.S.d.A., and S.d.S.e.M.; formal analysis, M.B.G. and T.M.F.; investigation, M.B.G., F.C.M., J.d.S.R.d.A., R.M.S.d.A., and T.M.F.; writing—original draft preparation, M.B.G. and T.M.F.; writing—review and editing, T.M.F., M.P.M., J.P.G.L., A.M.F., A.G.M., F.C.M., J.d.S.R.d.A., R.M.S.d.A., and S.d.S.e.M.; supervision, T.M.F.; project administration, T.M.F.; M.P.M., and J.P.G.L.; funding acquisition, T.M.F. and J.P.G.L. All authors have read and agreed to the published version of the manuscript.

**Acknowledgments:** We would like to thank the Rotavirus Surveillance System, coordinated by the Coordenação Geral de Laboratórios de Saúde Pública (CGLab), Brazilian Ministry of Health, and the State Central Laboratories involved in the study.

# References

1. WHO | Levels and Trends in Child Mortality Report 2019. Available online: https://www.who.int/maternal_child_adolescent/documents/levels_trends_child_mortality_2019/en/ (accessed on 2 May 2020).
2. Liu, L.; Qian, Y.; Zhang, Y.; Zhao, L.; Jia, L.; Dong, H. Epidemiological aspects of rotavirus and adenovirus in hospitalized children with diarrhea: A 5-year survey in Beijing. *BMC Infect. Dis.* **2016**, *16*, 508. [CrossRef] [PubMed]
3. Bányai, K.; Estes, M.K.; Martella, V.; Parashar, U.D. Viral gastroenteritis. *Lancet* **2018**, *392*, 175–186. [CrossRef]
4. Troeger, C.; Khalil, I.A.; Rao, P.C.; Cao, S.; Blacker, B.F.; Ahmed, T.; Armah, G.; Bines, J.E.; Brewer, T.G.; Colombara, D.V.; et al. Rotavirus Vaccination and the Global Burden of Rotavirus Diarrhea Among Children Younger Than 5 Years. *JAMA Pediatr.* **2018**, *172*, 958–965. [CrossRef]
5. Tate, J.E.; Burton, A.H.; Boschi-Pinto, C.; Parashar, U.D.; World Health Organization–Coordinated Global Rotavirus Surveillance Network. Global, Regional, and National Estimates of Rotavirus Mortality in Children <5 Years of Age, 2000–2013. *Clin. Infect. Dis* **2016**, *62*, S96–S105. [CrossRef]
6. Burnett, E.; Parashar, U.D.; Tate, J.E. Global impact of rotavirus vaccination on diarrhea hospitalizations and deaths among children <5 years old: 2006–2019. *J. Infect. Dis.* **2020**. [CrossRef]
7. Aliabadi, N.; Antoni, S.; Mwenda, J.M.; Weldegebriel, G.; Biey, J.N.M.; Cheikh, D.; Fahmy, K.; Teleb, N.; Ashmony, H.A.; Ahmed, H.; et al. Global impact of rotavirus vaccine introduction on rotavirus hospitalisations among children under 5 years of age, 2008–2016: Findings from the Global Rotavirus Surveillance Network. *Lancet Glob. Health* **2019**, *7*, e893–e903. [CrossRef]
8. Burke, R.M.; Tate, J.E.; Kirkwood, C.D.; Steele, A.D.; Parashar, U.D. Current and new rotavirus vaccines. *Curr. Opin. Infect. Dis.* **2019**, *32*, 435–444. [CrossRef] [PubMed]
9. Matthijnssens, J.; Van Ranst, M. Genotype constellation and evolution of group A rotaviruses infecting humans. *Curr. Opin. Virol.* **2012**, *2*, 426–433. [CrossRef]
10. Dóró, R.; Farkas, S.L.; Martella, V.; Bányai, K. Zoonotic transmission of rotavirus: Surveillance and control. *Expert Rev. Anti. Infect. Ther.* **2015**, *13*, 1337–1350. [CrossRef] [PubMed]
11. Matthijnssens, J.; Ciarlet, M.; Heiman, E.; Arijs, I.; Delbeke, T.; McDonald, S.M.; Palombo, E.A.; Iturriza-Gómara, M.; Maes, P.; Patton, J.T.; et al. Full genome-based classification of rotaviruses reveals a common origin between human Wa-Like and porcine rotavirus strains and human DS-1-like and bovine rotavirus strains. *J. Virol.* **2008**, *82*, 3204–3219. [CrossRef]
12. Rotavirus Classification Working Group: RCWG. Available online: https://rega.kuleuven.be/cev/viralmetagenomics/virus-classification/rcwg (accessed on 10 May 2020).
13. Dóró, R.; László, B.; Martella, V.; Leshem, E.; Gentsch, J.; Parashar, U.; Bányai, K. Review of global rotavirus strain prevalence data from six years post vaccine licensure surveillance: Is there evidence of strain selection from vaccine pressure? *Infect. Genet. Evol.* **2014**, *28*, 446–461. [CrossRef]
14. Bányai, K.; László, B.; Duque, J.; Steele, A.D.; Nelson, E.A.S.; Gentsch, J.R.; Parashar, U.D. Systematic review of regional and temporal trends in global rotavirus strain diversity in the pre rotavirus vaccine era: Insights for understanding the impact of rotavirus vaccination programs. *Vaccine* **2012**, *30*, A122–A130. [CrossRef] [PubMed]
15. Iturriza-Gómara, M.; Dallman, T.; Bányai, K.; Böttiger, B.; Buesa, J.; Diedrich, S.; Fiore, L.; Johansen, K.; Koopmans, M.; Korsun, N.; et al. Rotavirus genotypes co-circulating in Europe between 2006 and 2009 as determined by EuroRotaNet, a pan-European collaborative strain surveillance network. *Epidemiol. Infect.* **2011**, *139*, 895–909. [CrossRef] [PubMed]
16. de A. Mendes, P.S.; da C. Ribeiro, H.; Mendes, C.M.C. Temporal trends of overall mortality and hospital morbidity due to diarrheal disease in Brazilian children younger than 5 years from 2000 to 2010. *J. Pediatr. (Rio J.)* **2013**, *89*, 315–325. [CrossRef] [PubMed]
17. Gurgel, R.Q.; Alvarez, A.D.J.; Rodrigues, A.; Ribeiro, R.R.; Dolabella, S.S.; Da Mota, N.L.; Santos, V.S.; Iturriza-Gomara, M.; Cunliffe, N.A.; Cuevas, L.E. Incidence of Rotavirus and Circulating Genotypes in Northeast Brazil during 7 Years of National Rotavirus Vaccination. *PLoS ONE* **2014**, *9*. [CrossRef]
18. Gurgel, R.G.; Bohland, A.K.; Vieira, S.C.F.; Oliveira, D.M.P.; Fontes, P.B.; Barros, V.F.; Ramos, M.F.; Dove, W.; Nakagomi, T.; Nakagomi, O.; et al. Incidence of rotavirus and all-cause diarrhea in northeast Brazil following the introduction of a national vaccination program. *Gastroenterology* **2009**, *137*, 1970–1975. [CrossRef] [PubMed]

19. Linhares, A.C.; Velázquez, F.R.; Pérez-Schael, I.; Sáez-Llorens, X.; Abate, H.; Espinoza, F.; López, P.; Macías-Parra, M.; Ortega-Barría, E.; Rivera-Medina, D.M.; et al. Efficacy and safety of an oral live attenuated human rotavirus vaccine against rotavirus gastroenteritis during the first 2 years of life in Latin American infants: A randomised, double-blind, placebo-controlled phase III study. *Lancet* **2008**, *371*, 1181–1189. [CrossRef]
20. Carvalho-Costa, F.A.; de Assis, R.M.S.; Fialho, A.M.; Araújo, I.T.; Silva, M.F.; Gómez, M.M.; Andrade, J.S.; Rose, T.L.; Fumian, T.M.; Volotão, E.M.; et al. The evolving epidemiology of rotavirus A infection in Brazil a decade after the introduction of universal vaccination with Rotarix®. *BMC Pediatr.* **2019**, *19*, 42. [CrossRef]
21. Carvalho-Costa, F.A.; de M. Volotão, E.; de Assis, R.M.S.; Fialho, A.M.; da S.R. de Andrade, J.; Rocha, L.N.; Tort, L.F.L.; da Silva, M.F.M.; Gómez, M.M.; de Souza, P.M.; et al. Laboratory-based rotavirus surveillance during the introduction of a vaccination program, Brazil, 2005–2009. *Pediatr. Infect. Dis. J.* **2011**, *30*, S35–S41. [CrossRef]
22. Luchs, A.; do C.S.T. Timenetsky, M. Group A rotavirus gastroenteritis: Post-vaccine era, genotypes and zoonotic transmission. *Einstein (Sao Paulo)* **2016**, *14*, 278–287. [CrossRef] [PubMed]
23. da Silva Soares, L.; de Fátima Dos Santos Guerra, S.; do Socorro Lima de Oliveira, A.; da Silva Dos Santos, F.; de Fátima Costa de Menezes, E.M.; Mascarenhas, J.; d'Arc, P.; Linhares, A.C. Diversity of rotavirus strains circulating in Northern Brazil after introduction of a rotavirus vaccine: High prevalence of G3P[6] genotype. *J. Med. Virol.* **2014**, *86*, 1065–1072. [CrossRef]
24. Luchs, A.; da Costa, A.C.; Cilli, A.; Komninakis, S.C.V.; de C.C. Carmona, R.; Boen, L.; Morillo, S.G.; Sabino, E.C.; do C.S.T. Timenetsky, M. Spread of the emerging equine-like G3P[8] DS-1-like genetic backbone rotavirus strain in Brazil and identification of potential genetic variants. *J. Gen. Virol.* **2019**, *100*, 7–25. [CrossRef] [PubMed]
25. Jing, Z.; Zhang, X.; Shi, H.; Chen, J.; Shi, D.; Dong, H.; Feng, L. A G3P[13] porcine group A rotavirus emerging in China is a reassortant and a natural recombinant in the VP4 gene. *Transbound. Emerg. Dis.* **2018**, *65*, e317–e328. [CrossRef] [PubMed]
26. Komoto, S.; Tacharoenmuang, R.; Guntapong, R.; Ide, T.; Sinchai, P.; Upachai, S.; Fukuda, S.; Yoshikawa, T.; Tharmaphornpilas, P.; Sangkitporn, S.; et al. Identification and characterization of a human G9P[23] rotavirus strain from a child with diarrhoea in Thailand: Evidence for porcine-to-human interspecies transmission. *J. Gen. Virol.* **2017**, *98*, 532–538. [CrossRef] [PubMed]
27. Quaye, O.; Roy, S.; Rungsrisuriyachai, K.; Esona, M.D.; Xu, Z.; Tam, K.I.; Banegas, D.J.C.; Rey-Benito, G.; Bowen, M.D. Characterisation of a rare, reassortant human G10P[14] rotavirus strain detected in Honduras. *Mem. Inst. Oswaldo Cruz* **2018**, *113*, 9–16. [CrossRef]
28. Tacharoenmuang, R.; Komoto, S.; Guntapong, R.; Ide, T.; Singchai, P.; Upachai, S.; Fukuda, S.; Yoshida, Y.; Murata, T.; Yoshikawa, T.; et al. Characterization of a G10P[14] rotavirus strain from a diarrheic child in Thailand: Evidence for bovine-to-human zoonotic transmission. *Infect. Genet. Evol.* **2018**, *63*, 43–57. [CrossRef]
29. Gentsch, J.R.; Parashar, U.D.; Glass, R.I. Impact of rotavirus vaccination: The importance of monitoring strains. *Future Microbiol.* **2009**, *4*, 1231–1234. [CrossRef]
30. Matthijnssens, J.; Bilcke, J.; Ciarlet, M.; Martella, V.; Bányai, K.; Rahman, M.; Zeller, M.; Beutels, P.; Van Damme, P.; Van Ranst, M. Rotavirus disease and vaccination: Impact on genotype diversity. *Future Microbiol.* **2009**, *4*, 1303–1316. [CrossRef]
31. Roczo-Farkas, S.; Kirkwood, C.D.; Cowley, D.; Barnes, G.L.; Bishop, R.F.; Bogdanovic-Sakran, N.; Boniface, K.; Donato, C.M.; Bines, J.E. The Impact of Rotavirus Vaccines on Genotype Diversity: A Comprehensive Analysis of 2 Decades of Australian Surveillance Data. *J. Infect. Dis.* **2018**, *218*, 546–554. [CrossRef]
32. Esona, M.D.; Gautam, R.; Tam, K.I.; Williams, A.; Mijatovic-Rustempasic, S.; Bowen, M.D. Multiplexed one-step RT-PCR VP7 and VP4 genotyping assays for rotaviruses using updated primers. *J. Virol. Methods* **2015**, *223*, 96–104. [CrossRef]
33. Gómara, M.I.; Cubitt, D.; Desselberger, U.; Gray, J. Amino acid substitution within the VP7 protein of G2 rotavirus strains associated with failure to serotype. *J. Clin. Microbiol.* **2001**, *39*, 3796–3798. [CrossRef] [PubMed]
34. Gentsch, J.R.; Glass, R.I.; Woods, P.; Gouvea, V.; Gorziglia, M.; Flores, J.; Das, B.K.; Bhan, M.K. Identification of group A rotavirus gene 4 types by polymerase chain reaction. *J. Clin. Microbiol.* **1992**, *30*, 1365–1373. [CrossRef] [PubMed]

35. Kumar, S.; Stecher, G.; Li, M.; Knyaz, C.; Tamura, K. MEGA X: Molecular Evolutionary Genetics Analysis across Computing Platforms. *Mol. Biol. Evol.* **2018**, *35*, 1547–1549. [CrossRef] [PubMed]
36. Justino, M.C.A.; Campos, E.A.; Mascarenhas, J.D.P.; Soares, L.S.; de F.S. Guerra, S.; Furlaneto, I.P.; Pavão, M.J.C.; Maciel, T.S.; Farias, F.P.; Bezerra, O.M.; et al. Rotavirus antigenemia as a common event among children hospitalised for severe, acute gastroenteritis in Belém, northern Brazil. *BMC Pediatr.* **2019**, *19*, 193. [CrossRef] [PubMed]
37. Degiuseppe, J.I.; Stupka, J.A. First assessment of all-cause acute diarrhoea and rotavirus-confirmed cases following massive vaccination in Argentina. *Epidemiol. Infect.* **2018**, *146*, 1948–1954. [CrossRef]
38. Junaid, S.A.; Umeh, C.; Olabode, A.O.; Banda, J.M. Incidence of rotavirus infection in children with gastroenteritis attending Jos university teaching hospital, Nigeria. *Virol. J.* **2011**, *8*, 233. [CrossRef]
39. Nordgren, J.; Bonkoungou, I.J.O.; Nitiema, L.W.; Sharma, S.; Ouermi, D.; Simpore, J.; Barro, N.; Svensson, L. Rotavirus in diarrheal children in rural Burkina Faso: High prevalence of genotype G6P[6]. *Infect. Genet. Evol.* **2012**, *12*, 1892–1898. [CrossRef]
40. Umair, M.; Abbasi, B.H.; Sharif, S.; Alam, M.M.; Rana, M.S.; Mujtaba, G.; Arshad, Y.; Fatmi, M.Q.; Zaidi, S.Z. High prevalence of G3 rotavirus in hospitalized children in Rawalpindi, Pakistan during 2014. *PLoS ONE* **2018**, *13*, e0195947. [CrossRef]
41. Halasa, N.; Piya, B.; Stewart, L.S.; Rahman, H.; Payne, D.C.; Woron, A.; Thomas, L.; Constantine-Renna, L.; Garman, K.; McHenry, R.; et al. The Changing Landscape of Pediatric Viral Enteropathogens in the Post-Rotavirus Vaccine Era. *Clin. Infect. Dis.* **2020**. [CrossRef]
42. Rovida, F.; Nepita, E.V.; Giardina, F.; Piralla, A.; Campanini, G.; Baldanti, F. Rotavirus molecular epidemiology in hospitalized patients, Northern Italy, 2015–2018. *New Microbiol.* **2020**, *43*, 1–5.
43. Levy, K.; Hubbard, A.E.; Eisenberg, J.N.S. Seasonality of rotavirus disease in the tropics: A systematic review and meta-analysis. *Int. J. Epidemiol.* **2009**, *38*, 1487–1496. [CrossRef] [PubMed]
44. Samdan, A.; Ganbold, S.; Guntev, O.; Orosoo, S.; Javzandorj, N.; Gongor, A.; Enkhtuvshin, A.; Demberelsuren, S.; Abdul, W.; Jee, Y.; et al. Hospital-based surveillance for rotavirus diarrhea in Ulaanbaatar, Mongolia, April 2009 through March 2016. *Vaccine* **2018**, *36*, 7883–7887. [CrossRef] [PubMed]
45. Sadiq, A.; Bostan, N.; Bokhari, H.; Matthijnssens, J.; Yinda, K.C.; Raza, S.; Nawaz, T. Molecular characterization of human group A rotavirus genotypes circulating in Rawalpindi, Islamabad, Pakistan during 2015-2016. *PLoS ONE* **2019**, *14*. [CrossRef]
46. Luchs, A.; Cilli, A.; Morillo, S.G.; de C.C. Carmona, R.; do C.S.T. Timenetsky, M. ROTAVIRUS GENOTYPES CIRCULATING IN BRAZIL, 2007-2012: IMPLICATIONS FOR THE VACCINE PROGRAM. *Rev. Inst. Med. Trop. Sao Paulo* **2015**, *57*, 305–313. [CrossRef]
47. Huyen, D.T.T.; Hong, D.T.; Trung, N.T.; Hoa, T.T.N.; Oanh, N.K.; Thang, H.V.; Thao, N.T.T.; Hung, D.M.; Iijima, M.; Fox, K.; et al. Epidemiology of acute diarrhea caused by rotavirus in sentinel surveillance sites of Vietnam, 2012–2015. *Vaccine* **2018**, *36*, 7894–7900. [CrossRef]
48. Hull, J.J.; Teel, E.N.; Kerin, T.K.; Freeman, M.M.; Esona, M.D.; Gentsch, J.R.; Cortese, M.M.; Parashar, U.D.; Glass, R.I.; Bowen, M.D.; et al. United States rotavirus strain surveillance from 2005 to 2008: Genotype prevalence before and after vaccine introduction. *Pediatr. Infect. Dis. J.* **2011**, *30*, S42–S47. [CrossRef]
49. Desai, R.; Parashar, U.D.; Lopman, B.; de Oliveira, L.H.; Clark, A.D.; Sanderson, C.F.B.; Tate, J.E.; Matus, C.R.; Andrus, J.K.; Patel, M.M. Potential intussusception risk versus health benefits from rotavirus vaccination in Latin America. *Clin. Infect. Dis.* **2012**, *54*, 1397–1405. [CrossRef]
50. Clarke, E.; Desselberger, U. Correlates of protection against human rotavirus disease and the factors influencing protection in low-income settings. *Mucosal. Immunol.* **2015**, *8*, 1–17. [CrossRef]
51. Kang, G.; Iturriza-Gomara, M.; Wheeler, J.G.; Crystal, P.; Monica, B.; Ramani, S.; Primrose, B.; Moses, P.D.; Gallimore, C.I.; Brown, D.W.; et al. Quantitation of Group A Rotavirus by Real-Time Reverse-Transcription-Polymerase Chain Reaction. *J. Med. Virol.* **2004**, *73*, 118–122. [CrossRef]
52. da Silva, M.F.M.; Fumian, T.M.; de Assis, R.M.S.; Fialho, A.M.; Carvalho-Costa, F.A.; da Silva Ribeiro de Andrade, J.; Leite, J.P.G. VP7 and VP8* genetic characterization of group A rotavirus genotype G12P[8]: Emergence and spreading in the Eastern Brazilian coast in 2014. *J. Med. Virol.* **2017**, *89*, 64–70. [CrossRef]
53. Kirkwood, C.D.; Roczo-Farkas, S.; Australian Rotavirus Surveillance Group. Australian Rotavirus Surveillance Program annual report, 2013. *Commun. Dis. Intell. Q Rep.* **2014**, *38*, E334–E342.
54. Arana, A.; Montes, M.; Jere, K.C.; Alkorta, M.; Iturriza-Gómara, M.; Cilla, G. Emergence and spread of

G3P[8] rotaviruses possessing an equine-like VP7 and a DS-1-like genetic backbone in the Basque Country (North of Spain), 2015. *Infect. Genet. Evol.* **2016** *44*, 137–144. [CrossRef] [PubMed]

55. Dóró, R.; Marton, S.; Bartókné, A.H.; Lengyel, G.; Agócs, Z.; Jakab, F.; Bányai, K. Equine-like G3 rotavirus in Hungary, 2015–Is it a novel intergenogroup reassortant pandemic strain? *Acta. Microbiol. Immunol. Hung.* **2016**, *63*, 243–255. [CrossRef]

56. Perkins, C.; Mijatovic-Rustempasic, S.; Ward, M.L.; Cortese, M.M.; Bowen, M.D. Genomic Characterization of the First Equine-Like G3P[8] Rotavirus Strain Detected in the United States. *Genome. Announc.* **2017**, *5*. [CrossRef]

57. Kikuchi, W.; Nakagomi, T.; Gauchan, P.; Agbemabiese, C.A.; Noguchi, A.; Nakagomi, O.; Takahashi, T. Detection in Japan of an equine-like G3P[8] reassortant rotavirus A strain that is highly homologous to European strains across all genome segments. *Arch. Virol.* **2018**, *163*, 791–794. [CrossRef]

58. Komoto, S.; Ide, T.; Negoro, M.; Tanaka, T.; Asada, K.; Umemoto, M.; Kuroki, H.; Ito, H.; Tanaka, S.; Ito, M.; et al. Characterization of unusual DS-1-like G3P[8] rotavirus strains in children with diarrhea in Japan. *J. Med. Virol.* **2018**, *90*, 890–898. [CrossRef]

59. Pietsch, C.; Liebert, U.G. Molecular characterization of different equine-like G3 rotavirus strains from Germany. *Infect. Genet. Evol.* **2018**, *57*, 46–50. [CrossRef] [PubMed]

60. Guerra, S.F.S.; Soares, L.S.; Lobo, P.S.; Penha Júnior, E.T.; Sousa Júnior, E.C.; Bezerra, D.A.M.; Vaz, L.R.; Linhares, A.C.; Mascarenhas, J.D.P. Detection of a novel equine-like G3 rotavirus associated with acute gastroenteritis in Brazil. *J. Gen. Virol.* **2016**, *97*, 3131–3138. [CrossRef]

61. Maguire, J.E.; Glasgow, K.; Glass, K.; Roczo-Farkas, S.; Bines, J.E.; Sheppeard, V.; Macartney, K.; Quinn, H.E. Rotavirus Epidemiology and Monovalent Rotavirus Vaccine Effectiveness in Australia: 2010–2017. *Pediatrics* **2019**, *144*. [CrossRef]

62. Ianiro, G.; Delogu, R.; Camilloni, B.; Lorini, C.; Ruggeri, F.M.; Fiore, L. Detection of unusual G6 rotavirus strains in Italian children with diarrhoea during the 2011 surveillance season. *J. Med. Virol.* **2013**, *85*, 1860–1869. [CrossRef]

63. Mladenova, Z.; Nawaz, S.; Ganesh, B.; Iturriza-Gomara, M. Increased detection of G3P[9] and G6P[9] rotavirus strains in hospitalized children with acute diarrhea in Bulgaria. *Infect. Genet. Evol.* **2015**, *29*, 118–126. [CrossRef]

64. Ansari, S.; Sherchand, J.B.; Rijal, B.P.; Parajuli, K.; Mishra, S.K.; Dahal, R.K.; Shrestha, S.; Tandukar, S.; Chaudhary, R.; Kattel, H.P.; et al. Characterization of rotavirus causing acute diarrhoea in children in Kathmandu, Nepal, showing the dominance of serotype G12. *J. Med. Microbiol.* **2013**, *62*, 114–120. [CrossRef] [PubMed]

65. Dhital, S.; Sherchand, J.B.; Pokhrel, B.M.; Parajuli, K.; Shah, N.; Mishra, S.K.; Sharma, S.; Kattel, H.P.; Khadka, S.; Khatiwada, S.; et al. Molecular epidemiology of Rotavirus causing diarrhea among children less than five years of age visiting national level children hospitals, Nepal. *BMC Pediatr.* **2017**, *17*, 101. [CrossRef] [PubMed]

66. Santos, V.S.; Gurgel, R.Q.; Cavalcante, S.M.M.; Kirby, A.; Café, L.P.; Souto, M.J.; Dolabella, S.S.; de Assis, M.R.; Fumian, T.M.; Miagostovich, M.P.; et al. Acute norovirus gastroenteritis in children in a highly rotavirus-vaccinated population in Northeast Brazil. *J. Clin. Virol.* **2017**, *88*, 33–38. [CrossRef]

# Uncovering the First Atypical DS-1-like G1P[8] Rotavirus Strains That Circulated during Pre-Rotavirus Vaccine Introduction Era in South Africa

Peter N. Mwangi [1], Milton T. Mogotsi [1], Sebotsana P. Rasebotsa [1], Mapaseka L. Seheri [2], M. Jeffrey Mphahlele [3], Valantine N. Ndze [4], Francis E. Dennis [5], Khuzwayo C. Jere [6,7] and Martin M. Nyaga [1,*]

[1] Next Generation Sequencing Unit, Division of Virology, Faculty of Health Sciences, University of the Free State, Bloemfontein 9300, South Africa; 2017219839@ufs4life.ac.za (P.N.M.); tmogotsi16@gmail.com (M.T.M.); RasebotsaS@ufs.ac.za (S.P.R.)
[2] Diarrhoeal Pathogens Research Unit, Sefako Makgatho Health Sciences University, Medunsa 0204, Pretoria, South Africa; mapaseka.seheri@smu.ac.za
[3] South African Medical Research Council, 1 Soutpansberg Road, Pretoria 0001, South Africa; Jeffrey.Mphahlele@mrc.ac.za
[4] Faculty of Health Sciences, University of Buea, P.O. Box 63, Buea, Cameroon; valentinengum@yahoo.com
[5] Noguchi Memorial Institute for Medical Research, University of Ghana, P.O. Box LG581, Legon, Ghana; FDennis@noguchi.ug.edu.gh
[6] Centre for Global Vaccine Research, Institute of Infection and Global Health, University of Liverpool, Ronald Ross Building, 8 West Derby Street, Liverpool L69 7BE, UK; Khuzwayo.Jere@liverpool.ac.uk
[7] Malawi-Liverpool-Wellcome Trust Clinical Research Programme, College of Medicine, University of Malawi, Blantyre 312225, Malawi
* Correspondence: NyagaMM@ufs.ac.za;

**Abstract:** Emergence of DS-1-like G1P[8] group A rotavirus (RVA) strains during post-rotavirus vaccination period has recently been reported in several countries. This study demonstrates, for the first time, rare atypical DS-1-like G1P[8] RVA strains that circulated in 2008 during pre-vaccine era in South Africa. Rotavirus positive samples were subjected to whole-genome sequencing. Two G1P[8] strains (RVA/Human-wt/ZAF/UFS-NGS-MRC-DPRU1971/2008/G1P[8] and RVA/Human-wt/ZAF/UFS-NGS-MRC-DPRU1973/2008/G1P[8]) possessed a DS-1-like genome constellation background (I2-R2-C2-M2-A2-N2-T2-E2-H2). The outer VP4 and VP7 capsid genes of the two South African G1P[8] strains had the highest nucleotide (amino acid) nt (aa) identities of 99.6–99.9% (99.1–100%) with the VP4 and the VP7 genes of a locally circulating South African strain, RVA/Human-wt/ZAF/MRC-DPRU1039/2008/G1P[8]. All the internal backbone genes (VP1–VP3, VP6, and NSP1-NSP5) had the highest nt (aa) identities with cognate internal genes of another locally circulating South African strain, RVA/Human-wt/ZAF/MRC-DPRU2344/2008/G2P[6]. The two study strains emerged through reassortment mechanism involving locally circulating South African strains, as they were distinctly unrelated to other reported atypical G1P[8] strains. The identification of these G1P[8] double-gene reassortants during the pre-vaccination period strongly supports natural RVA evolutionary mechanisms of the RVA genome. There is a need to maintain long-term whole-genome surveillance to monitor such atypical strains.

**Keywords:** atypical strains; genome constellation; reassortment; rotavirus; whole-genome characterization

## 1. Introduction

Diarrhea persists as a leading infectious mortality cause in children under the age of five worldwide [1]. Group A rotavirus (RVA) is the primary viral etiologic agent for acute gastroenteritis in children under five years of age [2], resulting in annual mortality cases ranging from 122,322 to 215,757 with an estimated 81% reported in sub-Saharan Africa and Southeast Asia [3,4]. To combat RVA diarrhea, especially in countries with high RVA disease burden, the World Health Organization (WHO) recommends incorporation of RVA vaccines into the national immunization programs alongside other childhood vaccines [5]. The WHO has prequalified four vaccines (Rotarix®, GlaxoSmithKline, Rixenstart, Belgium; RotaTeq®, Merck & Co, USA; ROTAVAC®, Bharat Biotech, Hyderabad, India and ROTASIL®, Serum Institute of India, Pune, India) for global use [6]. Two vaccines (Rotavin-M1®, POLYVAC, Hanoi, Vietnam and Lanzhou lamb rotavirus, Lanzhou Institute of Biological Products, Lanzhou, China) have been approved for national use in Vietnam and China, respectively [7,8]. Human neonatal RVA vaccine (RV3-BB) and bovine human reassortant RVA vaccine candidates as well as neonatal and non-replicating injectable vaccines are in the pipeline [9]. South Africa was the first African country to adopt the monovalent RVA vaccine (Rotarix®) in September 2009 into its Expanded Program on Immunization (EPI) (WHO, 2009), which culminated in a 77% reduction in RVA disease during the first year that the vaccine was introduced [10,11].

Rotaviruses belong to the *Reoviridae* family. The RV genome is composed of 11 segments of double-stranded RNA (dsRNA) encapsulated in a three-layered protein capsid. Six structural proteins (VP1–VP4, VP6, and VP7) and five or sometimes six non-structural proteins (NSP1–NSP5/NSP6) that encode the RV genome [2]. The outer capsid proteins, VP7 and VP4, which act as neutralizing agents, are universally applied in the binary classification of RV strains into G and P types, respectively [2]. The contemporary classification of RVA strains is based on whole-genome composition underpinned by the nucleotide homology cutoff values that have been determined for the open reading frame (ORF) of each gene segment [12,13]. The numbers of currently described genotypes are 36 G (VP7), 51 P (VP4), 26 I (VP6), 22 R (VP1), 20 C (VP2), 20 M (VP3), 31 A (NSP1), 22 N (NSP2), 22T (NSP3), 27 E (NSP4), and 22 H (NSP5) (http://rega.kuleuven.be/cev/viralmetagenomics/virus-classification).

The globally predominant RVA genotypes are G1P[8], G2P[4], G3P[8], G4P[8], G9P[8], and G12P[8] [14]. However, RVA strains variability by region is well documented [15]. In Africa, RVA genotypes such as G1P[6], G8P[4], G8P[6], G8P[8], and G9P[6] are substantially prevalent but uncommon elsewhere [14–17]. Additionally, G3P[8] and G4P[8] genotypes have been on the decline in Africa and have not been detected in many African countries for almost a decade aside from an impromptu emergence of equine-like G3P[6] and G3P[8] in Botswana and Eswatini [18]. RVAs are classified further into three genogroups: Wa-like, which bears a genotype 1 constellation (I1-R1-C1-M1 A1-N1-T1-E1-H1), DS-1-like, which bears genotype 2 constellation (I2-R2-C2-M2-A2-N2-T2-E2-H2), and a relatively minor AU-1-like characterized by genotype 3 constellation (I3-R3-C3 M3-A3-N3-T3-E3-H3) [19]. Typically, G1P[8], G3P[8], G4P[8], G9P[8], and G12P[8] RVA have a Wa-like genotype constellation, whereas G2P[4], G8P[4], and G8P[6] strains usually have a DS-1-like genotype constellation [19]. G1P[8] is the world's most prevalent genotype accountable for an estimated 50% of RVA infections [20]. The vast antigenic and genetic heterogeneity of G1P[8] strains contributes to the persistent recurrence of VP4 and VP7 protein variants, and the epidemiological fitness of some of these variants might be accountable for their global prevalence [21].

The segmented RNA genome of RVA facilitates reassortment and recombination events, and the error-prone RNA-dependent RNA polymerase promotes high mutation rates [2]. These evolutionary mechanisms lead to the emergence of novel strains and distinct lineages [22]. Intergenogroup reassortment of G1P[8] gene segments has been reported in Africa, Asia, and the Americas [23–27]. These atypical G1P[8] strains were first reported in Okayama Prefecture, Japan during 2012–2013 post-RVA vaccine surveillance of acute gastroenteritis and then in other prefectures, including Aichi, Akita, Kyoto, and Osaka [25–27]. Subsequent incidences were then reported during 2013 post-RVA vaccine surveillance in Phetchabun and Sukhothai provinces in Thailand [28,29] and in 2012–2013 during the pre-RVA vaccine period in Hanoi, Vietnam [30]. Although unpublished, sequence data of G1P[8] DS-1-like sequence strains isolated during pre-vaccine period between August–November 2012 in Palawan, Southwestern region of Philippines have been deposited in the GenBank database. Recently, for the first time in the Americas, G1P[8] DS-1-like strains were reported in 2013 during post-RVA vaccination period from the states of Sao Paulo and Goias in Brazil [23]. In Africa, Jere and colleagues reported the emergence of atypical G1P[8] strains during the post-RVA vaccination period in Blantyre, Malawi [24]. It is not definitively resolved whether these atypical G1P[8] strains are widespread. In addition, there is a paucity of information on whole-genome sequences of G1P[8] strains post-vaccine era with only a few countries performing full-genome characterization of the strain [15,21,31–35]. The African Enteric Viruses Genome Initiative (AEVGI) is conducting whole-genome characterization of country-specific pre- and post-vaccine RVA strains in Africa and has identified, for the first time in South Africa, atypical G1P[8] strains that were circulating before vaccine introduction. This study aimed to determine the genetic relationship and the evolutionary origin of these pre-vaccine atypical G1P[8] RVA strains.

## 2. Results

### 2.1. Nucleotide Sequencing

Illumina® MiSeq sequencing yielded $14.7 \times 10^5$ reads (379 bp fragment size) and $11.3 \times 10^5$ reads (364 bp fragment size) for strains RVA/Human-wt/ZAF/UFS-NGS-MRC-DPRU1971/2008/G1P[8] and RVA/Human-wt/ZAF/UFS-NGS-MRC-DPRU1973/G1P[8], respectively. All the sequences had a phred score of $Q \geq 30$ (99.9% base calling accuracy).

### 2.2. Full-Genome Constellation Analysis

Whole-gene sequences of the 11 genes of strains, RVA/Human-wt/ZAF/UFS-NGS-MRC-DPRU1971/G1P[8] and RVA/Human-wt/ZAF/UFS-NGS-MRC-DPRU1973/G1P[8], were determined, and their genotype constellations were revealed as G1-P[8]-I2-R2-C2-M2-A2-N2-T2-E2-H2 (Table 1). The sizes of full-length segments 1 to 11 and their respective open reading frames (ORFs) for the two study strains were determined (Table 1). The ORF sequences for all the 11 genes of these two South African atypical G1P[8] strains were deposited in GenBank under accession numbers MT163245-MT163266.

**Table 1.** Whole genotype constellations of the South African DS-1-like G1P[8] rotavirus strains.

| Gene Segment | VP7 | VP4 | VP6 | VP1 | VP2 | VP3 | NSP1 | NSP2 | NSP3 | NSP4 | NSP5 |
|---|---|---|---|---|---|---|---|---|---|---|---|
| Base pair size for full length sequences | 1062 | 2359 | 1355 | 3302 | 2684 | 2591 | 1566 | 1059 | 1066 | 751 | 810 |
| Base pair size for the complete study strain ORF | 978 | 2325 | 1191 | 3264 | 2637 | 2505 | 1458 | 951 | 939 | 525 | 600 |
| RVA/Human-wt/ZAF/UFS-NGS-MRC-DPRU1971/2008/G1P[8] | G1 | P[8] | I2 | R2 | C2 | M2 | A2 | N2 | T2 | E2 | H2 |
| RVA/Human-wt/ZAF/UFS-NGS-MRC-DPRU1973/2008/G1P[8] | G1 | P[8] | I2 | R2 | C2 | M2 | A2 | N2 | T2 | E2 | H2 |

Color codes indicate genogroup attribution. Green color represents the genotype associated with the Wa-like genogroup, while red color represents the genotype belonging to the DS-1-like genogroup. The nomenclature of the RV strains indicates RV group, species where the strain was isolated, name of the country where the strain was originally isolated, common name, year of isolation, and genotypes for genome segments four and nine as proposed by the Rotavirus Classification Working Group (RCWG) [12]. ORF = open reading frame.

### 2.3. Sequence and Phylogenetic Analysis

#### 2.3.1. Phylogenetic Analysis of VP7

Phylogenetically, the diversity of the VP7 G1 genes has been established through seven known lineages (I-VII) [36] (Figure 1). The VP7 genes of the atypical G1P[8] study strains, RVA/

Human-wt/ZAF/UFS-NGS-MRC-DPRU1971/2008/G1P[8] and RVA/Human-wt/ZAF/UFS-NGS-MRC-DPRU1973/2008/G1P[8], clustered in genetic lineage I, which consisted of a global collection of G1 strains that circulated from 2002 to 2015 (Figure 1). In this lineage I, the two G1 study strains clustered closely together and shared almost absolute gene identities amongst themselves—nt (aa) 99.9% (100%) (Figure 1; Supplementary data 1 (S1)). Analysis of the G1 study strains with locally circulating South African strains retrieved from the GenBank identified the highest sequence identities of 99.8–99.9% (100%) with strain RVA/Human-wt/ZAF/MRC-DPRU1039/2008/G1P8 and clustered closely with this strain that was isolated the same year, 2008, as the two study strains (Figure 1). However, within the same lineage, the VP7 genes of the two G1 study strains from South Africa clustered distinctly away from the atypical G1P[8] strains reported in Brazil, Japan, Malawi, Philippines, Thailand, and Vietnam [22–26] and displayed overall nt (aa) similarities that ranged from 87.0–98.5% (87.1–98.8%) (Table S1 in Supplementary data 2 (S2)). Specifically, the nt (aa) similarities ranged from 96.9–97.0% (98.5%), 96.9–97.1% (98.5–98.8%), 87.0–98%5 (87.1–98.8), 96.5–96.8% (98.2–98.5%), 96.9–97.0% (98.8%), and 97.0–97.1% (96.9%) to the post-vaccination G1 atypical strains reported in Brazil, Japan, Philippines, Malawi, Thailand, and Vietnam, respectively (S1).

When the two South African G1 study strains were compared to the typical G1 strains selected globally, they displayed the highest nt (aa) similarities of 99.7–99.8% (100%) with a European strain, RVA/Human-wt/BEL/BEL00017/2006/G1P[8] (S1). The nt(aa) similarities comparison to representative strains from Africa (Eastern Africa, Southern Africa, and West Africa), America, Asia, Europe, and Oceania ranged from 93.9–97.6% (94.2–98.2%), 97.1–99.5% (98.2–100%), 97.1–97.9% (96.9–98.2%), 93.1.5–97.6% (94.8%–98.5%), 96.4–99.6% (97.8–99.7%), 99.7–99.8% (100%), and 93.7–98.4% (94.5–98.8%), respectively (Table S2 in S2). In addition, comparison of the VP7 genes of the two study strains to cognate gene sequence of the Rotarix® and RotaTeq® RV vaccine strains displayed nt (aa) identities that ranged from 94.2–94.3% (95.7%) and 91.0–91.1% (93.2%), respectively (S1).

Analysis of the VP7 Neutralization Epitopes

The VP7 genes contain three established neutralization epitopes: 7-1a, 7-1b, and 7-2. Twenty-nine amino acids (14 residues in 7-1a, 6 residues in 7-1b, and 9 residues in 7-2) define the three VP7 antigenic epitopes [37]. The VP7 neutralization epitope sites of the two South African study strains were aligned and mapped against cognate neutralization sites of the two RV vaccines, Rotarix®, and RotaTeq®. Four amino acid differences (N94S, S123N, K291R, and M217T) in the VP7 genes of the two South African study strains were identified relative to Rotarix® VP7 neutralization sites, while five amino acid differences (D97E, S123N, K291R, S147N, and M217T) were identified with comparison to RotaTeq® G1 antigenic sites (Figure 2). Antigenically, similar amino acid residues in the VP7 epitopes of the study strains were observed in the corresponding VP7 epitopes of the multiple atypical G1P[8] strains (Figure 2). The VP7 epitopes of the two South African G1 strains were contrasted with those of globally selected lineage I G1 strains. The analysis showed ten amino acid differences (T91N, S94N, D100N, D100E, N123S, R291K, T242A, N147D, L148F, and T217M) (Figure 2).

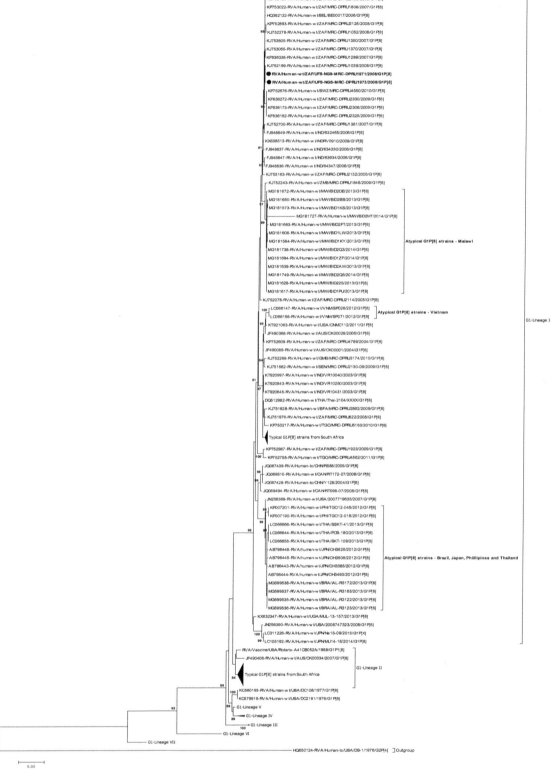

**Figure 1.** VP7 phylogenetic tree based on the full-length nucleotide sequences. Strains group A rotavirus (RVA)/Human-wt/ZAF/UFS-NGS-MRC-DPRU1971/2008/G1P[8] and RVA/Human-wt/ZAF/UFS-NGS-MRC-DPRU1973/2008/G1P[8] are identified by the black filled circular dots (•). Unusual G1P[8] strains from Malawi, Japan, Thailand, Vietnam, Brazil, and Philippine are indicated. Bootstrap values ≥ 70% are shown adjacent to each branch node. Each scale bar indicates the number of nucleotide substitutions per site.

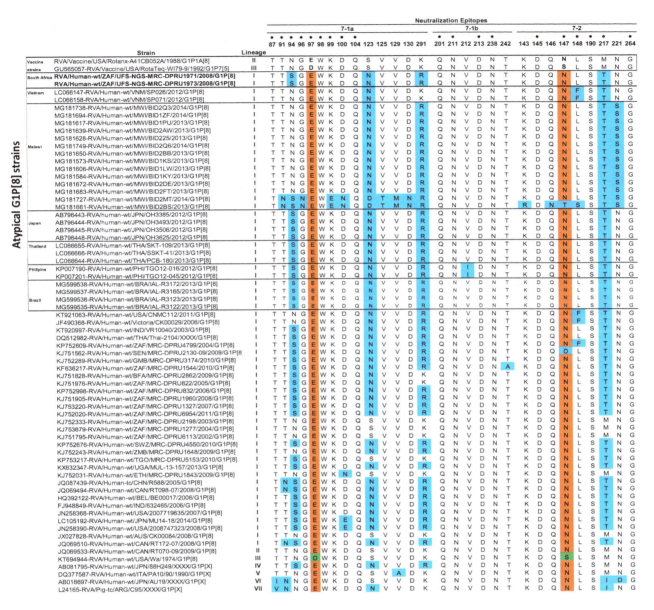

**Figure 2.** Alignment of antigenic residues in VP7 between the strains contained in Rotarix® and RotaTeq® and wild type G1 strains. Antigenic residues are divided in three epitopes (7-1a, 7-1b, and 7-2). Amino acids that differ between Rotarix® and RotaTeq® are indicated in boldface. Sky blue colored residues are residues that are different from both Rotarix® and RotaTeq®, green colored residues are different from Rotarix®, and brown colored residues are different from RotaTeq®. Amino acid changes that have been shown to escape neutralization with monoclonal antibodies are indicated with a black dot. Atypical G1P[8] and countries of detection are indicated on the left side of the figure. South Africa atypical G1P[8] strains are in boldface characters.

### 2.3.2. Phylogenetic analysis of VP4

The VP4 genes of the two atypical G1P[8] study strains were phylogenetically compared to the four established lineages (l-IV) of the P[8] genotypes [38] (Figure 3). The P[8] genes of the

South African strains, RVA/Human-wt/ZAF/UFS-NGS-MRC-DPRU1971/2008/G1P[8] and RVA/Human-wt/ZAF/UFS-NGS-MRC-DPRU1973/2008/G1P[8], clustered in lineage III, which consisted of a global collection of P[8] strains that circulated from 2002 to 2014 (Figure 3). Within the P[8]-lineage-III, the two atypical G1P[8] study strains clustered closely together and shared nt (aa) identities of 99.9% (99.7%) amongst themselves (Figure 3; S1). Homology analysis of the P[8] sequences of the two South African strains with sequences of South African strains retrieved from the GenBank demonstrated the highest nt (aa) sequence identities of 99.6% (99.1–99.4%) with strain RVA/Human-wt/ZAF/MRC-DPRU1039/2008/G1P[8] (Figure 3). However, within the same lineage, the VP4 genes of the two atypical strains from South Africa segregated distinctly away from the atypical strains that have been detected in Brazil, Japan, Malawi, Philippines, Thailand, and Vietnam. They exhibited overall nt (aa) similarities that ranged from 95.2–98.0% (95.1–98.6%) (Table S1 in S2). Specifically, the nt (aa) similarities ranged from 97.6–97.8% (98.1–98.6), 98.2–98.5% (98.5%), 95.2–98.0% (95.1–98.2%), 97.7–97.8% (98.1–98.5%), 97.8–98.0% (97.7–98.2%), and 98.1–98.2% (97.9–98.3%) to the post–vaccination atypical strains reported in Brazil, Japan, Malawi, Philippines, Thailand, and Vietnam, respectively (S1). A comparison of the South African P[8] study strains characterized in this study with a global collection of P[8] strains showed their closeness, and the study strains shared the highest nt (aa) similarity of 99.5% (99.1–99.4%) to a Belgian strain, RVA/Human–wt/BEL/BEL00017/2006/G1P[8] (S1). Overall, the nt (aa) similarities in comparison to representative strains from Africa (Eastern Africa, Southern Africa, Western Africa), America, Asia, Europe, and Oceania ranged from 97.4–97.8% (97.8–98.2%), 86.7–99.1% (91.1–99.2%), 86.7–99.1% (91.1–99.2%), 86.6–99.4% (91.0–99.2%), 86.5.–98.9% (91.1–98.7%), 86.8–99.5% (91.2–99.5%), and 86.5–98.5% (91.0%–98.6%), respectively. In addition, the comparison of the atypical VP4 genes to the P[8] genes of the Rotarix® and RotaTeq® vaccine strains displayed nt (aa) identities that ranged from 90.3–90.4% (93.9–94.2%) and 92.3% (95.2%), respectively (S1).

Analysis of the VP4 Neutralization Epitopes

The VP4 spike protein is cleaved by trypsin into two distinct structural proteins, VP8* and VP5* [2]. Analysis of the two South African study strains' VP4 sequences showed a conserved trypsin cleavage site (arginine) at positions 230, 240, and 581 [39]. Furthermore, the neutralization epitopes in the VP8* and the VP5* regions were analyzed. The VP8* region has four (8-1 to 8-4) neutralization epitopes, while VP5* has five (5-1 to 5-5) (Figure 4) [40]. Comparison of the two South African P[8] strains relative to the Rotarix® and the RotaTeq® P[8] sequences displayed 32 and 35 identical amino acid residues, respectively, spanning the VP4 antigenic epitopes (Figure 4). Amino acid differences between the two P[8] study strains and the P[8] component of vaccine strains were only identified in 8-1, 8-2, and 8-3 VP8* epitopes. Five amino acid differences (E150D, N195G, S125N, S131R, and N135D) were identified in the study strains in relation to Rotarix® P[8] strain, while two amino acid differences (E150D and D195G) were identified relative to P[8] strain of RotaTeq® (Figure 4). Analysis with VP4 epitopes of other atypical G1P[8] strains identified similar amino acid residues with the exception of position 113 in the 8-3 epitope, whereby asparagine was observed in the study strains while other atypical strains had either an aspartate or serine at this position (Figure 4). Further analysis of the study strain's VP4 neutralization epitopes with corresponding VP4 neutralization epitopes of globally selected P[8]-lineage-III strains identified two amino acid differences (S146G and N113D) (Figure 4).

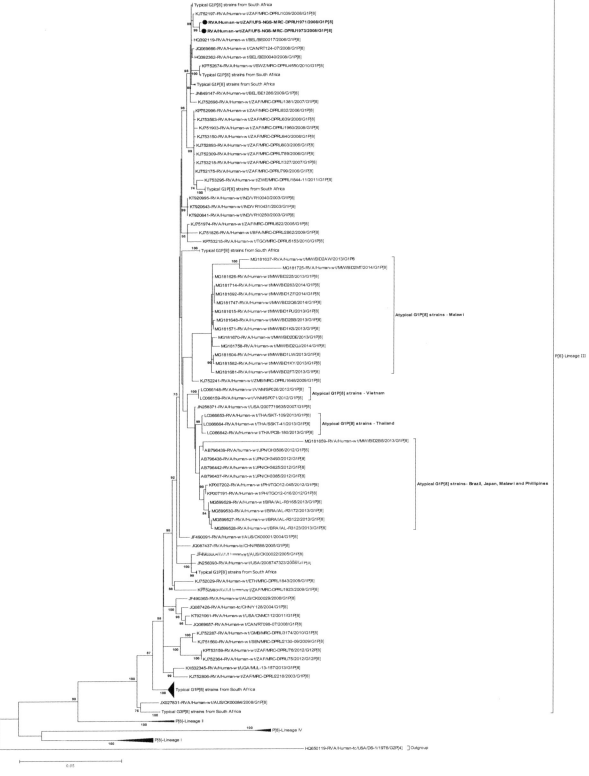

**Figure 3.** VP4 phylogenetic tree based on the full-length nucleotide sequences. Strains RVA/Human-wt/ZAF/UFS-NGS-MRC-DPRU1971/2008/G1P[8] and RVA/Human-wt/ZAF/UFS-NGS-MRC-DPRU1973/2008/G1P[8] are identified by the black filled circular dots (●). Unusual G1P[8] strains from Malawi, Japan, Thailand, Vietnam, Brazil, and Philippines are indicated. Bootstrap values ≥ 70% are shown adjacent to each branch node. Each scale bar indicates the number of nucleotide substitutions per site.

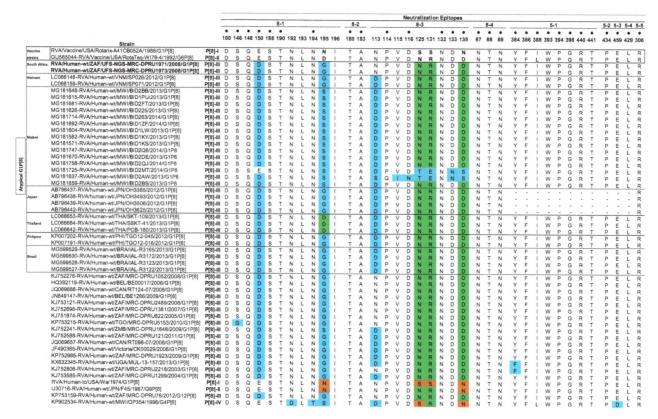

**Figure 4.** Alignment of antigenic residues in VP4 between the P[8] component of Rotarix® and RotaTeq® vaccines and wild type P[8] strains. Antigenic residues are divided in four antigenic epitopes in VP8* (8-1, 8-2, 8-3, and 8-4) and five antigenic epitopes in VP5* (5-1, 5-2, 5-3, 5-4, and 5-5). Amino acid changes that have been shown to escape neutralization with monoclonal antibodies are indicated with a black dot. Amino acids that differ between Rotarix® and RotaTeq® are indicated in boldface. Green colored residues are residues that are different from Rotarix®, brown colored residues are different from RotaTeq®, and residues colored in sky blue are different from both Rotarix® and RotaTeq®. Dashes (-) indicate no amino acid sequence.

### 2.3.3. Phylogenetic Analysis of VP1–VP3 and VP6

The evolutionary relationship of the VP1–VP3 and VP6 genes of the two South African study strains with a selection of global RVA strains was performed. The VP1–VP3 and VP6 genes of the two South African study strains clustered closely and displayed nearly absolute gene identities (≥99.9%) amongst each other (Figures S1–S4 in supplementary data 3 (S3)). The VP1–VP3 and VP6 genes of the two South African study strains clustered closely in sublineage composed mainly of locally circulating South African DS-1-like strains and were all found to cluster closely with cognate genes of strain RVA/Human-wt/ZAF/MRC-DPRU2344/2008/G2P[6], which was co-circulating in the population in the same year, 2008, as the study strains (Figures S1–S4 in S3). The VP1–VP3 and VP6 genes of the two study strains were closely related to cognate genes of strain RVA/Human-wt/ZAF/MRC-DPRU2344/2008/G2P[6] with nt (aa) identities ranging from ≥ 99.8–99.9% (≥99.9–100%) for VP1–VP3 and VP6 genes (S1). Phylogenetic relationship of the VP1–VP3 and VP6 genes of the atypical study strains with the cognate genes of the atypical G1P[8] strains reported in Brazil, Japan, Philippines, Thailand, Vietnam, and Malawi exhibited distinct clustering albeit belonging within the same lineage and displayed overall nt (aa) identities that ranged from ≥ 94.4–98.0% (≥ 97.1–100%) (Figure S1C–F in S3; Table S1 in S2). When VP1–VP3 and VP6 genes of the study strains were compared with selected global strains, highest genetic similarities ranging from ≥ 99.4–100% were identified with cognate genes of G3P[6] strains: RVA/Human-RVA/Human-wt/CMR/ES293/2011/G3P[6],

RVA/Human-wt/TGO/MRC-DPRU2206/2009/G3G9P[6], RVA/Human-wt/BEL/F01498/2009/G3P[6], and RVA/Human-wt/UGA/MUL-13-166/2013/G3P[6] for VP1–VP3 and VP6, respectively (S1).

### 2.3.4. Phlylogenetic Analysis of NSP1–NSP5

The NSP1–NSP5 genes of the two South African study strains were highly identical amongst each other with nt (aa) identity value of ≥99.8%, and clustered closely (Figures S5–S9). Close clustering with cognate genes of a locally circulating strain, RVA/Human-wt/ZAF/MRC-DPRU2344/2008/G2P[6], was observed for the all the NSP1–NSP5 genes, and they shared the highest nt (aa) similarities that ranged from ≥ 99.5–100% (99.4–100%) (S1). In contrast, the NSP1–NSP5 genes of the atypical study strains grouped distinctly away from cognate genes of atypical strains reported in Brazil, Japan, Philippines, Thailand, Vietnam, and Malawi and shared an overall nt (aa) similarities that ranged from ≥ 89.0–99.8% (≥94.3–100%) (Figures S5–S9 in S3; Table S1 in S2). Comparison of NSP1–NSP5 genes of the two South African study strains with corresponding selected reference strains collected globally demonstrated nt (aa) identities in the range of 98.6–100% (99.4–100%) with cognate A2, N2, T2, E2, and H2 genes of strains: RVA/Human-wt/BEL/F01498/2009/G3P[6], RVA/Human-wt/KEN/KDH1968/2014/G3P[6], RVA/Human-wt/GHA/GH018-08/2008/G8P[6], RVA/Human-wt/ZMB/MRC-DPRU1673/2009/G2P[4], and RVA/Human-wt/USA/2007769964/2007/G2P[4], respectively (S1).

### 2.4. Reassortment Analysis

The concatenated genomes of strains RVA/Human-wt/ZAF/UFS-NGS-MRC-DPRU1971/2008/G1P[8] and RVA/Human-wt/ZAF/UFS-NGS-MRC-DPRU1973/2008/G1P[8] were compared with two South African strains RVA/Human-wt/ZAF/MRC-DPRU1039/2008/G1P[8] and RVA/Human-wt/ZAF/MRC-DPRU2344/G2P[6] (Figure 5). The two atypical South African study strains shared a highly conserved backbone with all genes exhibiting > 99.8% nucleotide similarity. The VP7 and the VP4 genes of the two atypical strains shared the highest genetic similarities to RVA/Human-wt/ZAF/MRC-DPRU1039/2008/G1P[8]. However, the internal backbone genes were extremely diverse. The internal backbone genes of the atypical strains exhibited highest genetic similarity to RVA/Human-wt/ZAF/MRC-DPRU2344/G2P[6]. The results of this analysis suggest that the atypical G1P[8] strains were likely derived via reassortment events between contemporary, endemic South African strains.

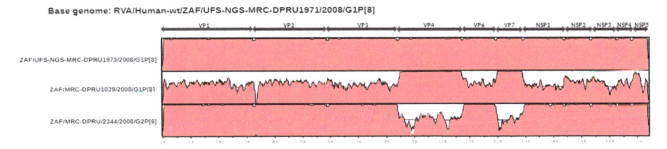

**Figure 5.** Nucleotide sequence similarities of the concatenated genome of RVA//Human-wt/ZAF/UFS-NGS-MRC-DPRU1971/2008/G1P[8] were compared with South African strains RVA//Human-wt/ZAF/UFS-NGS-MRC-DPRU1973/2008/G1P[8], RVA/Human-wt/ZAF/MRC-DPRU1039/2008/G1P[8], and RVA/Human-wt/ZAF/MRC-DPRU2344/2008/G2P[6]. The left axis displays the strains, and rotavirus genome segment is included in the top scale. The bottom scale shows distance in kb.

## 3. Discussion

This study described the first pre-vaccine era atypical reassortant G1P[8] strains, whose outer gene segments (VP7 and VP4) expressed a Wa-like genotype, whereas the backbone genes expressed a DS-1-like genotype constellation. Analysis of the whole-genome constellation showed that genetic reassortment mechanism generated the DS-1-like G1P[8] strains. Rotavirus reassortment events are mainly facilitated by the segmentation inherent in the RV genome [2], which can generate rare or novel RV strains and hence contribute to the vast RVA diversity [22]. Wa-like and DS-1-like intergenogroup reassortment events involving G1P[8] and DS-1-like genotype constellation have been described recently in six countries: Brazil, Japan, Philippines, Thailand, Vietnam, and Malawi [23–30]. According to literature, viable atypical reassortant strains can occur under natural conditions involving Wa-like G1P[8] or G3P[8] outer capsid genes expressing DS-1-like genetic background [41–44]. This study identified two DS-1-like G1P[8] strains in the course of the ongoing AEVGI whole-genome characterization of South African RVA strains. While reported in low frequencies and limited settings in Brazil (1.6% during 2013–2017 seasons) [22], Thailand (0.4% during 2012–2014 seasons) [27], and Vietnam (14% during 2012/2013 season) [28,29], 31–62% of these DS-1-like G1P[8] strains accounted for RVA positive strains circulating across selected regions in Japan [26], and 40% of randomly sampled post-vaccine samples were reported in Malawi [24]. Such atypical reassortant strains have the potential to predominate in circulation. G1P[4] strains suggested to have emerged from intergenogroup reassortment events accounted for 41% of RVA strains circulating in the peak months of the 2001 RVA season in Detroit, USA [45], whereas a surge in G3P[4] strains also presumed to have emerged from intergenogroup reassortment events were detected in Brazil at 36% [46] and in Ghana at 64% [47]. The two South African study strains were identified during the pre-RVA vaccination period in South Africa in contrast to the previously reported atypical strains found during the post-RVA vaccination period. This implies that the reassortment events that led to the emergence of the South African atypical G1P[8] strains may not necessarily be driven by vaccine-induced selective pressure but by natural evolutionary processes of RVA genome.

In order to identify the ancestral origin of these G1P[8] strains, assessment of whole-gene sequences and phylogenetic analysis showed that the outer capsid genes, VP7 and VP4, of strains RVA/Human-wt/ZAF/UFS-NGS-MRC-DPRU1971/2008/G1P[8] and RVA/Human-wt/ZAF/UFS-NGS-MRC-DPRU1973/2008/G1P[8] were 99.6–99.9% (99.1–100%) identical with South African strain RVA/Human-wt/ZAF/MRC-DPRU1039/2008/G1P[8] and clustered together in the same clade within the same. For the internal genes, the highest nucleotide identities were identified with cognate genes of another South African strain, RVA/Human-wt/ZAF/MRC-DPRU2344/2008/G2P[6], detected in the 2008 RVA season. Put together, it is probable that a locally circulating G2P[6] strain such as RVA/Human-wt/ZAF/MRC-DPRU2344/2008/G2P[6] with a DS-1-like backbone derived the VP7 and the VP4 genes from a locally co-circulating G1P[8] strain such as RVA/Human-wt/ZAF/MRC-DPRU1039/2008/G1P[8], generating the double-gene reassortants. Consequently, the results obtained in this study indicate that the two atypical South African G1P[8] strains were generated locally through genetic reassortment events. The generation of these reassortant double-gene strains tend to be independent of the events in which Brazilian, Japanese, Thai, Vietnamese, and Malawian DS-1-like G1P[8] strains were generated. The nine internal genes of the South African DS-1-like G1P[8] strains always clustered together with cognate genes of a locally circulating G2P[6] strain distinctly away from the cluster comprising Japanese, Thai, Philippines, and Malawi DS-1-like G1P[8] strains. Therefore, the South African DS-1-like G1P[8] strains emerged clonally from independent events, a phenomenon observed for the Malawian [24] and the Vietnamese [30] DS-1-like G1P[8] strains. In contrast, Brazilian, Japanese, and Thai G1P[8] DS-1-like strains were established to have been derived from a common ancestor [23,29].

Vaccine escape mutants can result due to mutations occurring in well-known VP7 neutralization epitope regions [48]. Host–antigen binding interactions involving human G1 strains are significantly impacted by mutations occurring at positions 94, 97, 147, and 291 [48]. The identified N94S substitution involving the substitution of asparagine (N) with a serine(S), which are both polar non-charged amino acid residues [49], may not significantly alter the overall morphology of the protein surface. However, since asparagine is usually N-glycosylated, there is a likely loss of glycosylation site, which could have a wide-ranging impact on the immunogenicity of the 7-1a epitope [50]. The D97E amino acid substitution involving polar negatively charged residues, aspartate (D) and glutamate (E), is likely to be a silent nucleotide change [49]. Similarly, a K291R substitution involving lysine (K), an amphipathic polar amino acid, and arginine (R), a positively charged amino acid, is unlikely to have a far-reaching structural effect on the VP7 protein surfaces. However, M217T substitution was identified resulting in substitution of methionine, a non-polar residue to threonine, a polar amino acid residue, which could likely result in significant changes in biochemical properties of VP7 [49]. This M217T substitution was also present in earlier strains as well as some post-vaccine strains that were included for analysis, and the role it plays in driving epidemiological fitness of G1 strains is not fully resolved. In the host cell, trypsin-like proteases cleave the VP4 spike protein into two structural domains (VP8* and VP5*) [2]. Four surface-exposed antigenic epitopes (8-1 to 8-4) have been described in the VP8* region, while five antigenic epitopes (5-1 to 5-5) in the VP5* region have been documented [40]. The amino acid changes E150D, N195G, S125N, and N135D that were observed relative to the vaccine strains were conservative. However, a S131R substitution that resulted in a change in polarity might play a role in escape of host immunity [49]. Another amino acid substitution R131S resulting in a change in charge from positively charged amino acid to non-charged amino acid that was identified when comparison was made against globally selected lineage-III VP4 strains might impact vaccine escape effect [49].

## 4. Materials and Methods

### 4.1. Ethics Approval

The study was approved under ethics number UFS-HSD2018/0510/3107 by the Health Sciences Research Ethics Committee (HSREC) of the University of Free State, Bloemfontein, South Africa. The patient identities and demographics were de-linked from their unique laboratory identifiers to ensure confidentiality.

### 4.2. Sample Collection

Rotavirus positive stool samples from children under five years of age treated for gastroenteritis at Dr. George Mukhari Hospital, Pretoria North, South Africa and conventionally genotyped as G1P[8] were sourced from archival storage (2002 to 2017) of South Africa Medical Research Council—Diarrheal Pathogens Research Unit (MRC-DPRU), a WHO Rotavirus Regional Reference Laboratory (WHO-RRL) in Pretoria, South Africa. The two stool samples that were later genotyped as DS-1-like G1P[8] strains were collected from 6-month female and 12-month male children on 15 and 16 May 2008, respectively, from Soshanguve, Pretoria.

### 4.3. Extraction and Purification of Double-Stranded RNA

The extraction of RV ds-RNA was conducted by utilizing a previously described method [51], albeit with modifications (UFS NCS unit extraction SOP). Briefly, a pea size (~100 mg) sample of stool was added to 200 µL of phosphate-buffered saline (PBS) solution, pH 7.2 (Sigma-Aldrich®, St Louis, MO, USA). The solution was mixed by pulse-vortexing for five seconds. A 1 mL volume of TRI-Reagent®-LS (Molecular Research Center, Inc, Cincinnati, OH, USA) was added and let to stand for five minutes. Phase separation was achieved by addition of 270 µL of chloroform (Sigma-Aldrich®, St Louis, MO, USA). Afterward, centrifugation for 13,000 revolutions per minute (RPM) was performed for 20 min at 4 °C in a temperature-controlled microcentrifuge (Eppendorf microcentrifuge 5427R, Hamburg, Germany). A volume of 1 mL isopropanol (Sigma-Aldrich®, St Louis, MO, USA) was added to the supernatant, and centrifugation was performed at 13,000 RPM for 30 min at room temperature. The supernatant was poured off, and the tubes were let to dry for 10 min, after which 95 µL of elution buffer (EB) from the MinElute Gel extraction kit (Qiagen, Hilden, Germany) was added. A 30 µL volume of of 8M LiCl2 (Sigma, St. Louis, MO, USA) was added, and the solution was precipitated for 16 h at 4 °C in a water bath in a Tupperware box. The MinElute gel extraction kit (Qiagen, Hilden, Germany) was used to purify the extracted RNA according to manufacturer's instructions, and 1% 0.5 X TBE agarose gel stained with Pronasafe (Condalab, UK) electrophoresis was used to verify the integrity and the enrichment of dsRNA, which was visualized on a G:Box Syngene UV transilluminator (Syngene, Cambridge, UK).

*4.4. Synthesis and Purification of Complementary DNA (cDNA)*

The Maxima H Minus Double-Stranded cDNA Synthesis Kit (Thermo Fischer Scientific, Waltham, MA) was utilized to synthesize cDNA from the extracted viral RNA. Briefly, denaturation at 95 °C for 5 min of the extracted RNA was performed followed by addition of 1 µL of 100 µM Random Hexamer primer. Incubation was performed in a thermocycler at 65 °C for five minutes. The First-Strand Reaction mix (5 µL) and the First Strand Enzyme Mix (1 µL) were added, and the solution was incubated at 25 °C for 10 min followed by 2 h at 50 °C, and then the reaction was terminated by heating at 85 °C for 5 min. A volume of 55 µL of nuclease-free water, 20 µL of 5X Second Strand Reaction Mix, and 5 µL of Second Strand Reaction Mix was then added. The solution was then incubated at 16 °C for 60 min, after which the reaction was stopped by adding 6 µL 0.5M EDTA. A volume of 10 µL RNAse I was then added, and the synthesized cDNA was incubated for five minutes at room temperature. Subsequently, the MSB® Spin PCRapace (Stratec) Purification Kit was used to purify the synthesized cDNA.

*4.5. DNA Library Preparation and Whole-Genome Sequencing*

The Nextera® XT DNA Library Preparation Kit (Illumina, San Diego, California, US) was utilized to prepare DNA libraries by following manufacturer's instructions. Briefly, the genomic DNA was tagmented by using the Nextera® transposome enzyme, and the tagmented DNA was subsequently amplified using a limited-cycle PCR program. The DNA libraries were cleaned-up using AMPure XP magnetic beads (Beckman Coulter, Pasadena, CA, USA) and 80% freshly prepared ethanol. The quantity of the DNA was determined using Qubit 2.0 fluorometer (Invitrogen, Carlsbad, CA, USA), and the quality of the libraries and the fragment sizes was assessed using Agilent 2100 BioAnalyzer® (Agilent Technologies, Waldbronn, Germany) by following the manufacturer's specified protocol. The Illumina MiSeq® sequencer (Illumina, San Diego, CA, USA) was utilized to perform paired-end nucleotide sequencing (301 × 2) for 600 cycles by using a MiSeq Reagent Kit v3 at the University of the Free State-Next Generation Sequencing (UFS-NGS) Unit, Bloemfontein, South Africa.

*4.6. Genome Assembly*

Geneious Prime® software, version 2019.1.1 (Biomatters, https://www.geneious.com/; [52]) was used for genome assembly. Briefly, for use with the reference mapping tools integrated in Geneious Prime version 2019.1.1, the default medium sensitivity parameter was selected to generate contigs from the FASTQ files data generated by the Illumina MiSeq® instrument. Complementary RV genome assembly was also performed using an in-house genome assembly pipeline and CLC Genomics Workbench 12 (https://www.qiagenbioinformatics.com/).

*4.7. Determination of Rotavirus Whole-Genotype Constellations*

The genotype of each gene segment was determined using Rota C, v 2.0 [13], an online server for genotyping RVA strains. This was used to generate the full genotype constellations for each RV strain.

*4.8. Phylogenetic Analyses*

Complete sequences for each gene segment were aligned and sequence comparisons performed as described previously [53–55]. Multiple sequence alignments were implemented utilizing the MUSCLE package in Molecular Evolutionary Genetics Analysis (MEGA) 6 software ([56]; http://www.megasoftware.net/). Upon alignment, the DNA Model Test program in MEGA 6 was used to determine the evolutionary model that best fits each gene sequence datasets. The models identified as best fitting with the sequence data for the indicated genes using the Corrected Akaike Information Criterion (AICc) were as follows: GTR+G+I (VP7, VP4, VP6, VP1, VP2, VP3, NSP1, NSP2, NSP3) and

HKY+G+I (NSP4 and NSP5). These models were utilized in maximum-likelihood trees' construction using MEGA 6 with 1000 bootstrap replicates to estimate branch support. Genetic distance matrices were prepared using the $p$-distance algorithm of MEGA 6 software [56]. In addition to the two whole-genome sequences of the strains in this study, other cognate sequences were acquired from GenBank ([57]; http://www.ncbi.nlm.gov/genbank). Further phylogenetic analysis by geographical regions Africa (Eastern Africa, Southern Africa, and West Africa), Asia, Americas, Europe, and Oceania was also performed. mVISTA software was used to visualize the comparative sequence similarities of concatenated whole-genome of genetically related strains [58].

## 5. Conclusions

Whole-gene analyses showed that the South African DS-1-like G1P[8] strains were generated involving locally circulating G2P[6] strains by acquiring the VP7 and the VP4 outer capsid proteins of locally co-circulating G1P[8] strains. Similar to their pre-vaccine era detection in Vietnam and Philippines, the identification of these atypical DS-1-like G1P[8] strains during the pre-vaccine period in South Africa, as opposed to their detection during post-vaccination era in selected settings in Brazil (Sao Paulo and Goias in 2013), Japan (Okayama, Aichi, Akita, Kyoto, and Osaka Prefectures in 2012), Thailand (Phetchabun and Sukhothai in 2013), and Malawi (Blantyre in 2013/2014), suggests that they originated from natural evolutionary processes of RVA genome. Whole-genome surveillance of RVA genotypes is imperative to understand the occurrence rate, the mechanisms that drive emergence of such atypical strains, and their epidemiological fitness as well as to assess the effect of vaccine selective pressure in shaping the antigenic landscape of RVA strains.

**Supplementary Materials:**
Supplementary data 1 (S1): Identity matrices analysis for VP1, VP2, VP3, VP4, VP6, NSP1, NSP2, NSP3, NSP5 and NSP5 nucleotide and deduced amino acid identities among strains calculated by distance matrices using P-distance algorithm in MEGA 6. Supplementary data 2 (S2): Homology analysis summary containing Table S1 and Table S2. Supplementary data 3 (S3): Additional phylograms containing Figure S1:VP1, S2:VP2, S3:VP3, S4:VP6, S5:NSP1, S6:NSP2, S7:NSP3, S8:NSP4 and S9:NSP5.

**Author Contributions:** M.M.N., K.C.J., F.E.D. and V.N.N. conceptualized the main project. P.N.M., M.T.M., M.M.N. and S.P.R. performed the laboratory experiments. M.J.M. and M.L.S. facilitated the sample resources. Formal analysis was done by P.N.M. and M.M.N. Data curation was performed by P.N.M., M.T.M., M.M.N. and S.P.R. Writing of the original draft preparation was performed by P.N.M. Review of the drafts was performed by all co-authors. Supervision, funding acquisition and project administration was performed by M.M.N. All authors have read and agreed to the published version of the manuscript.

**Acknowledgments:** Assistance in retrieval of the archived stool samples by Khutso Mothapo, Kebareng Rakau and Nonkululeko Magagula at the WHO-RRL in Pretoria, is hereby acknowledged. Assistance in laboratory work by Lesedi Mosime, Gilmore Pambuka and Teboho Mooko is duly acknowledged. Some aspects of data analysis guidance by Mathew Esona (CDC, Atlanta) and Felicity Burt is greatly acknowledged. Technical ICT support by Stephanus Riekert is also acknowledged.

## References

1. World Health Organization Causes of Mild Mortality. (WHO 2019). Available online: https://www.who.int/gho/child_health/mortality/causes/en/ (accessed on 20 August 2019).
2. Estes, M.K.; Greenberg, H.B. Rotaviruses. In *Fields Virology*; Knipe, D.M., Howley, P.M., Eds.; Wolters Kluwer Health/Lippincott, Williams and Wilkins: Philadelphia, PA, USA, 2013.
3. Troeger, C.; Khalil, I.A.; Rao, P.C.; Cao, S.; Blacker, B.F.; Ahmed, T.; Armah, G.; Bines, J.E.; Brewer, T.G.; Colombara, D.V.; et al. Rotavirus vaccination and the global burden of rotavirus diarrhea among children younger than 5 years. *JAMA Pediatr.* **2018**, *172*, 958–965. [CrossRef]
4. Tate, J.E.; Burton, A.H.; Boschi-Pinto, C.; Parashar, U.D.; World Health Organization–Coordinated Global Rotavirus Surveillance Network; Agocs, M.; Serhan, F.; de Oliveira, L.; Mwenda, J.M.; Mihigo, R.; et al. Global, regional, and national estimates of rotavirus mortality in children <5 years of age, 2000–2013. *Clin. Infect. Dis.* **2016** *62* (Suppl. 2), S96–S105.

5. World Health Organization. Meeting of the immunization Strategic Advisory Group of Experts. *Wkly. Epidemiol. Rec.* **2009**, *84*, 220–236.
6. World Health Organization. WHO Prequalifies New Rotavirus Vaccine. Available online: https://www.who.int/medicines/news/2018/prequalified_new-rotavirus_vaccine/en/ (accessed on 19 December 2019).
7. Anh, D.D.; Van Trang, N.; Thiem, V.D.; Anh, N.T.H.; Mao, N.D.; Wang, Y.; Jiang, B.; Hien, N.D.; Rotavin-M1 Vaccine Trial Group. A dose-escalation safety and immunogenicity study of a new live attenuated human rotavirus vaccine (Rotavin-M1) in Vietnamese children. *Vaccine* **2012**, *30*, A114–A121. [CrossRef]
8. Fu, C.; Wang, M.; Liang, J.; He, T.; Wang, D.; Xu, J. Effectiveness of Lanzhou lamb rotavirus vaccine against rotavirus gastroenteritis requiring hospitalization: A matched case-control study. *Vaccine* **2007**, *25*, 8756–8761. [CrossRef]
9. Kirkwood, C.D.; Steele, A.D. Rotavirus Vaccines in China. *Jama Netw. Open* **2018**, *1*, e181579. [CrossRef]
10. Madhi, S.A.; Cunliffe, N.A.; Steele, D.; Witte, D.; Kirsten, M.; Louw, C.; Ngwira, B.; Victor, J.C.; Gillard, P.H.; Cheuvart, B.B.; et al. Effect of human rotavirus vaccine on severe diarrhea in African infants. *N. Engl. J. Med.* **2010**, *362*, 289–298. [CrossRef]
11. Madhi, S.A.; Kirsten, M.; Louw, C.; Bos, P.; Aspinall, S.; Bouckenooghe, A.; Neuzil, K.M.; Steele, A.D. Efficacy and immunogenicity of two or three dose rotavirus-vaccine regimen in South African children over two consecutive rotavirus-seasons: A randomized, double-blind, placebo-controlled trial. *Vaccine* **2012**, *30*, A44–A51. [CrossRef]
12. Matthijnssens, J.; Ciarlet, M.; McDonald, S.M.; Attoui, H.; Bányai, K.; Brister, J.R.; Buesa, J.; Esona, M.D.; Estes, M.K.; Gentsch, J.R.; et al. Uniformity of rotavirus strain nomenclature proposed by the Rotavirus Classification Working Group (RCWG). *Arch. Virol.* **2011**, *156*, 1397–1413. [CrossRef]
13. Maes, P.; Matthijnssens, J.; Rahman, M.; Van Ranst, M. RotaC: A web-based tool for the complete genome classification of group A rotaviruses. *BMC Microbiol.* **2009**, *9*, 238. [CrossRef]
14. Dóró, R.; László, B.; Martella, V.; Leshem, E.; Gentsch, J.; Parashar, U.; Bányai, K. Review of global rotavirus strain prevalence data from six years post vaccine licensure surveillance: Is there evidence of strain selection from vaccine pressure? *Infect. Genet. Evol.* **2014**, *28*, 446–461. [CrossRef] [PubMed]
15. Banyai, K.; Mijatovic-Rustempasic, S.; Hull, J.J.; Esona, M.D.; Freeman, M.M.; Frace, A.M.; Bowen, M.D.; Gentsch, J.R. Sequencing and phylogenetic analysis of the coding region of six common rotavirus strains: Evidence for intragenogroup reassortment among co-circulating G1P[8] and G2P[4] strains from the United States. *J. Med. Virol.* **2011**, *83*, 532–539. [CrossRef] [PubMed]
16. Seheri, L.M.; Magagula, N.B.; Peenze, I.; Rakau, K.; Ndadza, A.; Mwenda, J.M.; Weldegebriel, G.; Steele, A.D.; Mphahlele, M.J. Rotavirus strain diversity in Eastern and Southern African countries before and after vaccine introduction. *Vaccine* **2018**, *36*, 7222–7230. [CrossRef]
17. Mwenda, J.M.; Ntoto, K.M.; Abebe, A.; Enweronu-Laryea, C.; Amina, I.; Mchomvu, J.; Kisakye, A.; Mpabalwani, E.M.; Pazvakavambwa, I.; Armah, G.E.; et al. Burden and epidemiology of rotavirus diarrhea in selected African countries: Preliminary results from the African Rotavirus Surveillance Network. *J. Infect. Dis.* **2010**, *202* (Suppl. 1), S5–S11. [CrossRef]
18. Seheri, L.M.; Ngomane, G.; Page, N.A.; Mokomane, M.; Maphalala, G.P.; Weldegebriel, G.; Peenze, I.; Magagula, N.B.; Nyaga, M.M.; Lisoga, J.; et al. Outbreak investigation of diarrheal disease in Botswana and Eswatini in 2018. In Proceedings of the 12th African Rotavirus Symposium, Johannesburg, South Africa, 30 July–1 August 2019.
19. Matthijnssens, J.; Van Ranst, M. Genotype constellation and evolution of group A rotaviruses infecting humans. *Curr. Opin. Virol.* **2012**, *2*, 426–433. [CrossRef]
20. Do, L.P.; Nakagomi, T.; Otaki, H.; Agbemabiese, C.A.; Nakagomi, O.; Tsunemitsu, H. Phylogenetic inference of the porcine Rotavirus A origin of the human G1 VP7 gene. *Infect. Genet. Evol.* **2016**, *40*, 205–213. [CrossRef]
21. Santos, F.S.; Junior, E.S.; Guerra, S.F.S.; Lobo, P.S.; Junior, E.P.; Lima, A.B.F.; Vinente, C.B.G.; Chagas, E.H.N.; Justino, M.C.A.; Linhares, A.C.; et al. G1P[8] Rotavirus in children with severe diarrhea in the post-vaccine introduction era in Brazil: Evidence of reassortments and structural modifications of the antigenic VP7 and VP4 regions. *Infect. Genet. Evol.* **2019**, *69*, 255–266. [CrossRef]
22. Kirkwood, C.D. Genetic and antigenic diversity of human rotaviruses: Potential impact on vaccination programs. *J. Infect. Dis.* **2010**, *202* (Suppl. 1), S43–S48. [CrossRef]
23. Luchs, A.; da Costa, A.C.; Cilli, A.; Komninakis, S.C.V.; Carmona, R.D.C.C.; Morillo, S.G.; Sabino, E.C.;

Timenetsky, M.D.C.S.T. First Detection of DS-1-like G1P[8] Double-gene Reassortant Rotavirus Strains on The American Continent, Brazil, 2013. *Sci. Rep.* **2019**, *9*, 2210. [CrossRef]

24. Jere, K.C.; Chaguza, C.; Bar-Zeev, N.; Lowe, J.; Peno, C.; Kumwenda, B.; Nakagomi, O.; Tate, J.E.; Parashar, U.D.; Heyderman, R.S.; et al. Emergence of double-and triple-gene reassortant G1P[8] rotaviruses possessing a DS-1-like backbone after rotavirus vaccine introduction in Malawi. *J. Virol.* **2018**, *92*, e01246-17. [CrossRef]

25. Fujii, Y.; Nakagomi, T.; Nishimura, N.; Noguchi, A.; Miura, S.; Ito, H.; Doan, Y.H.; Takahashi, T.; Ozaki, T.; Katayama, K.; et al. Spread and predominance in Japan of novel G1P[8] double-reassortant rotavirus strains possessing a DS-1-like genotype constellation typical of G2P[4] strains. *Infect. Genet. Evol.* **2014**, *28*, 426–433. [CrossRef]

26. Kuzuya, M.; Fujii, R.; Hamano, M.; Kida, K.; Mizoguchi, Y.; Kanadani, T.; Nishimura, K.; Kishimoto, T. Prevalence and molecular characterization of G1P[8] human rotaviruses possessing DS-1-like VP6, NSP4, and NSP5/6 in Japan. *J. Med. Virol.* **2014**, *86*, 1056–1064. [CrossRef] [PubMed]

27. Yamamoto, S.P.; Kaida, A.; Kubo, H.; Iritani, N. Gastroenteritis Outbreaks Caused by a DS-1–like G1P[8] Rotavirus Strain, Japan, 2012–2013. *Emerg. Infect. Dis.* **2014**, *20*, 1030. [CrossRef] [PubMed]

28. Komoto, S.; Tacharoenmuang, R.; Guntapong, R.; Ide, T.; Tsuji, T.; Yoshikawa, T.; Tharmaphornpilas, P.; Sangkitporn, S.; Taniguchi, K. Reassortment of human and animal rotavirus gene segments in emerging DS-1-like G1P[8] rotavirus strains. *PLoS ONE* **2016**, *11*, e0148416. [CrossRef] [PubMed]

29. Komoto, S.; Tacharoenmuang, R.; Guntapong, R.; Ide, T.; Haga, K.; Katayama, K.; Kato, T.; Ouchi, Y.; Kurahashi, H.; Tsuji, T.; et al. Emergence and characterization of unusual DS-1-like G1P[8] rotavirus strains in children with diarrhea in Thailand. *PLoS ONE* **2015**, *10*, e0141739. [CrossRef] [PubMed]

30. Nakagomi, T.; Nguyen, M.Q.; Gauchan, P.; Agbemabiese, C.A.; Kaneko, M.; Do, L.P.; Vu, T.D.; Nakagomi, O. Evolution of DS-1-like G1P[8] double-gene reassortant rotavirus A strains causing gastroenteritis in children in Vietnam in 2012/2013. *Arch. Virol.* **2017**, *162*, 739–748. [CrossRef] [PubMed]

31. Zeller, M.; Heylen, E.; Tamim, S.; McAllen, J.K.; Kirkness, E.F.; Akopov, A.; De Coster, S.; Van Ranst, M.; Matthijnssens, J. Comparative analysis of the Rotarix™ vaccine strain and G1P[8] rotaviruses detected before and after vaccine introduction in Belgium. *PeerJ* **2017**, *5*, e2733. [CrossRef]

32. Magagula, N.B.; Esona, M.D.; Nyaga, M.M.; Stucker, K.M.; Halpin, R.A.; Stockwell, T.B.; Seheri, M.L.; Steele, A.D.; Wentworth, D.E.; Mphahlele, M.J. Whole genome analyses of G1P[8] rotavirus strains from vaccinated and non-vaccinated South African children presenting with diarrhea. *J. Med. Virol.* **2015**, *87*, 79–101. [CrossRef]

33. Shintani, T.; Ghosh, S.; Wang, Y.H.; Zhou, X.; Zhou, D.J.; Kobayashi, N. Whole genomic analysis of human G1P[8] rotavirus strains from different age groups in China. *Viruses* **2012**, *4*, 1289–1304. [CrossRef]

34. Arora, R.; Chitambar, S.D. Full genomic analysis of Indian G1P[8] rotavirus strains. *Infect. Genet. Evol.* **2011**, *11*, 504–511. [CrossRef]

35. Rahman, M.; Matthijnssens, J.; Saiada, F.; Hassan, Z.; Heylen, E.; Azim, T.; Van Ranst, M. Complete genomic analysis of a Bangladeshi G1P[8] rotavirus strain detected in 2003 reveals a close evolutionary relationship with contemporary human Wa-like strains. *Infect. Genet. Evol.* **2010**, *10*, 746–754. [CrossRef] [PubMed]

36. Arista, S.; Giammanco, G.M.; De Grazia, S.; Ramirez, S.; Biundo, C.L.; Colomba, C.; Cascio, A.; Martella, V. Heterogeneity and temporal dynamics of evolution of G1 human rotaviruses in a settled population. *J. Virol.* **2006**, *80*, 10724–10733. [CrossRef] [PubMed]

37. Aoki, S.T.; Settembre, E.C.; Trask, S.D.; Greenberg, H.B.; Harrison, S.C.; Dormitzer, P.R. Structure of rotavirus outer-layer protein VP7 bound with a neutralizing Fab. *Science* **2009**, *324*, 1444–1447. [CrossRef] [PubMed]

38. Le, V.P.; Chung, Y.C.; Kim, K.; Chung, S.I.; Lim, I.; Kim, W. Genetic variation of prevalent G1P[8] human rotaviruses in South Korea. *J. Med. Virol.* **2010**, *82*, 886–896. [CrossRef] [PubMed]

39. Ciarlet, M.; Hyser, J.M.; Estes, M.K. Sequence Analysis of the VP4, VP6, VP7, and NSP4 Gene Products of the Bovine Rotavirus WC3. *Virus Genes* **2002**, *24*, 107–118. [CrossRef]

40. Zeller, M.; Patton, J.T.; Heylen, E.; De Coster, S.; Ciarlet, M.; Van Ranst, M.; Matthijnssens, J. Genetic analyses reveal differences in the VP7 and VP4 antigenic epitopes between human rotaviruses circulating in Belgium and rotaviruses in Rotarix and RotaTeq. *J. Clin. Microbiol.* **2012**, *50*, 966–976. [CrossRef]

41. Guntapong, R.; Tacharoenmuang, R.; Singchai, P.; Upachai, S.; Sutthiwarakom, K.; Komoto, S.; Tsuji, T.; Tharmaphornpilas, P.; Yoshikawa, T.; Sangkitporn, S.; et al. Predominant prevalence of human rotaviruses with the G1P[8] and G8P[8] genotypes with a short RNA profile in 2013 and 2014 in Sukhothai and

Phetchaboon provinces, Thailand. *J. Med. Virol.* **2017**, *89*, 615–620. [CrossRef]

42. Arana, A.; Montes, M.; Jere, K.C.; Alkorta, M.; Iturriza-Gómara, M.; Cilla, G. Emergence and spread of G3P[8] rotaviruses possessing an equine-like VP7 and a DS-1-like genetic backbone in the Basque Country (North of Spain), 2015. *Infect. Genet. Evol.* **2016**, *44*, 137–144. [CrossRef]

43. Cowley, D.; Donato, C.M.; Roczo-Farkas, S.; Kirkwood, C.D. Emergence of a novel equine-like G3P[8] inter-genogroup reassortant rotavirus strain associated with gastroenteritis in Australian children. *J. Gen. Virol.* **2016**, *97*, 403–410. [CrossRef]

44. Guerra, S.F.S.; Soares, L.S.; Lobo, P.S.; Júnior, E.T.P.; Júnior, E.C.S.; Bezerra, D.A.M.; Vaz, L.R.; Linhares, A.C.; Mascarenhas, J.D.A.P. Detection of a novel equine-like G3 rotavirus associated with acute gastroenteritis in Brazil. *J. Gen. Virol.* **2016**, *97*, 3131–3138. [CrossRef]

45. Abdel-Haq, N.M.; Thomas, R.A.; Asmar, B.I.; Zacharova, V.; Lyman, W.D. Increased prevalence of G1P[4] genotype among children with rotavirus-associated gastroenteritis in metropolitan Detroit. *J. Clin. Microbiol.* **2003**, *41*, 2680–2682. [CrossRef] [PubMed]

46. Rosa, M.E.S.; Pires, I.D.C.; Gouvea, V. 1998-1999 rotavirus seasons in Juiz de Fora, Minas Gerais, Brazil: Detection of an unusual G3P[4] epidemic strain. *J. Clin. Microbiol.* **2002**, *40*, 2837–2842. [CrossRef] [PubMed]

47. Asmah, R.H.; Green, J.; Armah, G.E.; Gallimore, C.I.; Gray, J.J.; Iturriza-Gómara, M.; Anto, F.; Oduro, A.; Binka, F.N.; Brown, D.W.; et al. Rotavirus G and P genotypes in rural Ghana. *J. Clin. Microbiol.* **2001**, *39*, 1981–1984. [CrossRef] [PubMed]

48. Coulson, B.S.; Kirkwood, C. Relation of VP7 amino acid sequence to monoclonal antibody neutralization of rotavirus and rotavirus monotype. *J. Virol.* **1991**, *65*, 5968–5974. [CrossRef]

49. Betts, M.J.; Russell, R.B. Amino acid properties and consequences of substitutions. *Bioinform. Genet.* **2003**, *317*, 289.

50. Caust, J.; Dyall-Smith, M.L.; Lazdins, I.; Holmes, I.H. Glycosylation, an important modifier of rotavirus antigenicity. *Arch. Virol.* **1987**, *96*, 123–134. [CrossRef]

51. Potgieter, A.C.; Page, N.A.; Liebenberg, J.; Wright, I.M.; Landt, O.; Van Dijk, A.A. Improved strategies for sequence-independent amplification and sequencing of viral double-stranded RNA genomes. *J. Gen. Virol.* **2009**, *90*, 1423–1432. [CrossRef]

52. Kearse, M.; Moir, R.; Wilson, A.; Stones-Havas, S.; Cheung, M.; Sturrock, S.; Buxton, S.; Cooper, A.; Markowitz, S.; Duran, C.; et al. Geneious Basic: An integrated and extendable desktop software platform for the organization and analysis of sequence data. *Bioinformatics* **2012**, *28*, 1647–1649. [CrossRef]

53. Esona, M.D.; Roy, S.; Rungsrisuriyachai, K.; Gautam, R.; Hermelijn, S.; Rey-Benito, G.; Bowen, M.D. Molecular characterization of a human G20P[28] rotavirus a strain with multiple genes related to bat rotaviruses. *Infect. Genet. Evol.* **2018**, *57*, 166–170. [CrossRef]

54. Esona, M.D.; Roy, S.; Rungsrisuriyachai, K.; Sanchez, J.; Vasquez, L.; Gomez, V.; Rios, L.A.; Bowen, M.D.; Vazquez, M. Characterization of a triple-recombinant, reassortant rotavirus strain from the Dominican Republic. *J. Gen. Virol.* **2017**, *98*, 134. [CrossRef]

55. Ward, M.L.; Mijatovic-Rustempasic, S.; Roy, S.; Rungsrisuriyachai, K.; Boom, J.A.; Sahni, L.C.; Baker, C.J.; Rench, M.A.; Wikswo, M.E.; Payne, D.C.; et al. Molecular characterization of the first G24P[14] rotavirus strain detected in humans. *Infect. Genet. Evol.* **2016**, *43*, 338–342. [CrossRef]

56. Tamura, K.; Stecher, G.; Peterson, D.; Filipski, A.; Kumar, S. MEGA6: Molecular evolutionary genetics analysis version 6.0. *Mol. Biol. Evol.* **2013**, *30*, 2725–2729. [CrossRef] [PubMed]

57. Benson, D.A.; Karsch-Mizrachi, I.; Lipman, D.J.; Ostell, J.; Rapp, B.A.; Wheeler, D.L. GenBank. *Nucleic Acids Res.* **2000**, *28*, 15–18. [CrossRef] [PubMed]

58. Mayor, C.; Brudno, M.; Schwartz, J.R.; Poliakov, A.; Rubin, E.M.; Frazer, K.A.; Pachter, L.S.; Dubchak, I. VISTA: Visualizing global DNA sequence alignments of arbitrary length. *Bioinformatics* **2000**, *16*, 1046–1047. [CrossRef] [PubMed]

# Whole Genome Characterization and Evolutionary Analysis of G1P[8] Rotavirus A Strains during the Pre- and Post-Vaccine Periods in Mozambique (2012–2017)

Benilde Munlela [1,2,*,†], Eva D. João [1,3,*,†], Celeste M. Donato [4,5,6], Amy Strydom [7], Simone S. Boene [1,2], Assucênio Chissaque [1,3], Adilson F. L. Bauhofer [1,3], Jerónimo Langa [1], Marta Cassocera [1,3], Idalécia Cossa-Moiane [1,8], Jorfélia J. Chilaúle [1], Hester G. O'Neill [7] and Nilsa de Deus [1,9]

[1] Instituto Nacional de Saúde (INS), Distrito de Marracuene, Maputo 3943, Mozambique; simone.boene@ins.gov.mz (S.S.B.); assucenio.chissaque@ins.gov.mz (A.C.); adilson.bauhofer@ins.gov.mz (A.F.L.B.); Jeronimo.Langa@ins.gov.mz (J.L.); marta.Cassocera@ins.gov.mz (M.C.); idalecia.moiane@ins.gov.mz (I.C.-M.); jorfelia.chilaule@ins.gov.mz (J.J.C.); nilsa.dedeus@ins.gov.mz (N.d.D.)
[2] Centro de Biotecnologia, Universidade Eduardo Mondlane, Maputo 3453, Mozambique
[3] Instituto de Higiene e Medicina Tropical (IHMT), Universidade Nova de Lisboa, UNL, Rua da Junqueira 100, 1349-008 Lisbon, Portugal
[4] Enteric Diseases Group, Murdoch Children's Research Institute, 50 Flemington Road, Parkville, Melbourne 3052, Australia; celeste.donato@mcri.edu.au
[5] Department of Paediatrics, the University of Melbourne, Parkville 3010, Australia
[6] Biomedicine Discovery Institute and Department of Microbiology, Monash University, Clayton 3800, Australia
[7] Department of Microbial, Biochemical and Food Biotechnology, University of the Free State, 205 Nelson Mandela Avenue, Bloemfontein 9301, South Africa; strydoma@ufs.ac.za (A.S.); oneillhg@ufs.ac.za (H.G.O.)
[8] Institute of Tropical Medicine (ITM), Kronenburgstraat 43, 2000 Antwerp, Belgium
[9] Departamento de Ciências Biológicas, Universidade Eduardo Mondlane, Maputo 3453, Mozambique
* Correspondence: benilde.munlela@ins.gov.mz or benildeantnio@gmail.com (B.M.); evadora1@hotmail.com (E.D.J.);
† These authors contributed equally in this work.

**Abstract:** Mozambique introduced the Rotarix® vaccine (GSK Biologicals, Rixensart, Belgium) into the National Immunization Program in September 2015. Although G1P[8] was one of the most prevalent genotypes between 2012 and 2017 in Mozambique, no complete genomes had been sequenced to date. Here we report whole genome sequence analysis for 36 G1P[8] strains using an Illumina MiSeq platform. All strains exhibited a Wa-like genetic backbone (G1-P[8]-I1-R1-C1-M1-A1-N1-T1-E1-H1). Phylogenetic analysis showed that most of the Mozambican strains clustered closely together in a conserved clade for the entire genome. No distinct clustering for pre- and post-vaccine strains were observed. These findings may suggest no selective pressure by the introduction of the Rotarix® vaccine in 2015. Two strains (HJM1646 and HGM0544) showed varied clustering for the entire genome, suggesting reassortment, whereas a further strain obtained from a rural area (MAN0033) clustered separately for all gene segments. Bayesian analysis for the VP7 and VP4 encoding gene segments supported the phylogenetic analysis and indicated a possible introduction from India around 2011.7 and 2013.0 for the main Mozambican clade. Continued monitoring of rotavirus strains in the post-vaccine period is required to fully understand the impact of vaccine introduction on the diversity and evolution of rotavirus strains.

**Keywords:** rotavirus group A; G1P[8]; whole genome sequencing; Rotarix®; Bayesian analysis; Mozambique

## 1. Introduction

Rotavirus is one of the leading causes of diarrheal disease in children under five years of age [1,2]. Worldwide, the number of deaths due to rotavirus infection in children under five years of age in 2016 was estimated to be 128,500, of which 104,733 occurred in sub-Saharan Africa [2]. Rotavirus is a member of the *Reoviridae* family. The genome is comprised of 11 double-stranded ribonucleic acid (dsRNA) segments. The mature virus has an icosahedral capsid formed by three concentric protein layers. The 11 segments of the rotavirus genome encode 12 viral proteins: 6 structural proteins VP1-VP4, VP6 and VP7and 6 non-structural proteins (NSP1-NSP6) [3–6].

The gene segments encoding the external capsid proteins, VP7 and VP4, are used in a binary classification system defining G and P genotypes, respectively [5,7]. Currently, 36 G and 51 P genotypes have been described in humans and various animal species [7–10]. At least 73 combinations of human rotavirus group A (RVA) G/P genotypes have been described, of which the most common combinations are G1P[8], G2P[4], G3P[8], G4P[8], G9P[8] and G12P[8] [10,11]. However, the implementation of whole genome sequencing has led to comprehensive sequence-based classification of all RVA genes into genotypes, which are identified and differentiated according to particular cut-off values of nucleotide sequence identities [9,11]. Currently, 26 I (VP6), 22 R (VP1), 20 C (VP2), 20 M (VP3), 31 A (NSP1), 22 N (NSP2), 22 T (NSP3), 27 E (NSP4) and 22 H (NSP5) genotypes have been described [8]. The whole genome constellation of a strain can be described following the nomenclature Gx-P[x]-Ix-Rx-Cx-Mx-Ax-Nx-Tx-Ex-Hx. Two major genotype constellations have been designated for strains that commonly infect humans: Wa-like (I1-R1-C1-M1-A1-N1-T1-E1-H1) and DS-1-like (I2-R2-C2-M2-A2-N2-T2-E2-H2). A third constellation also observed in human strains, called AU-1-like (I3-R3-C3-M3-A3-N3-T3-E3-H3), has been shown to have a feline/canine origin [9,11].

Four live oral vaccines, namely Rotarix® (GlaxoSmithKline Biologics, Rixensart, Belgium), RotaTeq® (Merck & Co., Kenilworth, NJ, USA), Rotavac® (Bharat Biotech, Hyderabad, India) and Rotasiil® (Serum Institute of India Pvt. Ltd., Pune, India) have been prequalified by the World Health Organization [12,13]. Rotarix® and RotaTeq® have been introduced into the immunization programs of more than 100 countries [13]. Rotarix® is a monovalent vaccine containing a single human G1P[8] strain and is administered from the age of six weeks [13]. Prior to vaccine introduction in Mozambique, a high burden of rotavirus disease was reported in children under five years old. The rate of rotavirus infection in urban (Maputo City) and rural (Manhiça District) areas between 2012 and 2013 was 42.4% [6]. In 2011, a 24.0% infection rate was reported in the Gaza province, another rural area in southern Mozambique [14]. In both studies G1P[8] was detected at a low frequency [14,15]. Data from the National Surveillance of Diarrhea (ViNaDia) revealed a high rotavirus infection rate of 40.2% and 38.3% in 2014 and 2015, respectively [16]. The Rotarix® vaccine was introduced in Mozambique in 2015 with increasing vaccine coverage of 70% and 80% in 2016 and 2017, respectively [16,17]. Post vaccine introduction, the rotavirus infection rate was reduced to 12.2% and 13.5% in 2016 and 2017, respectively [16]. During ViNaDia surveillance, G1P[8] strains were consistently observed in the pre- (2012–2015) and post-vaccination period (2016–2019). However, in the post-vaccine period a decrease in G1P[8] strains was observed which coincided with the emergence of other non-G1P[8] genotypes such as G3P[4] and G3P[8] [18].

The whole genomes of Mozambican G2P[4], G8P[4], G12P[6] and G12P[8] RVA strains from the pre-vaccination period have been described [19,20]. However, there are no reports of the whole genome analyses of G1P[8] strains from Mozambique. To address this, the consensus sequences of 36 G1P[8] strains collected between 2012–2017 from vaccinated and non-vaccinated children were analyzed to investigate the diversity and evolution of G1P[8] strains.

## 2. Results

*2.1. Genome Constellation*

A total of 36 G1P[8] (12 from the pre-vaccine period and 24 from the post-vaccine period) strains were successfully sequenced with an average coverage ranging from 450.0 to 46060.5 per sequence (Supplementary Table S1). Complete open reading frames (ORFs) were obtained for 393 of the 396 genome segments analyzed. A partial ORF (99.0%) for segment four of RVA/Human-wt/MOZ/HCN0690/2015/G1P[8] was obtained, while two genome segments (encoding VP2 and VP3, respectively) of RVA/Human-wt/MOZ/HGM0059/2014/G1P[8] could not be determined as insufficient data were generated for these two segments (Supplementary Table S1). The genotype constellations were determined and all strains exhibited a Wa-like genetic backbone (G1-P[8]-I1-R1-C1-M1-A1-N1-T1-E1-H1). The nucleotide (nt) identities among Mozambican strains varied from 92.5–100.0% and the comparison between Rotarix® and the 11 genes of the Mozambican strains revealed 84.0–97.9% nt identity (Supplementary Table S2).

*2.2. Phylogenetic Analyses*

2.2.1. Sequence Analyses of VP7 and VP4

The VP7 encoding sequences of the 36 Mozambican G1P[8] strains, collected between 2012 to 2017 from non-vaccinated and vaccinated children (Supplementary Table S3), were compared with human rotavirus sequences representing VP7 G1 lineages (I-VII) [21–28]. The Mozambican strains clustered into two distinct lineages, I and II (Figure 1a). The majority of Mozambican strains formed a highly conserved clade, and were closely related to various Indian strains circulating between 2012 and 2013. HGM0544 was moderately divergent to the rest of the strains in the clade sharing 99.2–99.7% nucleotide (nt) identity and 98.8–99.4% amino acid (aa) identity. Strains from the pre- and post-vaccine era were intermingled in lineage II. Only two Mozambican strains from this study clustered in the VP7 lineage I and were more diverse than the 34 strains clustering in lineage II. MAN0033, collected in a rural area in southern Mozambique before vaccine introduction, was closely related to Malawian strains from 2012 and to previously characterized Mozambican strains detected in 2011 [14]. HJM1646, collected in southern Mozambique after vaccine introduction, clustered distinctly and only shared 92.5–92.9% nt and 92.7–93.3% aa identity to the other Mozambican strains. HJM1646 clustered with contemporary Indian strains in a sub lineage of African and global strains (Figure 1a).

The P[8] encoding sequences of the 36 Mozambican strains were compared with human rotavirus sequences representing the four lineages (I–IV) [21–27] (Figure 1b). The Mozambican strains clustered in the major P[8] lineage III. Similar to the VP7 tree, the majority of Mozambican P[8] sequences formed a highly conserved clade, and were closely related to various Indian strains circulating between 2012 and 2013. The P[8] encoding sequence of HJM1646 clustered with HGM0544, despite clustering in different VP7 lineages. These two strains were moderately divergent to the rest of the study strains in the Mozambican clade and clustered close to another Mozambican strain, RVA/Human-wt/MOZ/0060a/2012/G12P[8]P[14], which was previously detected in the Manhiça district in southern Mozambique [19]. MAN0033 clustered distinctly to the rest of the Mozambican strains sharing 95.7–96.2% nt and 98.3–98.7% aa identity and was closely related to contemporary Malawian strains isolated in 2012 (Figure 1b, Supplementary Table S1).

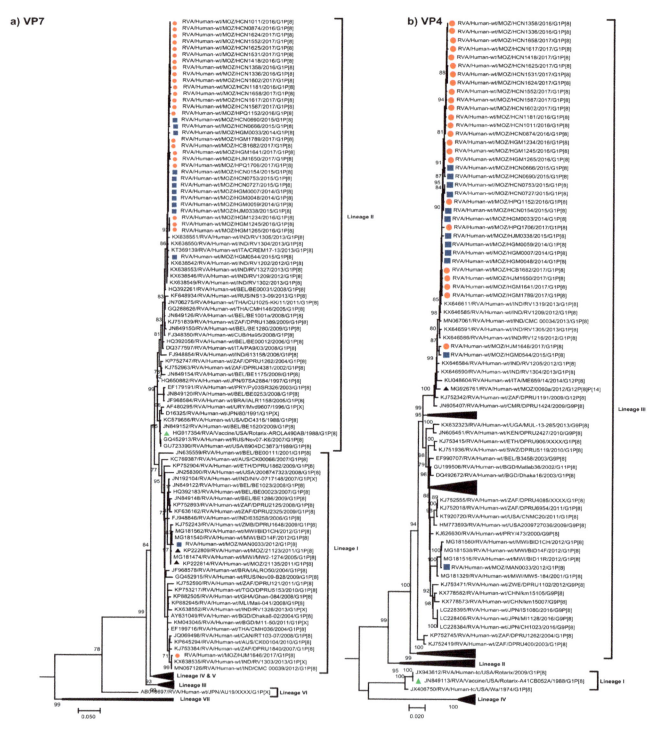

**Figure 1.** Phylogenetic trees based on the ORF (open reading frame) nucleotide sequence of the (**a**) VP7 and (**b**) VP4 genes of G1P[8] strains circulating in Mozambique and global strains obtained from GenBank. The trees were constructed based on the maximum likelihood method implemented in MEGA X [29], applying the best-fit nucleotide substitution model Tamura-3-parameter (T92+G+I) for VP7 and General Time Reversible (GTR-G) for VP4, determined by JModelTest [30]. Bootstrap values (1000 replicates) ≥70% are shown with DS-1 serving as an out-group (not shown in the final tree). Scale bar indicates genetic distance expressed as the number of nucleotide substitutions per site. Pre-vaccine Mozambican strains are indicated by blue squares, post-vaccine by red circles, the Rotarix® vaccine strain by a green triangle and Mozambican strains from previous studies [14,19] are indicated by black triangles. Lineages are defined from I-VIII for VP7 and I-IV for VP4 [21–23,25–28].

## 2.2.2. Sequence Analyses of VP1-VP3 and VP6

Thirty-three Mozambican strains formed conserved, monophyletic clades that were observed in the VP1, VP2 and VP3 trees, closely related to RVA/Human-wt/IND/CMC00034/2013/G1P[8], and within lineages comprising of contemporary African and global strains (Figure 2a–c). In the VP6 tree, the 35 Mozambican strains clustered together but did not form a discrete monophyletic clade, and were closely related to contemporary Indian G1P[8] strains (Figure 2d). HJM1646 and HGM0544 clustered together in the VP1 tree were moderately divergent from the main Mozambican clade (Figure 2a). In the VP2 tree, HJM1646 clustered close to the monophyletic clade while HGM0544 fell within the Mozambican clade (Figure 2b). In the VP3 tree, these strains clustered together, distinct from the Mozambican clade, adjacent to previously characterized G12P[6] Mozambican strains (Figure 2c) [19]. MAN0033 fell within the same lineage as the main Mozambican clade, showing minor divergence in the VP1 and VP2 tree and more pronounced divergence in the VP3 tree, closely related to contemporary Malawian G1P[8] strains (Figure 2a–c). This strain clustered within a different lineage in the VP6 tree, closely related to the same group of Malawian G1P[8] strains and adjacent to the Mozambican G12P[6] strains (Figure 2d).

## 2.2.3. Sequence Analyses of NSP1-NSP5/6

The conserved monophyletic clade, comprised of 33 Mozambican strains, was observed in the NSP1–NSP4 trees, with RVA/Human-wt/IND/CMC00034/2013/G1P[8] interspersed within the clade in the NSP2 tree (Figure 2e–h). HJM1646 and HGM0544 continued to show varied clustering patterns across the trees. In the NSP3 tree these strains clustered together and were divergent from the main Mozambican clade, clustering with Indian strains including RVA/Human-wt/IND/CMC00034/2013/G1P[8], and close to Mozambican G12P[6] strains (Figure 2g). HJM1646 was divergent to the Mozambican clade in the NSP1 and NSP4 trees, but clustered close to the monophyletic clade in the NSP2 tree. HGM0544 clustered with the main Mozambican clade in the NSP1, NSP2 and NSP4 trees. In the NSP5 tree, HJM1646 and HGM0544, along with 33 other Mozambican strains, formed a monophyletic clade that was interspersed with global strains (Figure 2i). MAN0033 clustered distinctly to the rest of the Mozambican strains and was closely related to contemporary Malawian strains isolated in 2012 across these trees (Figure 2e–i). The five G12P[6] [19] Mozambican strains fell within neighboring clusters to MAN0033 in the VP6 and NSP2 trees (Figure 2d,f).

## 2.3. Evolutionary Analysis of VP7 and VP4 Genes

A randomly subsampled dataset of 378 G1 genes that were representative of global strains temporally and genetically were analyzed (Supplementary Figure S1). The Mozambican strains detected between 2012 and 2017 shared a common ancestral strain circulating in 2009.9 (95% HPD 2008.1–2010.9). Of the Mozambican strains characterized in this study, 34 clustered within the same lineage and shared a most recent common ancestor in 2011.7 (95% HPD 2011.1–2012.0) and diverged from the closest related Indian strains around the same time. MAN0033 and HJM1646 clustered in the other major lineage present in the tree. MAN0033 and closely related Malawian strains shared a common ancestor in 2010.1 (95% HPD 2008.5–2010.9). These variants, circulating in Malawi, Zambia and Mozambique, diverged from a group of Indian G1P[8] strains in 2001.3 (95% HPD 1998.4–2003.5). HJM1646 was divergent to the other G1 strains from Mozambique in this lineage and shared its most recent common ancestor with Indian strains in 2012.9 (95% HPD 2012.4–2013.0) (Supplementary Figure S1).

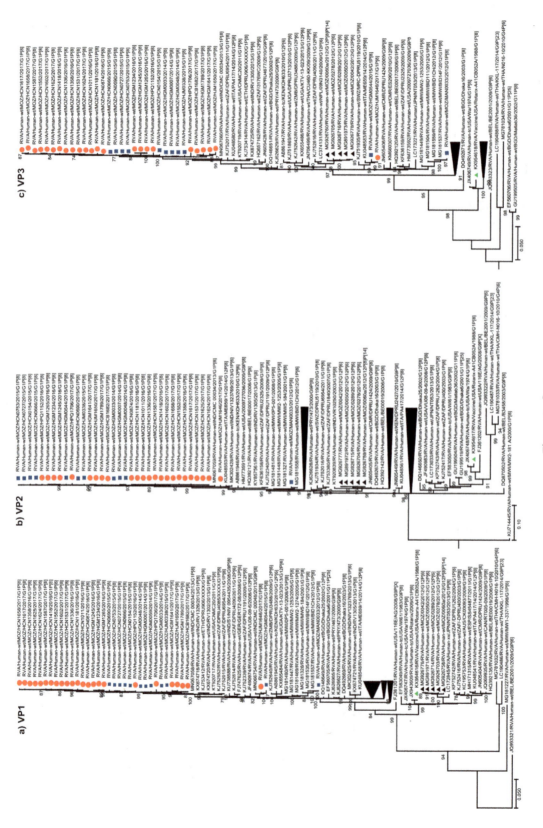

Figure 2. Cont.

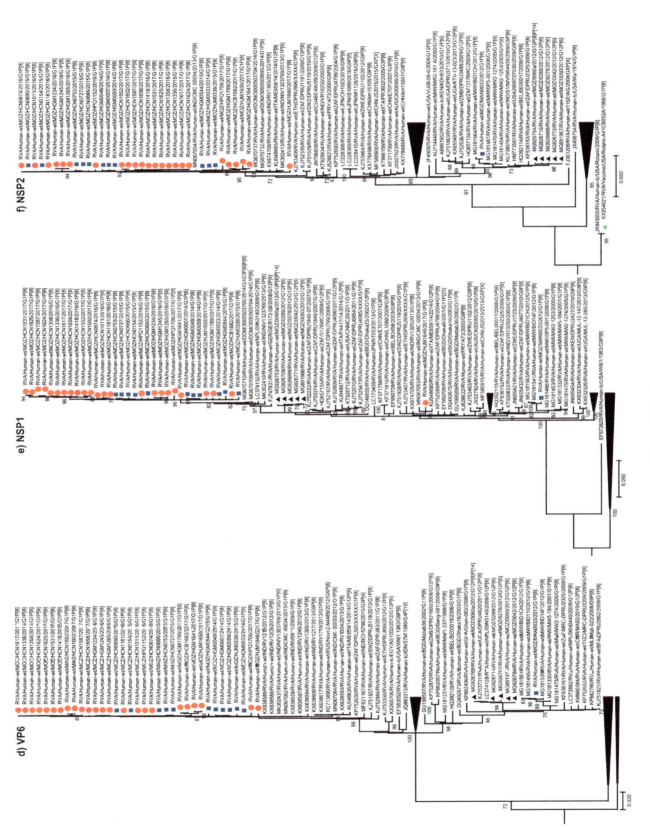

**Figure 2.** *Cont.*

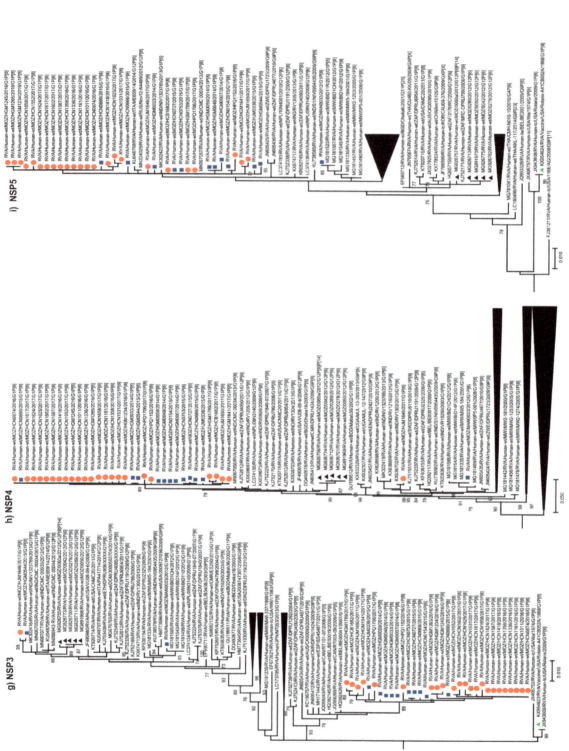

**Fig. 2** Phylogenetic trees based on the ORF nucleotide sequences of the (**a**) VP1, (**b**) VP2, (**c**) VP3, (**d**) VP6, (**e**) NSP1, (**f**) NSP2, (**g**) NSP3, (**h**) NSP4 and (**i**) NSP5 genes of G1P[8] strains circulating in Mozambique and global strains obtained from GenBank. The trees were constructed based on the maximum likelihood method implemented in MEGA X [29], using the best-fit nucleotide substitution model General Time Reversible (GTR+G+I) for VP3, GTR+G for VP2, NSP2 and NSP3, Hasegawa Kishino Yano (HKY+G+I) for VP6 and NSP1, HKY+G for VP1, NSP4 and NSP5/6, determined by JModelTest [30]. Bootstrap values (1000 replicates) ≥70% are shown with DS-1 serving as an out-group (not shown in the final tree). Scale bar indicates genetic distance expressed as the number of nucleotide substitutions per site. Pre-vaccine Mozambican strains are indicated by blue squares, post-vaccine by red circles, the Rotarix® vaccine strain by a green triangle and Mozambican strains from a previous study [19] are indicated by black triangles.

A subsampled dataset of 235 P[8] genes, representative of global strains temporally and genetically, was also analyzed. Thirty-three Mozambican strains characterized in this study clustered within the same lineage and shared a common ancestor in 2013.0 (95% HPD 2012.1–2013.6) and diverged from the closest related Indian strains around 2011.6 (95% HPD 2011.2–2011.9) (Supplementary Figure S2). The most recent common ancestor of HGM0544 and HJM1646 (that was moderately divergent to the rest of the Mozambican strains in the major clade), was estimated to be 2014.1 (95% HPD 2013.0–2014.9). Clustering in a separate lineage to the other Mozambican G1P[8] strains, MAN0033 diverged from the closest Malawian strain in 2010.9 (95% HPD 2009.5–2011.7) (Supplementary Figure S2).

### 2.4. Comparative Analysis of Neutralizing Antigenic Epitopes of the VP7 and VP4 Genes of Mozambican Strains and the Rotarix® Vaccine Strain

The rotavirus VP7 protein consists of two antigenic epitopes, 7-1 and 7-2, with 7-1 subdivided into 7-1a and 7-1b [31]. The comparative analysis of the VP7 antigenic epitopes between Mozambican strains and the Rotarix® vaccine strain revealed amino acid substitutions in all three antigenic sites. However, most of the amino acid substitutions were observed in antigenic region 7-2. A total of 30 strains shared conserved amino acid differences at positions N147D and 25 strains at M217I. Sporadic mutations were observed in MAN0033 (unvaccinated) and HJM1646 (fully vaccinated) (S123N, K291R and M217T). The HJM1646 strain contained an additional amino acid substitution at N96S (Figure 3).

| Antigenic regions | 7-1a | | | | | | | | | | | | | | 7-1b | | | | | | | 7-2 | | | | | | | |
|---|---|---|---|---|---|---|---|---|---|---|---|---|---|---|---|---|---|---|---|---|---|---|---|---|---|---|---|---|---|
| | 87 | 91 | 94 | 96 | 97 | 98 | 99 | 100 | 104 | 123 | 125 | 129 | 130 | 291 | 201 | 211 | 212 | 213 | 238 | 242 | 143 | 145 | 146 | 147 | 148 | 190 | 217 | 221 | 264 |
| Rotarix® | T | T | N | G | E | W | K | D | Q | S | V | V | D | K | Q | N | V | D | N | T | K | D | Q | N | L | S | M | N | G |
| HCB1682 | . | . | . | . | . | . | . | . | . | . | . | . | . | . | . | . | . | . | . | . | . | . | . | D | . | . | . | . | . |
| HCN0154 | . | . | . | . | . | . | . | . | . | . | . | N | . | . | . | . | . | . | . | . | . | . | . | D | . | . | I | . | . |
| HCN0666 | . | . | . | . | . | . | . | . | . | . | . | . | . | . | . | . | . | . | . | . | . | . | . | D | . | . | I | . | . |
| HCN0690 | . | . | . | . | . | . | . | . | . | . | . | . | . | . | . | . | . | . | . | . | . | . | . | D | . | . | I | . | . |
| HCN0727 | . | . | . | . | . | . | . | . | . | . | . | . | . | . | . | . | . | . | . | . | . | . | . | D | . | . | I | . | . |
| HCN0753 | . | . | . | . | . | . | . | . | . | . | . | . | . | . | . | . | . | . | . | . | . | . | . | D | . | . | I | . | . |
| HCN0874 | . | . | . | . | . | . | . | . | . | . | . | . | . | . | . | . | . | . | . | . | . | . | . | D | . | . | I | . | . |
| HCN1011 | . | . | . | . | . | . | . | . | . | . | . | . | . | . | . | . | . | . | . | . | . | . | . | D | . | . | I | . | . |
| HCN1181 | . | . | . | . | . | E | . | . | . | . | . | . | . | . | . | . | . | . | . | . | . | . | . | D | . | . | I | . | . |
| HCN1336 | . | . | . | . | . | . | . | . | . | . | . | . | . | . | . | . | . | . | . | . | . | . | . | D | . | . | I | . | . |
| HCN1358 | . | . | . | . | . | . | . | . | . | . | . | . | . | . | . | . | . | . | . | . | . | . | . | D | . | . | I | . | . |
| HCN1418 | . | . | . | . | . | . | . | . | . | . | . | . | . | . | . | . | . | . | . | . | . | . | . | D | . | . | I | . | . |
| HCN1531 | . | . | . | . | . | . | . | . | . | . | . | . | . | . | . | . | . | . | . | . | . | . | . | D | . | . | I | . | . |
| HCN1552 | . | . | . | . | . | . | . | . | . | . | . | . | . | . | . | . | . | . | . | . | . | . | . | D | . | . | I | . | . |
| HCN1587 | . | . | . | . | . | . | . | . | . | . | . | . | . | . | . | . | . | . | . | . | . | . | . | D | . | . | I | . | S |
| HCN1602 | . | . | . | . | . | . | . | . | . | . | . | . | . | . | . | . | . | . | . | . | . | . | . | D | . | . | I | . | . |
| HCN1617 | . | . | . | . | . | . | . | . | . | . | . | . | . | . | . | . | . | . | . | . | . | . | . | D | . | . | I | . | . |
| HCN1624 | . | . | . | . | . | . | . | . | . | . | . | . | . | . | . | . | . | . | . | . | . | . | . | D | . | . | I | . | . |
| HCN1625 | . | . | . | . | . | . | . | . | . | . | . | . | . | . | . | . | . | . | . | . | . | . | . | D | . | . | I | . | . |
| HCN1658 | . | . | . | . | . | . | . | . | . | . | . | . | . | . | . | . | . | . | . | . | . | . | . | D | . | . | I | . | . |
| HGM0007 | . | . | . | . | . | . | . | . | . | . | . | . | . | . | . | . | . | . | . | . | . | . | . | D | . | . | . | . | . |
| HGM0033 | . | . | . | . | . | . | . | . | . | . | . | . | . | . | . | . | . | . | . | . | . | . | . | D | . | . | . | . | . |
| HGM0048 | . | . | . | . | . | . | . | . | . | . | . | . | . | . | . | . | . | . | . | . | . | . | . | D | . | . | . | . | . |
| HGM0059 | . | . | . | . | . | . | . | . | . | . | . | . | . | . | . | . | . | . | . | . | . | . | . | D | . | . | . | . | . |
| HGM0544 | . | . | . | . | . | . | . | . | . | . | . | . | . | . | . | . | . | . | I | . | . | . | . | . | . | . | . | . | . |
| HGM1234 | . | . | . | . | . | . | . | . | . | . | . | . | . | . | . | . | . | . | . | . | . | . | . | . | . | . | I | . | . |
| HGM1245 | . | . | . | . | . | . | . | . | . | . | . | . | . | . | . | . | . | . | . | . | . | . | . | . | . | . | I | . | . |
| HGM1265 | . | . | . | . | . | . | . | . | . | . | . | . | . | . | . | . | . | . | . | . | . | . | . | . | . | . | I | . | . |
| HGM1641 | . | . | . | . | . | . | . | . | . | . | . | . | . | . | . | . | . | . | . | . | . | . | . | D | . | . | . | . | . |
| HGM1789 | . | . | . | . | . | . | . | . | . | . | . | . | . | . | . | . | . | . | . | . | . | . | . | D | . | . | . | . | . |
| HJM0338 | . | . | . | . | . | . | . | . | . | . | . | . | . | . | . | . | . | . | . | . | . | . | . | D | . | . | . | . | . |
| HJM1646 | . | . | S | . | . | . | . | . | . | N | . | . | . | R | . | . | . | . | . | . | . | . | . | . | . | . | T | . | . |
| HJM1650 | . | . | . | . | . | . | . | . | . | . | . | . | . | . | . | . | . | . | . | . | . | . | . | D | . | . | . | . | . |
| HPQ1152 | . | . | . | . | . | . | . | . | . | . | . | . | . | . | . | . | . | . | . | . | . | . | . | D | . | . | I | . | . |
| HPQ1706 | . | . | . | . | . | . | . | . | . | . | . | . | . | . | . | . | . | . | . | . | . | . | . | D | . | . | . | . | . |
| MAN0033 | . | . | . | . | . | . | . | . | . | N | . | . | . | R | . | . | . | . | . | . | . | . | . | . | . | . | T | . | . |

**Figure 3.** The alignment of amino acids corresponding to three VP7 antigenic epitopes (7-1a, 7-1b and 7-2). The amino acid sequence of Rotarix® is the reference strain and the conserved residues between the Rotarix® to Mozambican strains are indicated by dots (.) and residues that differ are in bold.

Activation of the protein VP4 requires proteolytic cleavage to produce the VP8* and VP5* subunits. These regions contain four (8-1 to 8-4) and five (5-1 to 5-5) antigenic epitopes, respectively [32,33]. The amino acid substitutions between the Rotarix® vaccine strain and Mozambican P[8] strains were concentrated in the 8-1 and 8-3 epitopes. There were five conserved amino acid substitutions, at positions E150D, N195D/G, S125N, S131R and N135D. Sporadic mutations were observed in MAN0033 (N195S and N113D), HJM0338 (S146N) and HGM1789 (P114T) (Figure 4).

| Antigenic region | 8-1 | | | | | | | | | | | 8-2 | | 8-3 | | | | | | | 8-4 | | | 5-1 | | | | | | | | | 5-2 | 5-3 | 5-4 | 5-5 |
|---|---|---|---|---|---|---|---|---|---|---|---|---|---|---|---|---|---|---|---|---|---|---|---|---|---|---|---|---|---|---|---|---|---|---|---|---|
| | 100 | 146 | 148 | 150 | 188 | 190 | 192 | 193 | 194 | 195 | 196 | 180 | 183 | 113 | 114 | 115 | 116 | 125 | 131 | 132 | 133 | 135 | 87 | 88 | 89 | 384 | 386 | 388 | 393 | 394 | 398 | 440 | 441 | 434 | 459 | 429 | 306 |
| Rotarix® | D | S | Q | E | S | T | M | L | N | N | I | T | A | N | P | V | D | S | S | N | D | N | N | T | N | Y | F | I | W | P | G | R | T | P | E | L | R |
| HCN1181 | . | . | . | . | . | . | . | . | . | . | . | . | . | . | . | . | . | . | . | . | . | . | . | . | . | . | . | . | . | . | . | . | . | . | . | . | . |
| HCN1011 | . | . | . | D | . | . | . | . | . | . | D | . | . | . | . | . | . | . | N | R | . | D | . | . | . | . | . | . | . | . | . | . | . | . | . | . | . |
| HCN0874 | . | . | . | D | . | . | . | . | . | . | D | . | . | . | . | . | . | . | N | R | . | D | . | . | . | . | . | . | . | . | . | . | . | . | . | . | . |
| HCN1418 | . | . | . | D | . | . | . | . | . | . | D | . | . | . | . | . | . | . | N | R | . | D | . | . | . | . | . | . | . | . | . | . | . | . | . | . | . |
| HCN1531 | . | . | . | D | . | . | . | . | . | . | D | . | . | . | . | . | . | . | N | R | . | D | . | . | . | . | . | . | . | . | . | . | . | . | . | . | . |
| HCN1624 | . | . | . | D | . | . | . | . | . | . | D | . | . | . | . | . | . | . | N | R | . | D | . | . | . | . | . | . | . | . | . | . | . | . | . | . | . |
| HCN1625 | . | . | . | D | . | . | . | . | . | . | D | . | . | . | . | . | . | . | N | R | . | D | . | . | . | . | . | . | . | . | . | . | . | . | . | . | . |
| HCN0753 | . | . | . | D | . | . | . | . | . | . | D | . | . | . | . | . | . | . | N | R | . | D | . | . | . | . | . | . | . | . | . | . | . | . | . | . | . |
| HCN1358 | . | . | . | D | . | . | . | . | . | . | D | . | . | . | . | . | . | . | N | R | . | D | . | . | . | . | . | . | . | . | . | . | . | . | . | . | . |
| HCN1336 | . | . | . | D | . | . | . | . | . | . | D | . | . | . | . | . | . | . | N | R | . | D | . | . | . | . | . | . | . | . | . | . | . | . | . | . | . |
| HCN1552 | . | . | . | D | . | . | . | . | . | . | D | . | . | . | . | . | . | . | N | R | . | D | . | . | . | . | . | . | . | . | . | . | . | . | . | . | . |
| HCN1587 | . | . | . | D | . | . | . | . | . | . | D | . | . | . | . | . | . | . | N | R | . | D | . | . | . | . | . | . | . | . | . | . | . | . | . | . | . |
| HCN1602 | . | . | . | D | . | . | . | . | . | . | D | . | . | . | . | . | . | . | N | R | . | D | . | . | . | . | . | . | . | . | . | . | . | . | . | . | . |
| HCN1617 | . | . | . | D | . | . | . | . | . | . | D | . | . | . | . | . | . | . | N | R | . | D | . | . | . | . | . | . | . | . | . | . | . | . | . | . | . |
| HCN1658 | . | . | . | D | . | . | . | . | . | . | D | . | . | . | . | . | . | . | N | R | . | D | . | . | . | . | . | . | . | . | . | . | . | . | . | . | . |
| HGM1234 | . | . | . | D | . | . | . | . | . | . | D | . | . | . | . | . | . | . | N | R | . | D | . | . | . | . | . | . | . | . | . | . | . | . | . | . | . |
| HGM1245 | . | . | . | D | . | . | . | . | . | . | D | . | . | . | . | . | . | . | N | R | . | D | . | . | . | . | . | . | . | . | . | . | . | . | . | . | . |
| HGM1265 | . | . | . | D | . | . | . | . | . | . | D | . | . | . | . | . | . | . | N | R | . | D | . | . | . | . | . | . | . | . | . | . | . | . | . | . | . |
| HCN0666 | . | . | . | D | . | . | . | . | . | . | D | . | . | . | . | . | . | . | N | R | . | D | . | . | . | . | . | . | . | . | . | . | . | . | . | . | . |
| HCN0690 | . | . | . | D | . | . | . | . | . | . | G | . | . | . | . | . | . | . | N | R | . | D | . | . | . | . | . | . | . | . | . | . | . | . | . | . | . |
| HCN0727 | . | . | . | D | . | . | . | . | . | . | G | . | . | . | . | . | . | . | N | R | . | D | . | . | . | . | . | . | . | . | . | . | . | . | . | . | . |
| HCN0154 | . | . | . | D | . | . | . | . | . | . | G | . | . | . | . | . | . | . | N | R | . | D | . | . | . | . | . | . | . | . | . | . | . | . | . | . | . |
| HPQ1152 | . | . | . | D | . | . | . | . | . | . | G | . | . | . | . | . | . | . | N | R | . | D | . | . | . | . | . | . | . | . | . | . | . | . | . | . | . |
| HGM1641 | . | . | . | D | . | . | . | . | . | . | G | . | . | . | . | . | . | . | N | R | . | D | . | . | . | . | . | . | . | . | . | . | . | . | . | . | . |
| HGM0007 | . | . | . | D | . | . | . | . | . | . | G | . | . | . | . | . | . | . | N | R | . | D | . | . | . | . | . | . | . | . | . | . | . | . | . | . | . |
| HGM0048 | . | . | . | D | . | . | . | . | . | . | G | . | . | . | . | . | . | . | N | R | . | D | . | . | . | . | . | . | . | . | . | . | . | . | . | . | . |
| HGM0059 | . | . | . | D | . | . | . | . | . | . | G | . | . | . | . | . | . | . | N | R | . | D | . | . | . | . | . | . | . | . | . | . | . | . | . | . | . |
| HJM1650 | . | . | . | D | . | . | . | . | . | . | G | . | . | . | . | . | . | . | N | R | . | D | . | . | . | . | . | . | . | . | . | . | . | . | . | . | . |
| HCB1682 | . | . | . | D | . | . | . | . | . | . | G | . | . | . | . | . | . | . | N | R | . | D | . | . | . | . | . | . | . | . | . | . | . | . | . | . | . |
| HGM0033 | . | . | . | D | . | . | . | . | . | . | G | . | . | . | . | . | . | . | N | R | . | D | . | . | . | . | . | . | . | . | . | . | . | . | . | . | . |
| HGM1789 | . | . | . | D | . | . | . | . | . | . | G | . | . | T | . | . | . | . | N | R | . | D | . | . | . | . | . | . | . | . | . | . | . | . | . | . | . |
| HJM0338 | . | N | . | D | . | . | . | . | . | . | G | . | . | . | . | . | . | . | N | R | . | D | . | . | . | . | . | . | . | . | . | . | . | . | . | . | . |
| HPQ1706 | . | . | . | D | . | . | . | . | . | . | G | . | . | . | . | . | . | . | N | R | . | D | . | . | . | . | . | . | . | . | . | . | . | . | . | . | . |
| HJM1646 | . | . | . | D | . | . | . | . | . | . | G | . | . | . | . | . | . | . | N | R | . | D | . | . | . | . | . | . | . | . | . | . | . | . | . | . | . |
| HGM0544 | . | . | . | D | . | . | . | . | . | . | G | . | . | . | . | . | . | . | N | R | . | D | . | . | . | . | . | . | . | . | . | . | . | . | . | . | . |
| MAN0033 | . | . | . | D | . | . | . | . | . | . | S | . | . | D | . | . | . | . | N | R | . | D | . | . | . | . | . | . | . | . | . | . | . | . | . | . | . |

**Figure 4.** The alignment of the amino acids corresponding to the VP4 antigenic epitopes (8-1, 8-2, 8-3, 8-4 for VP8* and 5-1, 5-2, 5-3, 5-4, 5-5 for VP5). The amino acid sequence of Rotarix® is the reference strain and the conserved residues between the Rotarix® to Mozambican strains are indicated by dots (.) and residues that differ are in bold.

## 3. Discussion

In the present study, whole genome sequencing was performed for 36 G1P[8] RVA strains obtained from Mozambican children with gastroenteritis between 2012–2017 (12 from the pre-vaccine period and 24 from the post-vaccine period). This is the first study to perform whole genome analysis of G1P[8] strains in Mozambique, facilitating the description of genetic diversity and the origins of Mozambican strains.

Of the 36 strains characterized, 33 clustered within the same conserved Mozambican clade across all trees. Two strains, HGM0544 and HJM1646, showed varied patterns by clustering within and were distinct from the Mozambican clade across trees, suggesting these strains had undergone reassortment events. The strain, MAN0033, clustered distinctly from the rest of the Mozambican strains in all trees. This strain was closely related to a conserved group of Malawian G1P[8] strains suggesting that this strain may have been recently introduced from a neighboring country. No distinct clustering patterns were observed based on the year of isolation or vaccination status, which suggests that strains with limited sequence diversity may have circulated among children in the country over the five year period investigated (2012–2017). The homogeneous population of G1P[8] strains suggests that the introduction of Rotarix®has not resulted in a dramatic shift in the diversity of G1P[8] strains circulating in Mozambique. A similar finding was reported in South Africa where no distinct clustering was observed for strains from the pre- and post-vaccine introduction period [26]. Analysis of G1P[8] strains in Brazil over a 27 year period also did not detect any evidence of a selective pressure exerted by the mass introduction of Rotarix® [34]. In contrast, Australia and Belgium reported some unique clusters of G1P[8] strains following vaccine introduction, which may have been due to natural fluctuation or the first signs of vaccine-driven evolution [35]. In Rwanda, unique clusters of G1P[8] strains were identified following RotaTeq introduction [36]. Although neighboring countries reported the widespread (Malawi) and sporadic (South Africa) detection of G1P[8] strains that had undergone reassortment with DS-1 like strains [28,37], all Mozambican strains characterized in this study exhibited a typical Wa-like genetic backbone. Despite some reports of vaccine-derived G1P[8] strains detected in Australia and England, none of the strains identified in this study were derived from the Rotarix® vaccine [38,39].

Although there are seven recognized lineages described for global G1 sequences [40], the majority of Mozambican strains from this study clustered in lineage II, with only two strains clustering in lineage I. However, one strain that clustered in lineage I represented the oldest Mozambican strain sequenced in this study from 2012, which clustered with previously characterized G1P[8] Mozambican strains from 2011 [14]. This may suggest that lineage I strains were replaced in later years by G1 strains associated with lineage II [26,41]. The VP7 lineage I strains were detected in the south of Mozambique which may suggest geographical restriction in the circulation of strains. However, these results can be in part due to the short sampling period of this study. Of the four established lineages of the P[8] genotype [21], all Mozambican strains clustered in lineage III and shared a high level of genetic similarity, except strain MAN0033 which clustered in a distinct sub-lineage.

Maximum likelihood phylogenetic analysis showed that the majority of the Mozambican strains, with the exception of MAN0033, were most closely related to a conserved group of Indian strains across most genes. Even the two reassortant strains (HJM1646 and HGM0544) were most closely related to Indian strains. This suggests that there may have been multiple, contemporary introductions of diverse strains from a similar origin, perhaps India, into Mozambique. This was further supported by the results of the Bayesian analysis, where the time to the most recent common ancestor for the VP7 and VP4 genes of the main Mozambican clade were 2011.7 and 2013.0, respectively, and which had diverged from the closest Indian strain in 2011.7 and 2011.6, respectively. This suggests that the strains became endemic shortly after being introduced and became the dominant variant circulating in the population. These Indian strains were submitted directly to the GenBank database and no associated manuscripts were found, so it is unclear if these strains were associated with any particular outbreak or were detected as part of routine surveillance.

Overall, the VP7 and VP4 antigenic epitopes exhibited conserved substitutions among the Mozambican strains when compared to Rotarix®. The substitutions in the 7-2 VP7 epitope at position M217I, N147D and 8-1, 8-3 VP4 at positions E150D, N195D and S125N, S131R, N135D were observed in pre- and post-vaccine introduction strains, suggesting that these substitutions are not due to the vaccine introduction.

The main limitation of the study was the limited number of strains successfully sequenced, and that fewer strains were sequenced from the pre-vaccine period.

There is a need to expand the whole genome analysis to other strains detected in Mozambique such as G3, G9 in combination with P[4], P[6] and P[8] genotypes reported previously [18] in order to evaluate the possible influence of vaccine introduction on other rotavirus genotypes.

Mozambique has introduced the Rotarix® vaccine, however cases of rotavirus infection associated with G1P[8] strains resulting in hospitalization of children are still being reported. The present analysis showed that G1P[8] strains detected in the post-vaccine period did not undergo significant mutations in the epitope regions that could result in vaccine escape. However, the short post vaccine period analyzed (three years) may have influenced these results, as it may be too early to see major genetic changes associated with vaccine pressure. These results highlight the need for future studies to understand host factors such as the role of histo-blood group antigen status, nutritional status and enteric co-infections that can influence the vaccine effectiveness in Mozambique.

## 4. Materials and Methods

### 4.1. Ethics Approval

The ViNaDia Protocol was approved by the National Health Bioethics Committee of Mozambique (CNBS) under number (IRB00002657, reference Nr: 348/CNBS/13). Participants' anonymity and confidentiality were guaranteed.

### 4.2. Sample Collection

Forty-three fecal samples, collected between 2012 and 2017 that were positive for RVA by ELISA (Prospect EIA rotavirus, Basingstoke, UK) and identified as genotype G1P[8] by multiplex RT-PCR according to described protocols [42,43], were selected for sequencing according to year of isolation, location of collection (region of Mozambique) and the child's vaccination status. The samples were obtained from children <5 years of age, hospitalized with acute gastroenteritis, and collected at five sentinel sites of the National Diarrheal Surveillance (ViNaDia), which are Hospital Geral de Mavalane (HGM), Hospital Geral Jose Macamo (HJM), Hospital Central da Beira (HCB), Hospital Geral de Quelimane (HGQ) and Hospital Central de Nampula (HCN), and from a previous study of Centro de Investigação em Saúde da Manhiça (CISM) in Mozambique between 2012 and 2013 (Supplementary Figure S3) [15]. Clinical information was collected through a structured questionnaire from ViNaDia which included metadata such as age, gender, site and vaccination status.

### 4.3. RNA Extraction and cDNA Synthesis

Total RNA was extracted from stool samples with TRI-reagent (Sigma, Darmstadt, Germany) and single-stranded RNA was precipitated with lithium chloride. The self-priming PC3-T7 loop primer (Integrated DNA Technologies, Coralville, IA, USA) was ligated to dsRNA in order to obtain full-length sequences and cDNA was synthesized using the Maxima H Minus double-stranded cDNA kit (Thermo Fisher Scientific, Massachusetts, MA, USA) as previously described [20,44].

### 4.4. Next Generation Sequencing

The whole genome sequencing was performed using an Illumina MiSeq sequencing platform (Illumina, Inc. San Diego, CA, USA) at the Next Generation Sequencing Unit at the University of the

Free State (NGS-UFS). Sequencing was completed using the Nextera XT DNA Library Preparation Kit (Illumina, Inc., San Diego, CA, USA) using protocols previously describe [19].

*4.5. Data Analyses*

A de novo assembly was performed for all samples using CLC Bio Genomics Workbench (12.0.3; Qiagen, Aarhus, Denmark); all contigs with an average coverage above 100 were identified on the Nucleotide Basic Local Alignment Search Tool (BLASTn at the National Center for Biotechnology information (NCBI). References were chosen based on the Blastn results for reference mapping and extraction of consensus sequences for each segment. The genotyping tools, Virus Pathogenic database and analysis resource (ViPR) [45] and RotaC v2.0 [46], were used to determine the genotype of each gene. The sequences were submitted to GenBank and accession numbers MT737379-MT737772 were assigned.

*4.6. Phylogenetic Analysis*

Multiple nucleotide sequence alignments with strains obtained from GenBank [24] were made with multiple sequence alignment program (MAFFT v7.450) [47] on Geneious prime v2020.0.3 and Multiple Sequence Comparison by Log Expectation (MUSCLE) [48] alignment available in Molecular Evolutionary Genetic Analysis X (MEGA X) [29]. The optimal nucleotide substitution model for phylogenetic analysis was selected based upon the Akaike information criterion (corrected) (AICc) ranking implemented in the model selection algorithm available on JModelTest [30] and the models selected for each segment were: Tamura-3 parameter (T92+G+I) [49] for VP7; General Time Reversible (GTR+G+I) [50] for VP3; GTR+G for VP2, VP4, NSP2 and NSP3; Hasegawa Kishino Yano (HKY+G+I) for VP6 and NSP1; and HKY+G for VP1, NSP4 and NSP5/6 [51]. The maximum-likelihood trees were generated using MEGA X [29] using 1000 bootstrap replicates to estimate branch support. Pairwise distance matrix nucleotides were obtained in MEGA X using the p-distance algorithm [29]. Amino acid sequences of the VP7 and VP4 Mozambican strains were aligned and epitopes were identified and compared to those of the vaccine strain Rotarix® (A41CB052A, with accession numbers JN849114 and JN849113 for VP7 and VP4) using MEGA X [23,31].

*4.7. Evolutionary Analysis*

Maximum likelihood trees were generated using the Randomized Accelerated Maximum Likelihood (RAxML) program (v2.0.0) [52], applying the nucleotide substitution model GTR+G. The trees were used as the input for TempEst 1.5.3 to plot root-to-tip genetic distances, and sequences not conforming to a linear evolutionary pattern were discarded [53]. Time-measured evolutionary histories were reconstructed using the Bayesian Evolutionary Analysis Sampling Trees (BEAST) Program package (v 1.7.5) [54]. The nucleotide substitution model Hasegawa-Kishino-Yano model (HKY+G) for VP7 and GTR+G for VP4 were selected based on AICc raking in jModelTest [30].

The parameters applied included a relaxed uncorrelated lognormal molecular clock to account for varied evolutionary rates among lineages and a coalescent Gaussian Markov random field (GMRF) Bayesian Skyride tree prior. Three independent Markov chain Monte Carlo (MCMC) chains were run for 200 million generations with sampling every 20,000 generations, with the first 10% discarded as burn-in. Convergence and mixing of the chains was assessed using Tracer (v1.7.1) and all parameters yielded effective sample sizes $\geq$ 200 [55]. The Maximum Clade Credibility (MCC) trees were summarized using TreeAnnotator (v1.10.4) [54]. The time-ordered MCC trees were visualized in FigTree (v1.4.4) (http://tree.bio.ed.ac.uk/software/figtree/).

## 5. Conclusions

This study provides important insights into the whole genome sequences of G1P[8] strains in Mozambique. Whilst similar strains were detected prior to and following vaccine introduction, multiple introductions of diverse strains from India highlight the importance of continuously monitoring the strains detected in Mozambique to determine if the strains are evolving by vaccine-induced selection or by natural evolutionary pressures.

**Supplementary Materials:**
Table S1: Genome assembly of Mozambican Wa-like G1P[8] strains from 2012 to 2017. The percentage identity was determined with BLASTn; Table S2: Nucleotide identities of the Mozambican and Rotarix® vaccine strains; Table S3: Mozambican G1P[8] strains. Figure S1: A simplified maximum clade credibility trees (MCC) for the G1 VP7 strains characterized between 1978 and 2017; Figure S2: A simplified maximum clade credibility trees (MCC) for the P[8] VP4 strains characterized between 2000 and 2017; Figure S3: Mozambique Map with the geographical location of study sentinel sites.

**Author Contributions:** Conceptualization: N.d.D., B.M. and E.D.J.; methodology: B.M., C.M.D., A.S. and E.D.J.; validation: N.d.D., C.M.D. and H.G.O.; formal analysis: B.M., E.D.J., C.M.D. and A.S.; investigation: B.M., E.D.J., J.J.C., J.L., A.C., A.F.L.B., M.C., I.C.-M. and S.S.B.; resources: N.d.D.; data curation: C.M.D. and A.S.; writing—original draft preparation: B.M. and E.D.J.; writing—review and editing: B.M., E.D.J., C.M.D., N.d.D., A.S., H.G.O., A.F.L.B. and A.C.; visualization: B.M., E.D.J., C.M.D., N.d.D., A.S. and H.G.O.; supervision: C.M.D. and N.d.D.; project administration: J.J.C. and funding acquisition: N.d.D. and H.G.O. All authors have read and agreed to the published version of the manuscript.

**Acknowledgments:** We want to thank the caretakers who consented for their children to be enrolled in the surveillance. For their efforts with recruitment, data collection and shipment of specimens to Maputo, we would like to thank Elda Anapakala, Esperança Guimarães, Júlia Sambo, Diocreciano Bero, Lena Manhique, Judite Salência, Félix Gundane, Aunésia Marurele, Délcio Muteto, Angelina Pereira, Mulaja Kabeya Étienne, Celso Gabriel, Titos Maulate, Julieta Ernesto, Francisca Ricardo, Siasa Mendes, Hércio Simbine, Susete de Carvalho, Marcos Joaquim, Elvira Sarguene, Fernando Vilanculos, Felicidade Martins, Dulce Graça, Edma Samuel, Vivaldo Pedro, Lúcia Matabel, Maria Safrina, Natércia Abreu, Vanessa da Silva, Nazareth Mabutana, Carlos Guilamba and Celina Nhamuave and Rui Cossa for providing the map illustration. For technical ICT support we thank Stephanus Riekert.

## References

1. Tate, J.E.; Burton, A.H.; Boschi-Pinto, C.; Parashar, U.D. Global, Regional, and National Estimates of Rotavirus Mortality in Children <5 Years of Age, 2000–2013. *Clin. Infect. Dis.* **2016**, *62* (Suppl. 2), S96–S105. [CrossRef] [PubMed]
2. Troeger, C.; Khalil, I.A.; Rao, P.C.; Cao, S.; Blacker, B.F.; Ahmed, T.; Armah, G.; Bines, J.E.; Brewer, T.G.; Colombara, D.V.; et al. Rotavirus Vaccination and the Global Burden of Rotavirus Diarrhea Among Children Younger Than 5 Years. *JAMA Pediatr.* **2018**, *172*, 958–965. [CrossRef] [PubMed]
3. Estes, M.K.; Cohen, J. Rotavirus gene structure and function. *Microbiol. Rev.* **1989**, *53*, 410–449. [CrossRef] [PubMed]
4. Jayaram, H.; Estes, M.; Prasad, B.V. Emerging themes in rotavirus cell entry, genome organization, transcription and replication. *Virus Res.* **2004**, *101*, 67–81. [CrossRef]
5. Desselberger, U. Rotaviruses. *Virus Res.* **2014**, *190*, 75–96. [CrossRef]
6. De Deus, N.; João, E.; Cuamba, A.; Cassocera, M.; Luís, L.; Acácio, S.; Mandomando, I.; Augusto, O.; Page, N. Epidemiology of Rotavirus Infection in Children from a Rural and Urban Area, in Maputo, Southern Mozambique, before Vaccine Introduction. *J. Trop. Pediatr.* **2017**, *64*, 141–145. [CrossRef]
7. Matthijnssens, J.; Ciarlet, M.; McDonald, S.M.; Attoui, H.; Banyai, K.; Brister, J.R.; Buesa, J.; Esona, M.D.; Estes, M.K.; Gentsch, J.R.; et al. Uniformity of rotavirus strain nomenclature proposed by the Rotavirus Classification Working Group (RCWG). *Arch. Virol.* **2011**, *156*, 1397–1413. [CrossRef]
8. Rotavirus Classification Working Group. Virus Classification. Available online: https://rega.kuleuven.be/cev/viralmetagenomics/virus-classification (accessed on 5 June 2020).
9. Matthijnssens, J.; Ciarlet, M.; Heiman, E.; Arijs, I.; Delbeke, T.; McDonald, S.M.; Palombo, E.A.; Iturriza-Gómara, M.; Maes, P.; Patton, J.T.; et al. Full Genome-Based Classification of Rotaviruses Reveals a Common Origin between Human Wa-Like and Porcine Rotavirus Strains and Human DS-1-Like and Bovine Rotavirus Strains. *J. Virol.* **2008**, *82*, 3204–3219. [CrossRef]
10. Mwenda, J.M.; Tate, J.E.; Parashar, U.D.; Mihigo, R.; Agócs, M.; Serhan, F.; Nshimirimana, D. African Rotavirus Surveillance Network. *Pediatr. Infect. Dis. J.* **2014**, *33*, S6–S8. [CrossRef]
11. Matthijnssens, J.; Van Ranst, M. Genotype constellation and evolution of group A rotaviruses infecting humans. *Curr. Opin. Virol.* **2012**, *2*, 426–433. [CrossRef]

12. World Health Organization. WHO Prequalifies New Rotavirus Vaccine. Available online: http://www.who.int/medicines/news/2018/prequalified_new-rotavirus_vaccine/en/ (accessed on 5 June 2020).
13. Burke, R.M.; Tate, J.E.; Kirkwood, C.D.; Steele, A.D.; Parashar, U.D. Current and new rotavirus vaccines. *Curr. Opin. Infect. Dis.* **2019**, *32*, 435–444. [CrossRef] [PubMed]
14. Langa, J.S.; Thompson, R.; Arnaldo, P.; Resque, H.R.; Rose, T.; Enosse, S.M.; Fialho, A.; De Assis, R.M.S.; Da Silva, M.F.M.; Leite, J.P.G. Epidemiology of rotavirus A diarrhea in Chókwè, Southern Mozambique, from February to September, 2011. *J. Med. Virol.* **2016**, *88*, 1751–1758. [CrossRef] [PubMed]
15. João, E.D.; Strydom, A.; O'Neill, H.G.; Cuamba, A.; Cassocera, M.; Acácio, S.; Mandomando, I.; Motanyane, L.; Page, N.; De Deus, N. Rotavirus A strains obtained from children with acute gastroenteritis in Mozambique, 2012–2013: G and P genotypes and phylogenetic analysis of VP7 and partial VP4 genes. *Arch. Virol.* **2017**, *163*, 153–165. [CrossRef] [PubMed]
16. De Deus, N.; Chilaúle, J.J.; Cassocera, M.; Bambo, M.; Langa, J.S.; Sitoe, E.; Chissaque, A.; Anapakala, E.; Sambo, J.; Guimarães, E.L.; et al. Early impact of rotavirus vaccination in children less than five years of age in Mozambique. *Vaccine* **2018**, *36*, 7205–7209. [CrossRef]
17. World Health Organization. WHO and UNICEF Estimates of National Immunization Coverage. Available online: http://www.who.int/immunization/monitoring_surveillance/routine/coverage/en/index4.html (accessed on 1 April 2020).
18. João, E.; Munlela, B.; Chissaque, A.; Chilaúle, J.; Langa, J.S.; Augusto, O.; Boene, S.; Anapakala, E.; Sambo, J.; Guimarães, E.; et al. Molecular Epidemiology of Rotavirus A Strains Pre- and Post-Vaccine (Rotarix®) Introduction in Mozambique, 2012–2019: Emergence of Genotypes G3P[4] and G3P[8]. *Pathogens* **2020**, *9*, 671. [CrossRef]
19. Strydom, A.; Motanyane, L.; Nyaga, M.M.; João, E.D.; Cuamba, A.; Mandomando, I.; Cassocera, M.; De Deus, N.; O'Neill, H.G. Whole-genome characterization of G12 rotavirus strains detected in Mozambique reveals a co-infection with a GXP[14] strain of possible animal origin. *J. Gen. Virol.* **2019**, *100*, 932–937. [CrossRef]
20. Strydom, A.; João, E.D.; Motanyane, L.; Nyaga, M.M.; Potgieter, A.C.; Cuamba, A.; Mandomando, I.; Cassocera, M.; De Deus, N.; O'Neill, H.G. Whole genome analyses of DS-1-like Rotavirus A strains detected in children with acute diarrhoea in southern Mozambique suggest several reassortment events. *Infect. Genet. Evol.* **2019**, *69*, 68–75. [CrossRef]
21. Le, V.P.; Chung, Y.-C.; Kim, K.; Chung, S.-I.; Lim, I.; Kim, W. Genetic variation of prevalent G1P[8] human rotaviruses in South Korea. *J. Med. Virol.* **2010**, *82*, 886–896. [CrossRef]
22. Arista, S.; Giammanco, G.M.; De Grazia, S.; Ramirez, S.; Biundo, C.L.; Colomba, C.; Cascio, A.; Martella, V. Heterogeneity and Temporal Dynamics of Evolution of G1 Human Rotaviruses in a Settled Population. *J. Virol.* **2006**, *80*, 10724–10733. [CrossRef]
23. Zeller, M.; Patton, J.T.; Heylen, E.; De Coster, S.; Ciarlet, M.; Van Ranst, M.; Matthijnssens, J. Genetic Analyses Reveal Differences in the VP7 and VP4 Antigenic Epitopes between Human Rotaviruses Circulating in Belgium and Rotaviruses in Rotarix and RotaTeq. *J. Clin. Microbiol.* **2012**, *50*, 966–976. [CrossRef]
24. Ianiro, G.; Delogu, R.; Fiore, L.; Ruggeri, F.M. Genetic variability of VP7, VP4, VP6 and NSP4 genes of common human G1P[8] rotavirus strains circulating in Italy between 2010 and 2014. *Virus Res.* **2016**, *220*, 117–128. [CrossRef] [PubMed]
25. Almeida, T.N.V.; De Sousa, T.T.; Da Silva, R.A.; Fiaccadori, F.S.; Souza, M.; Badr, K.R.; de Paula Cardoso, D.d.D. Phylogenetic analysis of G1P[8] and G12P[8] rotavirus A samples obtained in the pre- and post-vaccine periods, and molecular modeling of VP4 and VP7 proteins. *Acta Trop.* **2017**, *173*, 153–159. [CrossRef] [PubMed]
26. Magagula, N.B.; Esona, M.D.; Nyaga, M.M.; Stucker, K.M.; Halpin, R.A.; Stockwell, T.B.; Seheri, M.L.; Steele, A.D.; Wentworth, D.E.; Mphahlele, M.J. Whole genome analyses of G1P[8] rotavirus strains from vaccinated and non-vaccinated South African children presenting with diarrhea. *J. Med. Virol.* **2015**, *87*, 79–101. [CrossRef] [PubMed]
27. Damanka, S.; Kwofie, S.; Dennis, F.E.; Lartey, B.L.; Agbemabiese, C.A.; Doan, Y.H.; Adiku, T.K.; Katayama, K.; Enweronu-Laryea, C.C.; Armah, G.E. Whole genome characterization and evolutionary analysis of OP354-like P[8] Rotavirus A strains isolated from Ghanaian children with diarrhoea. *PLoS ONE* **2019**, *14*, e0218348. [CrossRef] [PubMed]

28. Jere, K.C.; Chaguza, C.; Bar-Zeev, N.; Lowe, J.; Peno, C.; Kumwenda, B.; Nakagomi, O.; Tate, J.E.; Parashar, U.D.; Heyderman, R.S.; et al. Emergence of Double- and Triple-Gene Reassortant G1P[8] Rotaviruses Possessing a DS-1-Like Backbone after Rotavirus Vaccine Introduction in Malawi. *J. Virol.* **2017**, *92*, e01246-17. [CrossRef] [PubMed]
29. Kumar, S.; Stecher, G.; Li, M.; Knyaz, C.; Tamura, K. MEGA X: Molecular Evolutionary Genetics Analysis across Computing Platforms. *Mol. Biol. Evol.* **2018**, *35*, 1547–1549. [CrossRef]
30. Darriba, D.; Taboada, G.L.; Doallo, R.; Posada, D. jModelTest 2: More models, new heuristics and parallel computing. *Nat. Methods* **2012**, *9*, 772. [CrossRef]
31. Aoki, S.T.; Settembre, E.C.; Trask, S.D.; Greenberg, H.B.; Harrison, S.C.; Dormitzer, P.R. Structure of Rotavirus Outer-Layer Protein VP7 Bound with a Neutralizing Fab. *Science* **2009**, *324*, 1444–1447. [CrossRef]
32. Dormitzer, P.R.; Sun, Z.J.; Wagner, G.; Harrison, S.C. The rhesus rotavirus VP4 sialic acid binding domain has a galectin fold with a novel carbohydrate binding site. *EMBO J.* **2002**, *21*, 885–897. [CrossRef]
33. Dormitzer, P.R.; Nason, E.B.; Prasad, B.V.V.; Harrison, S.C. Structural rearrangements in the membrane penetration protein of a non-enveloped virus. *Nat. Cell Biol.* **2004**, *430*, 1053–1058. [CrossRef]
34. Da Silva, M.F.M.; Rose, T.L.; Gómez, M.M.; Carvalho-Costa, F.A.; Fialho, A.M.; De Assis, R.M.; Sde Andrade, J.d.S.R.; Volotão, E.D.M.; Leite, J.P.G. G1P[8] species A rotavirus over 27 years–Pre- and post-vaccination eras–in Brazil: Full genomic constellation analysis and no evidence for selection pressure by Rotarix® vaccine. *Infect. Genet. Evol.* **2015**, *30*, 206–218. [CrossRef] [PubMed]
35. Zeller, M.; Donato, C.; Trovão, N.S.; Cowley, D.; Heylen, E.; Donker, N.C.; McAllen, J.K.; Akopov, A.; Kirkness, E.F.; Lemey, P.; et al. Genome-Wide Evolutionary Analyses of G1P[8] Strains Isolated Before and After Rotavirus Vaccine Introduction. *Genome Biol. Evol.* **2015**, *7*, 2473–2483. [CrossRef] [PubMed]
36. Rasebotsa, S.; Mwangi, P.N.; Mogotsi, M.T.; Sabiu, S.; Magagula, N.B.; Rakau, K.; Uwimana, J.; Mutesa, L.; Muganga, N.; Murenzi, D.; et al. Whole genome and in-silico analyses of G1P[8] rotavirus strains from pre- and post-vaccination periods in Rwanda. *Sci. Rep.* **2020**, *10*, 1–22. [CrossRef] [PubMed]
37. Mwangi, P.N.; Mogotsi, M.; Rasebotsa, S.P.; Seheri, M.L.; Mphahlele, M.J.; Ndze, V.N.; Dennis, F.E.; Jere, K.C.; Nyaga, M.M. Uncovering the First Atypical DS-1-like G1P[8] Rotavirus Strains That Circulated during Pre-Rotavirus Vaccine Introduction Era in South Africa. *Pathogens* **2020**, *9*, 391. [CrossRef]
38. Donato, C.M.; Ch'Ng, L.S.; Boniface, K.F.; Crawford, N.W.; Buttery, J.P.; Lyon, M.; Bishop, R.F.; Kirkwood, C.D. Identification of Strains of RotaTeq Rotavirus Vaccine in Infants With Gastroenteritis Following Routine Vaccination. *J. Infect. Dis.* **2012**, *206*, 377–383. [CrossRef]
39. Gower, C.M.; Dunning, J.; Nawaz, S.; Allen, D.; Ramsay, M.E.; Ladhani, S.N. Vaccine-derived rotavirus strains in infants in England. *Arch. Dis. Child.* **2019**, *105*, 553–557. [CrossRef]
40. Arora, R.; Chitambar, S. Full genomic analysis of Indian G1P[8] rotavirus strains. *Infect. Genet. Evol.* **2011**, *11*, 504–511. [CrossRef]
41. Kulkarni, R.; Arora, R.; Arora, R.; Chitambar, S.D. Sequence analysis of VP7 and VP4 genes of G1P[8] rotaviruses circulating among diarrhoeic children in Pune, India: A comparison with Rotarix and RotaTeq vaccine strains. *Vaccine* **2014**, *32*, A75–A83. [CrossRef]
42. Gouvea, V.; Glass, R.I.; Woods, P.; Taniguchi, K.; Clark, H.F.; Forrester, B.; Fang, Z.Y. Polymerase chain reaction amplification and typing of rotavirus nucleic acid from stool specimens. *J. Clin. Microbiol.* **1990**, *28*, 276–282. [CrossRef]
43. Gentsch, J.R.; Glass, R.I.; Woods, P.; Gouvea, V.; Gorziglia, M.; Flores, J.; Das, B.K.; Bhan, M.K. Identification of group A rotavirus gene 4 types by polymerase chain reaction. *J. Clin. Microbiol.* **1992**, *30*, 1365–1373. [CrossRef]
44. Potgieter, A.C.; Page, N.A.; Liebenberg, J.; Wright, I.M.; Landt, O.; Van Dijk, A. Improved strategies for sequence-independent amplification and sequencing of viral double-stranded RNA genomes. *J. Gen. Virol.* **2009**, *90*, 1423–1432. [CrossRef] [PubMed]
45. Pickett, B.E.; Sadat, E.L.; Zhang, Y.; Noronha, J.M.; Squires, R.B.; Hunt, V.; Liu, M.; Kumar, S.; Zaremba, S.; Gu, Z.; et al. ViPR: An open bioinformatics database and analysis resource for virology research. *Nucleic Acids Res.* **2012**, *40*, D593–D598. [CrossRef] [PubMed]
46. Maes, P.; Matthijnssens, J.; Rahman, M.; Van Ranst, M. RotaC: A web-based tool for the complete genome classification of group A rotaviruses. *BMC Microbiol.* **2009**, *9*, 238. [CrossRef]
47. Katoh, K.; Standley, D.M. MAFFT multiple sequence alignment software version 7: Improvements in performance and usability. *Mol. Biol. Evol.* **2013** *30*, 772–780. [CrossRef] [PubMed]

48. Edgar, R.C. MUSCLE: Multiple sequence alignment with high accuracy and high throughput. *Nucleic Acids Res.* **2004**, *32*, 1792–1797. [CrossRef]
49. Hazkani-Covo, E.; Graur, D. A Comparative Analysis of numt Evolution in Human and Chimpanzee. *Mol. Biol. Evol.* **2006**, *24*, 13–18. [CrossRef]
50. Nei, M.; Kumar, S. *Molecular Evolution and Phylogenetics*; Oxford University Press: Oxford, UK, 2000.
51. Hasegawa, M.; Kishino, H.; Yano, T.-A. Dating of the human-ape splitting by a molecular clock of mitochondrial DNA. *J. Mol. Evol.* **1985**, *22*, 160–174. [CrossRef]
52. Stamatakis, A. RAxML version 8: A tool for phylogenetic analysis and post-analysis of large phylogenies. *Bioinformatics* **2014**, *30*, 1312–1313. [CrossRef]
53. Rambaut, A.; Lam, T.T.; Carvalho, L.M.; Pybus, O.G. Exploring the temporal structure of heterochronous sequences using TempEst (formerly Path-O-Gen). *Virus Evol.* **2016**, *2*, vew007. [CrossRef]
54. Suchard, M.A.; Lemey, P.; Baele, G.; Ayres, D.L.; Drummond, A.J.; Rambaut, A. Bayesian phylogenetic and phylodynamic data integration using BEAST 1.10. *Virus Evol.* **2018**, *4*, vey016. [CrossRef]
55. Rambaut, A.; Drummond, A.J.; Xie, D.; Baele, G.; Suchard, M.A. Posterior Summarization in Bayesian Phylogenetics Using Tracer 1.7. *Syst. Biol.* **2018**, *67*, 901–904. [CrossRef] [PubMed]

# Retrospective Case-Control Study of 2017 G2P[4] Rotavirus Epidemic in Rural and Remote Australia

Bianca F. Middleton [1,2,*], Margie Danchin [3,4,5], Helen Quinn [6,7], Anna P. Ralph [1,8], Nevada Pingault [9], Mark Jones [10], Marie Estcourt [10] and Tom Snelling [1,11,12]

1. Global and Tropical Health, Menzies School of Health Research, Charles Darwin University, Darwin 0810, Australia; Anna.Ralph@menzies.edu.au (A.P.R.); tom.snelling@sydney.edu.au (T.S.)
2. Division of Women, Children and Youth, Royal Darwin Hospital, Darwin 0810, Australia
3. Department of Paediatrics, University of Melbourne, Melbourne 3052, Australia; margie.danchin@rch.org.au
4. Murdoch Children's Research Institute, Melbourne 3052, Australia
5. Department of General Medicine, Royal Children's Hospital, Melbourne 3052, Australia
6. The National Centre for Immunisation Research and Surveillance (NCIRS), The Children's Hospital at Westmead, Sydney 2145, Australia; helen.quinn@health.nsw.gov.au
7. Faculty of Medicine and Health, Westmead Clinical School, The University of Sydney, Westmead 2145, Australia
8. Division of Medicine, Royal Darwin Hospital, Darwin 0810, Australia
9. Department of Health Western Australia, Communicable Disease Control Directorate, Perth 6004, Australia; nevada.pingault@health.wa.gov.au
10. Health and Clinical Analytics, School of Public Health, The University of Sydney, Sydney 2006, Australia; mark.jones1@sydney.edu.au (M.J.); marie.estcourt@sydney.edu.au (M.E.)
11. Wesfarmers Centre for Vaccine and Infectious Diseases, Telethon Kids Institute, Perth 6009, Australia
12. School of Public Health, Curtin University, Perth 6102, Australia
* Correspondence: bianca.middleton@menzies.edu.au;

**Abstract:** Background: A widespread G2P[4] rotavirus epidemic in rural and remote Australia provided an opportunity to evaluate the performance of Rotarix and RotaTeq rotavirus vaccines, ten years after their incorporation into Australia's National Immunisation Program. Methods: We conducted a retrospective case-control analysis. Vaccine-eligible children with laboratory-confirmed rotavirus infection were identified from jurisdictional notifiable infectious disease databases and individually matched to controls from the national immunisation register, based on date of birth, Aboriginal status and location of residence. Results: 171 cases met the inclusion criteria; most were Aboriginal and/or Torres Strait Islander (80%) and the median age was 19 months. Of these cases, 65% and 25% were fully or partially vaccinated, compared to 71% and 21% of controls. Evidence that cases were less likely than controls to have received a rotavirus vaccine dose was weak, OR 0.79 (95% CI, 0.46–1.34). On pre-specified subgroup analysis, there was some evidence of protection among children <12 months (OR 0.48 [95% CI, 0.22–1.02]), and among fully vs. partially vaccinated children (OR 0.65 [95% CI, 0.42–1.01]). Conclusion: Despite the known effectiveness of rotavirus vaccination, a protective effect of either rotavirus vaccine during a G2P[4] outbreak in these settings among predominantly Aboriginal children was weak, highlighting the ongoing need for a more effective rotavirus vaccine and public health strategies to better protect Aboriginal children.

**Keywords:** rotavirus; rotavirus vaccines; vaccine effectiveness; case control

## 1. Introduction

Rotavirus is a leading cause of severe dehydrating diarrhoeal illness in children and continues to be responsible for the deaths of 118,000 to 183,000 children every year [1]. Many of these deaths occur in resource-poor settings [2].

In 2006, two oral rotavirus vaccines, Rotarix and RotaTeq, were licensed for use and in 2009 the World Health Organization endorsed their use globally [3]. Subsequent epidemiological studies have confirmed a strong protective effect of vaccination on rotavirus morbidity in high- and upper middle-income countries (vaccine efficacy [VE] >84%) [2]. However, in low-income countries, despite a large reduction in the absolute number of cases of gastroenteritis, measured vaccine efficacy has been lower (45–57%) and in some settings there is evidence of decreased protection in the second year of life [2,4–6].

The incorporation of rotavirus vaccines into the Northern Territory immunisation schedule in 2006 and then into the Australian National Immunisation Program (NIP) in 2007, resulted in a substantial and sustained decrease in rotavirus hospitalisations [7]. However, among Aboriginal and Torres Strait Islander children living in the hyperendemic settings of rural and remote Australia, the decrease in rotavirus hospitalisation was less dramatic and not sustained, with Aboriginal children living in the Northern Territory (NT) remaining more than 20 times more likely to be hospitalised with rotavirus than their non-Aboriginal counterparts [7]. An early vaccine effectiveness study in this setting also suggested reduced effectiveness against heterotypic strains and poor protection in the second year of life [8].

In 2017, an epidemic of G2P[4] rotavirus arose in the Northern Territory and subsequently spread to adjoining rural and remote regions of Western Australia (WA). These two jurisdictions cover a large geographic area which is sparsely populated; they have a higher proportion of resident Aboriginal and Torres Strait Islander people, many of whom live in rural and remote communities. The rotavirus epidemic occurred at a time when the Northern Territory exclusively administered Rotarix and Western Australia exclusively administered RotaTeq as part of the jurisdictional implementation of the NIP. We evaluated the protective effectiveness of both vaccines in these high-burden settings, ten years after the incorporation of rotavirus vaccines into the NIP.

## 2. Materials and Methods

### 2.1. Study Setting

The Alice Springs and Barkly regions of the Northern Territory, and the Kimberley, Pilbara and Goldfields regions of Western Australia are large but sparsely populated administrative health regions. Ranging from the semi-arid south, to the arid center and tropical north, these five regions encompass more than 2,500,000 km$^2$, but are home to a combined total of just 174,000 people [9]. Children aged <5 years represent between 7–9% of the population, and between 5 and 41% of the population in each of these regions identify as being Aboriginal and/or Torres Strait Islander (hereafter respectfully referred to as 'Aboriginal') [9]. Many of these children live in towns or small remote communities. Rotarix and RotaTeq rotavirus vaccines have been licensed for use in Australia since June 2006. The Northern Territory immunisation program has funded the administration of Rotarix exclusively since October 2006. The Western Australian immunisation program funded the administration of Rotarix from July 2007 to June 2009, RotaTeq from July 2009 to June 2017, and Rotarix from July 2017.

### 2.2. Study Design

We conducted a retrospective, population-based, case control study of children age-eligible for at least 1 dose of rotavirus vaccine (those born after the introduction of Rotarix rotavirus vaccine to the NT schedule—after 1 July 2006 and aged ≥6 weeks, and those born after the introduction of RotaTeq rotavirus vaccine to the WA schedule—after 1 May 2009 and aged ≥6 weeks) who had laboratory positive and notified rotavirus infection during the 2017 G2P[4] rotavirus epidemic in the NT and WA.

Cases were individually matched to controls sampled from the national immunisation register. As a secondary analysis, we also compared cases who were age-eligible for full rotavirus vaccination (those born after 1 July 2006 and aged ≥24 weeks in the NT and those born after 1 May and aged ≥32 weeks in WA) with un-matched control children diagnosed with non-rotavirus gastrointestinal infections sampled from disease notification registers.

*2.3. Data Sources*

Rotavirus is a notifiable disease in the NT and WA. Data regarding rotavirus cases and disease register controls were ascertained from the two jurisdictional-based notifiable infectious disease databases—The Northern Territory Notifiable Disease System (NTNDS) managed by the NT Centre for Disease Control, and the Western Australian Notifiable Infectious Disease Database (WANIDD) managed by the WA Department of Health.

To estimate baseline vaccine coverage in the case-referent population, matched population controls were sampled from the Australian Immunisation Register (AIR), a comprehensive population-based register which contains vaccination data for all children registered with Australia's universal health insurance scheme, Medicare (~99% of the population).

*2.4. Participants*

2.4.1. Population-Based Analysis

Rotavirus cases were vaccine-eligible children aged ≥6 weeks with laboratory positive and notified rotavirus infection between 1 March and 30 June 2017. Cases were drawn from the Alice Springs and Barkly regions of the NT, and the Kimberley, Pilbara and Goldfields regions of WA. To be vaccine-eligible, children had to be born on or after 1 July 2006 in the NT (for Rotarix) and on or after 1 May 2009 in WA (for RotaTeq).

De-identified population controls were selected from the Australian Immunisation Register and matched to each case by date of birth (±14 days), Aboriginal status and location of residence (listed residential postcode within either the Alice Springs, Barkly, Pilbara, Goldfields or Kimberley regions). Up to 10 eligible controls were randomly selected for each case.

2.4.2. Disease Register Analysis

Rotavirus cases were selected as above, but because individual matching was not feasible, the analysis was restricted to children old enough to be fully vaccinated: age ≥24 weeks (for Rotarix) in the NT and ≥32 weeks (for RotaTeq) in WA.

Disease register controls were vaccine-eligible children (aged ≥24 weeks or ≥32 weeks in the NT and WA respectively), with microbiologically confirmed, non-rotavirus and non-vaccine preventable, notifiable gastrointestinal infections, notified between 1 January and 31 December 2017. Controls were selected form the Alice Springs and Barkly regions of the NT, and the Kimberley, Pilbara and Goldfields regions of WA. Non-rotavirus notifiable gastrointestinal infections included campylobacter, shigella, salmonella and cryptosporidium, and controls were excluded if they were also identified as a rotavirus case. Age, Aboriginal status, sex and location of residence were obtained from the disease register for inclusion in the regression analysis.

*2.5. Immunisation Status*

The immunisation status of all rotavirus cases, population controls and disease register controls were determined from the Australian Immunisation Register (AIR). Full vaccination was defined as AIR-documented receipt of at least two doses of Rotarix for children living in the NT and at least three doses of RotaTeq for children living in WA. Partial vaccination was defined as AIR-documented receipt of one dose only of Rotarix for children living in the NT and either one or two doses only of RotaTeq for children living in WA. Unvaccinated children were defined as those registered on the

AIR, but without documented receipt of any rotavirus vaccines. In circumstances where a child had a vaccine dose recorded as dose two or dose three on the register, but where an earlier dose was not recorded, it was assumed the missing dose had been given [10]. A vaccine dose was considered administered on the date recorded as administered on the register (i.e., without any post-vaccination censoring). A vaccine dose was considered invalid if (1) administered too early (before six weeks of age or <28 days from prior vaccine dose), (2) it exceeded the recommended number of vaccine doses in the schedule (>2 doses of Rotarix or >3 doses of RotaTeq) or (3) the administered vaccine was different to the prior vaccine (mixed Rotarix/RotaTeq vaccination schedule). Children were excluded from selection as cases and controls if they had an invalid vaccine dose. Children were also excluded from the analysis if they were recorded as having received the non-programmatic vaccine for their resident jurisdiction (i.e., RotaTeq but living in the NT, or Rotarix but living in WA).

*2.6. Statistical Analysis*

Conditional logistic regression was used to determine the odds ratio (OR) of vaccination for rotavirus cases compared with matched population controls from the immunisation register. Additional models were fit to compute the OR for any dose of vaccine (full and/or partial vaccination) vs none, full vaccination vs none, partial vaccination vs none, and full vs partial vaccination. Subgroup analyses were by jurisdiction (NT versus WA), and by age (<12 months versus ≥12 months).

For the disease register analysis, ordinary logistic regression was used to determine the odds ratio of vaccination for rotavirus cases compared with disease register controls. Age (months), sex, Aboriginal status (Aboriginal vs non-Aboriginal) and jurisdiction of residence (NT vs WA) were included in the model, together with an interaction term for Aboriginal status and jurisdiction of residence.

Assuming a baseline population vaccine coverage of 80%, we estimated that 80 matched sets of cases and population controls, with 10 controls for each case, would have at least 80% power to detect a significant real-world vaccine effectiveness of 45% (OR = 0.55).

All analysis was performed using Stata, version 15.1 (Stata).

*2.7. Ethics Committee Approvals*

Approval was granted by the Central Australian Human Research Ethics Committee (CAHREC 18-3219), the Human Research Ethics Committee of the Northern Territory Department of Health and Menzies School of Health Research (HREC 18-3248), the Department of Health Western Australian Human Research Ethics Committee (DOH HREC 2018/30), the Western Australian Aboriginal Health Ethics Committee (HREC 891) and the Charles Darwin University Human Research Ethics Committee (H19040). Approval to access data held by the Australian Immunisation Register was granted by the Australian Government Department of Health.

## 3. Results

The rotavirus epidemic occurred between 1 March and 30 June 2017. A total of 194 vaccine-eligible children aged ≥6 weeks were identified as rotavirus cases from which 171 were eligible for inclusion in the study (see Figure 1).

The median age of rotavirus infection was 19 months (range from 1 to 94 months). Most rotavirus cases were among children who identified as Aboriginal and/or Torres Strait Islander (NT 86%, WA 75%). Genotype results were available for only 60% of rotavirus cases, however, of those typed, all were G2P[4] strains. A total of 99 children were documented as having been hospitalised with rotavirus infection—78% of rotavirus cases in the NT and 39% of rotavirus cases in WA. Hospitalisation status was unknown for 15% of WA rotavirus cases (see Table 1).

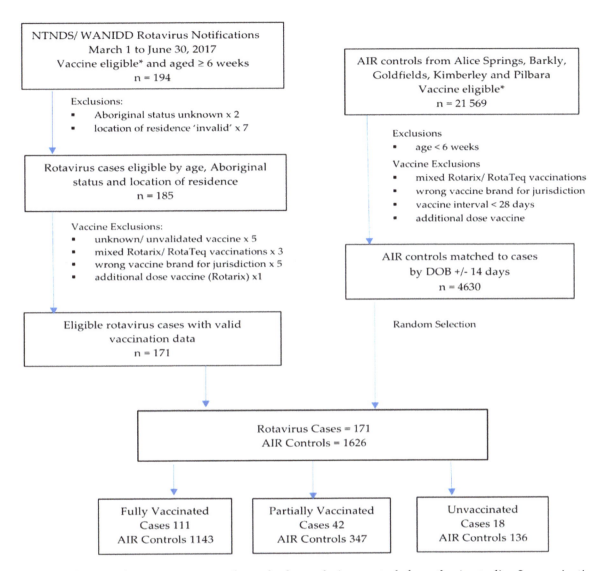

**Figure 1.** Selection of rotavirus cases and matched population controls from the Australian Immunisation Register. * Vaccine-Eligible: children eligible by date of birth to have received at least one dose of Rotarix vaccine (those born after 1 July 2006 in the Northern Territory) or at least one dose of RotaTeq vaccine (those born after 1 May 2009 in Western Australia).

Among rotavirus cases, 65% were fully vaccinated, 25% partially vaccinated and 10% unvaccinated; among matched population controls from the immunisation register, 71% were fully vaccinated, 21% partially vaccinated and 8% unvaccinated. In the population-based analysis, the odds ratio of receipt of any doses of rotavirus vaccine versus none was 0.79 (95% CI, 0.46–1.34). For the NT and WA, the OR of any doses versus none was 1.10 (95% CI, 0.50–2.41) and 0.56 (95% CI, 0.27–1.16), respectively. For children aged <12 months and for children aged ≥12 months, the ORs were 0.48 (95% CI, 0.22–1.02) and 1.22 (95% CI, 0.55–2.73), respectively. The OR of full versus partial vaccination was 0.65 (95% CI, 0.42–1.01) (see Table 2 and Figure 2).

Of the 171 notified rotavirus cases above, 149 were age eligible for inclusion in the disease register analysis (aged ≥24 weeks or ≥32 weeks in the NT and WA, respectively). A total of 347 vaccine-eligible children were identified as having non-rotavirus gastrointestinal infections in the twelve-month period from 1 January and 31 December 2017. Of these children, 299 were eligible for inclusion (Supplementary Materials Figure S1). The median age of disease register controls was older than that of rotavirus cases, 29 months vs. 20 months (Supplementary Materials Table S1). Disease register controls were less likely to be hospitalised than rotavirus cases (35% vs 58%) and, in WA, were less likely to identify as Aboriginal (41% vs 74%).

In the disease register analysis, 73%, 19% and 8% of cases were fully vaccinated, partially vaccinated and unvaccinated, respectively, compared with 83%, 12% and 5% of controls. The adjusted OR of any doses of rotavirus vaccine versus none was 0.58 (95% CI, 0.24–1.39); for WA and NT children, the adjusted ORs were 0.30 (95% CI, 0.09–0.98) and 1.40 (95% CI, 0.34–5.80), respectively, and for children aged <12 months and ≥12 months old, the adjusted ORs were 0.28 (95% CI, 0.03–2.83) and 0.81 (95% CI, 0.29–2.28), respectively. The adjusted OR of full vs. partial vaccination was 0.63 (95% CI, 0.35–1.13) (see Table 2 and Supplementary Materials Table S2).

Table 1. Baseline characteristics of rotavirus cases.

| Characteristic | Rotavirus Cases | |
| --- | --- | --- |
| | NT | WA |
| | n = 83 | n = 88 |
| **Age** | | |
| Median age (months) | 18 | 19 |
| Age range (months) | 1 to 72 | 1 to 94 |
| 6 weeks to <24 wks (NT only) | 12 (14%) | |
| 6 weeks to <32 wks (WA only) | | 10 (11%) |
| 6 weeks to <1 year | 25 (30%) | 23 (26%) |
| 1 year to <2 years | 36 (44%) | 34 (39%) |
| 2 years to <3 years | 11 (13%) | 15 (17%) |
| 3 years to <4 years | 7 (8%) | 5 (6%) |
| 4 years to <5 years | 3 (4%) | 5 (6%) |
| ≥5 years | 1 (1%) | 6 (6%) |
| **Sex** | | |
| Female | 42 (51%) | 43 (49%) |
| Male | 41 (49%) | 45 (51%) |
| **Aboriginal Status** | | |
| Aboriginal | 71 (86%) | 66 (75%) |
| Non-Aboriginal | 12 (14%) | 22 (25%) |
| **Location of Residence** | | |
| Alice Springs | 70 (84%) | |
| Barkly | 13 (16%) | |
| Goldfields | | 17 (19%) |
| Kimberley | | 49 (56%) |
| Pilbara | | 22 (25%) |
| **Genotype** | | |
| G2P[4] | 44 (53%) | 59 (67%) |
| Unknown | 39 (47%) | 29 (33%) |
| **Hospitalisation** | | |
| Yes | 65 (78%) | 34 (39%) |
| No | 18 (22%) | 41 (46%) |
| Unknown | | 13 (15%) |
| **Vaccination** | | |
| 0 doses | 8 (10%) | 10 (11%) |
| 1 doses | 15 (18%) | 8 (9%) |
| 2 doses | 60 (72%) | 19 (22%) |
| 3 doses | | 51 (58%) |

**Table 2.** Odds ratio of vaccination in rotavirus cases versus controls in the population-based analysis and the disease register analysis.

| | Immunisation Register Analysis | | | Disease Register Analysis | | |
|---|---|---|---|---|---|---|
| **Immunisation Status** | Cases | Controls | Odds Ratio (95% CI) | Cases | Controls | Odds Ratio (95% CI) |
| **Any Dose vs. None** | n = 171 | n = 1626 | 0.79 (0.46, 1.34) | n = 149 | n = 299 | 0.58 (0.24, 1.39) |
| ≥One Dose Vaccine | 153 | 1490 | | 137 | 283 | |
| Unvaccinated | 18 | 136 | | 12 | 16 | |
| **Any Dose vs. None NT (Rotarix)** | n = 83 | n = 753 | 1.10 (0.50, 2.41) | n = 71 | n = 123 | 1.40 (0.34, 5.80) |
| ≥One Dose Vaccine | 75 | 676 | | 68 | 114 | |
| Unvaccinated | 8 | 77 | | 3 | 9 | |
| **Any Dose vs. None WA (RotaTeq)** | n = 88 | n = 873 | 0.56 (0.27, 1.16) | n = 78 | n = 176 | 0.30 (0.09, 0.98) |
| ≥One Dose Vaccine | 78 | 814 | | 69 | 169 | |
| Unvaccinated | 10 | 59 | | 9 | 7 | |
| **Any Dose vs. None < 12 mths** | n = 48 | n = 449 | 0.48 (0.22, 1.02) | n = 26 | n = 37 | 0.28 (0.03, 2.83) |
| ≥One Dose Vaccine | 37 | 392 | | 21 | 36 | |
| Unvaccinated | 11 | 57 | | 5 | 1 | |
| **Any Dose vs. None ≥12mths** | n = 123 | n = 1177 | 1.22 (0.55, 2.73) | n = 123 | n = 262 | 0.81 (0.29, 2.28) |
| ≥One Dose Vaccine | 116 | 1098 | | 116 | 247 | |
| Unvaccinated | 7 | 79 | | 7 | 15 | |
| **Full Dose vs. None** | n = 129 | n = 1008 | 0.83 (0.43, 1.58) | n = 121 | n = 264 | 0.55 (0.23, 1.32) |
| Fully Vaccinated | 111 | 913 | | 109 | 248 | |
| Unvaccinated | 18 | 95 | | 12 | 16 | |
| **Full Dose vs. None NT (Rotarix)** | n = 68 | n = 529 | 2.06 (0.62, 6.83) | n = 61 | n = 117 | 1.27 (0.31, 5.23) |
| Fully Vaccinated | 60 | 469 | | 58 | 108 | |
| Unvaccinated | 8 | 60 | | 3 | 9 | |
| **Full Dose vs. None WA (RotaTeq)** | n = 61 | n = 479 | 0.40 (0.18, 0.93) | n = 60 | n = 147 | 0.29 (0.09, 0.96) |
| Fully Vaccinated | 51 | 444 | | 51 | 140 | |
| Unvaccinated | 10 | 35 | | 9 | 7 | |
| **Full Dose vs. Partial Dose** | n = 153 | n = 1350 | 0.65 (0.42, 1.01) | n = 137 | n = 283 | 0.63 (0.35, 1.13) |
| Fully Vaccinated | 111 | 1060 | | 109 | 248 | |
| Partially Vaccinated | 42 | 290 | | 28 | 35 | |

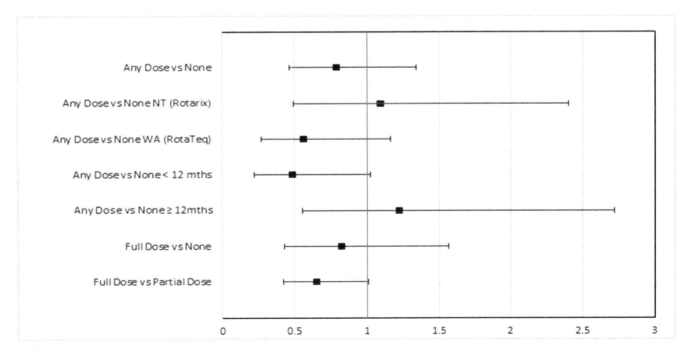

**Figure 2.** Odds ratio of vaccination in rotavirus cases versus controls in the population-based analysis.

Additional analyses were performed as requested after peer review—including restricting the population-based analysis to children age-eligible for full vaccination only (aged ≥24 weeks in the NT and ≥32 weeks in WA), restricting the population-based analysis to children aged <5 years and restricting the population-based analysis to Aboriginal children only. An additional analysis was also run without the 'missing dose assumption', i.e., in circumstances where a child had a vaccine dose recorded as dose two or three on the register but where an earlier dose was not recorded, the cases and controls were reclassified as 'partially vaccinated' (Supplementary Materials Table S3). This resulted in the reclassification of 26 population controls as partially vaccinated, but no change to the classification of rotavirus cases. The results of the additional analyses were broadly in keeping with the per-protocol analysis.

## 4. Discussion

In the context of a G2P[4] rotavirus epidemic with 171 laboratory confirmed rotavirus notifications, we failed to find evidence that either rotavirus vaccine provided strong protection against rotavirus gastroenteritis. This contrasts with the large decrease in rotavirus morbidity and mortality observed globally in young children following the licensing of the oral two rotavirus vaccines, Rotarix and RotaTeq, in 2006 [2,7,11].

The 2017 G2P[4] rotavirus epidemic in the Northern Territory and adjoining regions of rural and remote Western Australia predominantly affected Aboriginal and Torres Strait Islander children (NT 86%, WA 75%). Two thirds of cases (65%) were fully vaccinated, and cases were only slightly less likely to have received a vaccine dose than matched population controls sampled from the immunisation register (OR of 0.79 is equivalent to a VE of 21% where VE = 1—OR). There was some evidence of protection among the subgroup of children <12 months old, although all 95% confidence intervals included one (no effect) and there was significant overlap in the confidence intervals across the subgroup analyses. We found little evidence of a protective effect for full vaccination overall (OR of full vs. no vaccination 0.83 (95% CI, 0.43, 1.58)), although there was some evidence that fully vaccinated children were better protected than unvaccinated children in Western Australia (OR of full vs no vaccination for WA 0.40 (95% CI, 0.18–0.93)). We also found some evidence that fully vaccinated children were moderately better protected than partially vaccinated children (OR of full vs. partial vaccination 0.65 (95% CI, 0.42–1.01)). These findings are consistent with recently published vaccine effectiveness studies evaluating the performance of Rotarix in New South Wales and both Rotarix/RotaTeq in Western Australia. In both studies, VE estimates were highest for fully vaccinated children aged <12 months, and there was evidence of increasing vaccine effectiveness with increasing doses of both Rotarix and RotaTeq vaccines [12,13].

Rotarix is a live, monovalent, attenuated oral rotavirus vaccine derived from the most common human rotavirus strain G1P[8], and RotaTeq is a pentavalent (G1, G2, G3, G4, P[8]) human–bovine reassortant vaccine [14]. While post-licensure studies have reported similar vaccine effectiveness levels for Rotarix and RotaTeq [2], very few studies have directly compared the effectiveness of each vaccine in the same setting or during the same outbreak [15–17]. While there is good evidence that RotaTeq is protective against G2P[4] strains [18], post-licensure studies have shown mixed results for the effectiveness of Rotarix against G2 strains [8,19] and in some jurisdictions using Rotarix, G2P[4] has emerged as the dominant circulating genotype [20–23]. An earlier study of a 2009 G2P[4] outbreak amongst NT Aboriginal infants failed to show that the rotavirus vaccine provided strong protection (OR 0.81 (95% CI, 0.32–2.05)) [8]. In our study, all rotavirus samples sent for genotypic analysis from the five administrative health regions between March and June 2017 were identified as G2P[4]. Given the epidemic was well-defined in time and geography, it is reasonable to assume that G2P[4] accounted for all epidemic cases; this study provides a unique opportunity to evaluate the performance of both Rotarix and RotaTeq during the same G2P[4] epidemic and in similar, albeit geographically distinct, populations. While the point estimate of the OR was consistently lower in the jurisdiction using Rotateq (consistent with better effectiveness), the confidence intervals were wide and overlapping.

Small rotavirus case numbers in both jurisdictions and programmatic differences in how cases are ascertained limit our ability to draw conclusions about the comparative effectiveness of the vaccines in this study.

While there was evidence of a protective effect among younger children, our estimates suggest that a strong protective effect of vaccination is unlikely among older children. The median age of rotavirus infection was 19 months with a substantial proportion of cases occurring among children aged 12–23 months (NT 44%, WA 39%). Decreased vaccine protection in the second year of life and persistent burden of rotavirus disease have been reported in other high-burden low-resource settings [2,5,24]. Possible determinants of poor vaccine response include high levels of maternally-derived, vaccine-neutralising anti-rotavirus antibodies, poor infant nutrition, intestinal microbiota imbalance, environmental enteropathy, comorbid infections such as HIV and a high diversity of circulating rotavirus strains [25]. In the population included in this study, children are very unlikely to have been HIV infected, but other infective comorbidities are common. Apart from reduced vaccine-induced protection, programmatic restrictions, including upper age-limits for rotavirus vaccine administration may also diminish the program. An early rotavirus vaccine, RRV-TV, caused intussusception in a small number of vaccinated older infants [26] and despite reassuring phase 3 clinical trial safety results, the manufacturers of Rotarix and RotaTeq have conservatively recommended upper age limits on the administration of their vaccines—24 weeks for Rotarix and 32 weeks for RotaTeq. In practice, this limits opportunity to complete the full vaccination schedule and eliminates the possibility of catch-up of missed vaccinations in later childhood [25]. Delayed and/or incomplete vaccination is more common among Australian Aboriginal children [27] and in one observational study, two-dose DTPa coverage increased by a further 16% after the upper age limit of rotavirus vaccine administration (from 75% to 91% in Aboriginal infants), whereas two-dose rotavirus vaccine coverage increased by only 3% (from 75% to 78% in Aboriginal infants) [28]. This suggests that relaxing the upper age restrictions for rotavirus vaccines, as recommended by WHO for countries with high rotavirus burden [3], could be considered as a strategy for improving vaccine uptake and schedule completion.

The validity of case-control methods is largely dependent on adequate control of confounders, that is, factors which are causally related to both vaccination and baseline risk of disease [29]. In our setting, vaccination coverage is influenced by age, Aboriginal status, geographical location and calendar time; age and Aboriginal status remain the two strongest baseline risk factors for rotavirus gastroenteritis requiring hospitalisation [7], and epidemics are clustered in geographic space and time. Our study therefore sought to control for these potential confounders by directly matching cases to population controls on age (date of birth), Aboriginal status and location of residence, and by confining the analysis to the defined outbreak period. In the disease register analysis, these factors were not matched but were captured and adjusted for in the regression analysis. This study could not directly measure socio-economic status for individual cases and controls, although Indigenous status and remoteness of residence may be considered surrogate measures, with the Alice Springs, Barkly, Kimberley and Goldfields regions encompassing some of the most socially disadvantaged regions in Australia, as measured by the Index of Relative Socioeconomic Advantage and Disadvantage.

While the jurisdiction-based notifiable infectious disease databases are believed to capture all laboratory-confirmed rotavirus cases during the epidemic, we acknowledge that not all children with rotavirus gastroenteritis present for medical care, are referred for testing, or complete testing when it is recommended. Rotavirus vaccines have been found to be more effective in preventing severe disease requiring hospitalisation than asymptomatic and other less severe forms of infection [2]. While we were not able to directly ascertain disease severity, most cases in this study are likely to have had either moderate or severe gastroenteritis because all sought medical care (in order to be hospitalised), and 78% and 39% were hospitalised in the NT and WA respectively.

It is also acknowledged that the propensity to seek medical care for rotavirus gastroenteritis symptoms may be associated with the propensity to access medical care for other reasons, including vaccination, and this is a potential source of bias in the population-based analysis which may have caused us to underestimate vaccine protection. The disease register analysis is less likely to be affected by this bias because the vaccination status of rotavirus cases was compared to that of other children with (non-vaccine preventable), notifiable gastrointestinal clinical infections, i.e., children with clinical presentations which are likely to have been indistinguishable from rotavirus infection and who also underwent microbiological testing. The results of the disease register nested analysis were limited by small numbers, especially in the subgroup analyses, but were in broad agreement with the population-based analysis.

Rotavirus gastroenteritis cannot be reliably distinguished from other causes of non-bloody diarrhea on clinical grounds, and so only laboratory confirmed cases reported to the notifiable infectious disease databases were included. The sensitivity and specificity for detecting rotavirus in stool samples using commercially available EIA is high, although false positives and false negatives have been reported [30]. This is noted as a limitation of the nested disease register case-control study, where an assay error may result in misclassification of a case as a control, or vice versa, which would have caused us to underestimate vaccine protection.

While the Australian Immunisation Register provides credible individual and population-level data regarding vaccine coverage by vaccine type, date-of-birth, location of residence and Aboriginal status, controls were matched to cases based on their location of residence, as recorded on the register in October 2019, which may or may not accurately reflect their jurisdiction of residence between March and June 2017. It is unclear what, if any, bias this may have caused.

## 5. Conclusions

The incorporation of two rotavirus vaccines into the Australian NIP in 2007 has resulted in a substantial and sustained decrease in rotavirus morbidity across most of Australia, although Aboriginal and Torres Strait Islander children remain at increased risk of severe rotavirus disease requiring hospitalisation [7]. Our evaluation of the 2017 G2P[4] rotavirus epidemic in remote Australia suggests that rotavirus vaccination provided little protection against notifiable rotavirus disease for children living in rural and remote Australia, with the likely exception of children aged <12 months for whom moderate evidence of protection was found.

The admission of an additional 99 children with gastroenteritis to small regional and remote hospitals over fourteen weeks highlights the ongoing public health importance of rotavirus and the need for strategies to better protect Aboriginal children. Our data indicate a likely benefit from full rather than partial vaccination, underscoring the importance of completing the rotavirus schedule. Schedule completion could be enhanced by relaxing the upper age limit of rotavirus vaccination as has been recommended by the World Health Organisation for high-burden settings [3].

Our study also reports a high percentage of rotavirus cases in children aged 12–23 months and decreased vaccine protection among children older than 12 months. It is plausible that administering an additional or booster dose of rotavirus vaccine to slightly older children (beyond manufacturer upper age limit restrictions) may extend protection into the second year of life. Scheduling a third dose of Rotarix vaccine (at between 6 and 11 months old) is currently under investigation in the NT [31].

**Supplementary Materials:**
Figure S1: Selection of rotavirus cases and un-matched disease register controls for disease register nested case-control study. Table S1. Baseline characteristics of rotavirus cases and disease register controls for the unmatched disease-register nested case-control study. Table S2. Odds Ratio of vaccination in rotavirus cases versus controls in the matched population-based analysis and the disease register nested analysis (full results). Table S3. Odds Ratio of vaccination in rotavirus cases versus controls in additional population-based analysis (i) children age-eligible for full vaccination only (aged ≥ 24 weeks in the NT and ≥32 weeks in WA), (ii) children aged <5 years only, (iii) Aboriginal children only, and (iv) 'missing dose assumption' removed.

**Author Contributions:** Conceptualization, T.S., M.D. and B.F.M.; methodology, T.S., M.D., H.Q., A.P.R. and M.E.; formal analysis, T.S. and B.F.M.; data curation, B.F.M. and H.Q.; writing—original draft preparation, B.F.M.; writing—review and editing, T.S., M.D., H.Q., A.P.R., M.E., N.P. and M.J.; supervision, T.S. and M.D.; project administration, B.F.M.; funding acquisition, B.F.M. All authors have read and agreed to the published version of the manuscript.

**Acknowledgments:** We acknowledge the support of the Menzies Child Health Indigenous Reference Group, the Kimberley Aboriginal Health Planning Forum and the Pilbara Aboriginal Health Planning Forum. We also acknowledge the support and assistance of Peter Markey and Heather Cook at the Northern Territory Centre for Disease Control, Paul Effler, Robyn Gibbs, Carolien Giele and Clare Huppatz from the Western Australian Communicable Disease Control Directorate, Rob Baird from Territory Pathology, and Julie Bines and Susie Roczo-Farkas from the Enteric Diseases Group, Murdoch Children's Research Institute.

## References

1. Troeger, C.; Khalil, I.A.; Rao, P.C.; Cao, S.; Blacker, B.F.; Ahmed, T.; Armah, G.; Bines, J.E.; Brewer, T.G.; Colombara, D.V.; et al. Rotavirus Vaccination and the Global Burden of Rotavirus Diarrhea among Children Younger Than 5 Years. *JAMA Pediatr.* **2018**, *172*, 958–965. [CrossRef] [PubMed]
2. Burnett, E.; Parashar, U.D.; Tate, J.E. Real-world effectiveness of rotavirus vaccines, 2006–2019: A literature review and meta-analysis. *Lancet Glob. Health* **2020**, *8*, e1195–e1202. [CrossRef]
3. WHO. Rotavirus vaccines WHO position paper: January 2013—Recommendations. *Vaccine* **2013**, *31*, 6170–6171. [CrossRef] [PubMed]
4. Armah, G.E.; Sow, S.O.; Breiman, R.F.; Dallas, M.J.; Tapia, M.D.; Feikin, D.R.; Binka, F.N.; Steele, A.D.; Laserson, K.F.; Ansah, N.A.; et al. Efficacy of pentavalent rotavirus vaccine against severe rotavirus gastroenteritis in infants in developing countries in sub-Saharan Africa: A randomised, double-blind, placebo-controlled trial. *Lancet* **2010**, *376*, 606–614. [CrossRef]
5. Madhi, S.A.; Cunliffe, N.A.; Steele, D.; Witte, D.; Kirsten, M.; Louw, C.; Ngwira, B.; Victor, J.C.; Gillard, P.H.; Cheuvart, B.B.; et al. Effect of human rotavirus vaccine on severe diarrhea in African infants. *N. Engl. J. Med.* **2010**, *362*, 289–298. [CrossRef]
6. Zaman, K.; Anh, D.D.; Victor, J.C.; Shin, S.; Yunus; Dallas, M.J.; Podder, G.; Thiem, V.D.; Mai, L.T.P.; Luby, S.P.; et al. Efficacy of pentavalent rotavirus vaccine against severe rotavirus gastroenteritis in infants in developing countries in Asia: A randomised, double-blind, placebo-controlled trial. *Lancet* **2010**, *376*, 615–623. [CrossRef]
7. Dey, A.; Wang, H.; Menzies, R.; Macartney, K. Changes in hospitalisations for acute gastroenteritis in Australia after the national rotavirus vaccination program. *Med. J. Aust.* **2012**, *197*, 453–4547. [CrossRef]
8. Snelling, T.L.; Andrews, R.M.; Kirkwood, C.D.; Culvenor, S.; Carapetis, J.R. Case-control evaluation of the effectiveness of the G1P[8] human rotavirus vaccine during an outbreak of rotavirus G2P[4] infection in central Australia. *Clin. Infect. Dis.* **2011**, *52*, 191–199. [CrossRef]
9. ABS. *2016 Census QuickStats (SA3)*; Australian Bureau of Statistics: Canberra, Australia, 2017. Available online: https://www.abs.gov.au/websitedbs/censushome.nsf/home/quickstats?opendocument&navpos=220 (accessed on 20 July 2020).
10. Hull, B.P.; Lawrence, G.; MacIntyre, C.R.; McIntyre, P.B. Estimating immunisation coverage: Is the 'third dose assumption' still valid? *Commun. Dis. Intell. Q. Rep.* **2003**, *27*, 357–361.
11. Field, E.J.; Vally, H.; Grimwood, K.; Lambert, S. Pentavalent rotavirus vaccine and prevention of gastroenteritis hospitalizations in Australia. *Pediatrics* **2010**, *126*, e506–e512. [CrossRef]
12. Fathima, P.; Snelling, T.L.; Gibbs, R.A. Effectiveness of rotavirus vaccines in an Australian population: A case-control study. *Vaccine* **2019**, *37*, 6048–6053. [CrossRef] [PubMed]
13. Maguire, J.E.; Glasgow, K.; Glass, K.; Roczo-Farkas, S.; Bines, J.E.; Sheppeard, V.; Macartney, K.; Quinn, H.E. Rotavirus Epidemiology and Monovalent Rotavirus Vaccine Effectiveness in Australia: 2010–2017. *Pediatrics* **2019**, *144*, 1–10. [CrossRef] [PubMed]
14. Australian Technical Advisory Group on Immunisation (ATAGI). *Australian Immunisation Handbook*; Australian Government Department of Health: Canberra, Australia, 2018.
15. Payne, D.C.; Boom, J.A.; Staat, M.A.; Edwards, K.M.; Szilagyi, P.G.; Klein, E.J.; Selvarangan, R.; Azimi, P.H.; Harrison, C.; Moffatt, M.; et al. Effectiveness of pentavalent and monovalent rotavirus vaccines in concurrent use among US children <5 years of age, 2009–2011. *Clin. Infect. Dis.* **2013**, *57*, 13–20. [PubMed]
16. Castilla, J.; Beristain, X.; Martínez-Artola, V.; Ortega, A.N.; Cenoz, M.G.; Álvarez, N.; Polo, I.; Mazón, A.; Gil-Setas, A.; Barricarte, A. Effectiveness of rotavirus vaccines in preventing cases and hospitalizations due to rotavirus gastroenteritis in Navarre, Spain. *Vaccine* **2012**, *30*, 539–543. [CrossRef]
17. Muhsen, K.; Shulman, L.; Kasem, E.; Rubinstein, U.; Shachter, J.; Kremer, A.; Goren, S.; Zilberstein, I.; Chodick, G.; Ephros, M.; et al. Effectiveness of rotavirus vaccines for prevention of rotavirus gastroenteritis-associated hospitalizations in Israel: A case-control study. *Hum. Vaccines* **2010**, *6*, 450–454. [CrossRef]

18. Leshem, E.; Lopman, B.; Glass, R.; Gentsch, J.; Banyai, K.; Parashar, U.; Patel, M. Distribution of rotavirus strains and strain-specific effectiveness of the rotavirus vaccine after its introduction: A systematic review and meta-analysis. *Lancet Infect. Dis.* **2014**, *14*, 847–856. [CrossRef]
19. Correia, J.B.; Patel, M.M.; Nakagomi, O.; Montenegro, F.M.U.; Germano, E.M.; Correia, N.B.; Cuevas, L.E.; Parashar, U.D.; Cunliffe, N.A.; Nakagomi, T. Effectiveness of monovalent rotavirus vaccine (Rotarix) against severe diarrhea caused by serotypically unrelated G2P[4] strains in Brazil. *J. Infect. Dis.* **2010**, *201*, 363–369. [CrossRef]
20. Zeller, M.; Rahman, M.; Heylen, E.; De Coster, S.; De Vos, S.; Arijs, I.; Novo, L.; Verstappen, N.; Van Ranst, M.; Matthijnssens, J. Rotavirus incidence and genotype distribution before and after national rotavirus vaccine introduction in Belgium. *Vaccine* **2010**, *28*, 7507–7513. [CrossRef]
21. Doro, R.; László, B.; Martella, V.; Leshem, E.; Gentsch, J.; Parashar, U.; Banyai, K. Review of global rotavirus strain prevalence data from six years post vaccine licensure surveillance: Is there evidence of strain selection from vaccine pressure? *Infect. Genet. Evol.* **2014**, *28*, 446–461. [CrossRef]
22. Roczo-Farkas, S.; Kirkwood, C.D.; Cowley, D.; Barnes, G.L.; Bishop, R.F.; Bogdanovic-Sakran, N.; Boniface, K.; Donato, C.M.; E Bines, J. The Impact of Rotavirus Vaccines on Genotype Diversity: A Comprehensive Analysis of 2 Decades of Australian Surveillance Data. *J. Infect. Dis.* **2018**, *218*, 546–554. [CrossRef]
23. Santos, V.S.; Nóbrega, F.A.; Soares, M.W.S.; Moreira, R.D.; Cuevas, L.E.; Gurgel, R.Q. Rotavirus Genotypes Circulating in Brazil Before and After the National Rotavirus Vaccine Program: A Review. *Pediatr. Infect. Dis. J.* **2018**, *37*, e63–e65. [CrossRef] [PubMed]
24. Patel, M.; Glass, R.I.; Jiang, B.; Santosham, M.; Lopman, B.; Parashar, U. A systematic review of anti-rotavirus serum IgA antibody titer as a potential correlate of rotavirus vaccine efficacy. *J. Infect. Dis.* **2013**, *208*, 284–294. [CrossRef] [PubMed]
25. Velasquez, D.E.; Parashar, U.; Jiang, B. Decreased performance of live attenuated, oral rotavirus vaccines in low-income settings: Causes and contributing factors. *Expert Rev. Vaccines* **2018**, *17*, 145–161. [CrossRef] [PubMed]
26. Peter, G.; Myers, M.G. Intussusception, rotavirus, and oral vaccines: Summary of a workshop. *Pediatrics* **2002**, *110*, e67. [CrossRef]
27. Moore, H.C.; Fathima, P.; Gidding, H.F.; De Klerk, N.; Liu, B.; Sheppeard, V.; Effler, P.V.; Snelling, T.L.; McIntyre, P.; Blyth, C.C.; et al. Assessment of on-time vaccination coverage in population subgroups: A record linkage cohort study. *Vaccine* **2018**, *36*, 4062–4069. [CrossRef]
28. Fathima, P.; Gidding, H.F.; Snelling, T.L.; McIntyre, P.; Blyth, C.C.; Sheridan, S.; Liu, B.; De Klerk, N.; Moore, H.C. Timeliness and factors associated with rotavirus vaccine uptake among Australian Aboriginal and non-Aboriginal children: A record linkage cohort study. *Vaccine* **2019**, *37*, 5835–5843. [CrossRef]
29. Orenstein, W.A.; Bernier, R.H.; Hinman, A.R. Assessing vaccine efficacy in the field. Further observations. *Epidemiol. Rev.* **1988**, *10*, 212–241. [CrossRef]
30. Izzo, M.M.; Kirkland, P.D.; Gu, X.; Lele, Y.; Gunn, A.A.; House, J. Comparison of three diagnostic techniques for detection of rotavirus and coronavirus in calf faeces in Australia. *Aust. Vet. J.* **2012**, *90*, 122–129. [CrossRef] [PubMed]
31. Middleton, B.F.; Jones, M.A.; Waddington, C.S.; Danchin, M.; McCallum, C.; Gallagher, S.; Leach, A.J.; Andrews, R.; Kirkwood, C.; Cunliffe, N.; et al. The ORVAC trial protocol: A phase IV, double-blind, randomised, placebo-controlled clinical trial of a third scheduled dose of Rotarix rotavirus vaccine in Australian Indigenous infants to improve protection against gastroenteritis. *BMJ Open* **2019**, *9*, e032549. [CrossRef]

# Group A Rotavirus Detection and Genotype Distribution before and after Introduction of a National Immunisation Programme in Ireland: 2015–2019

Zoe Yandle *, Suzie Coughlan, Jonathan Dean, Gráinne Tuite, Anne Conroy and Cillian F. De Gascun

UCD National Virus Reference Laboratory, University College Dublin, Dublin 4, Ireland; suzie.coughlan@ucd.ie (S.C.); jonathan.dean@ucd.ie (J.D.); grainne.tuite@ucd.ie (G.T.); anne.conroy@ucd.ie (A.C.); cillian.degascun@ucd.ie (C.F.D.G.)
* Correspondence: zyandle@ucd.ie;

**Abstract:** Immunisation against rotavirus infection was introduced into Ireland in December 2016. We report on the viruses causing gastroenteritis before (2015–2016) and after (2017–2019) implementation of the Rotarix vaccine, as well as changes in the diversity of circulating rotavirus genotypes. Samples from patients aged ≤ 5 years (n = 11,800) were received at the National Virus Reference Laboratory, Dublin, and tested by real-time RT-PCR for rotavirus, Rotarix, norovirus, sapovirus, astrovirus, and enteric adenovirus. Rotavirus genotyping was performed either by multiplex or hemi-nested RT-PCR, and a subset was characterised by sequence analysis. Rotavirus detection decreased by 91% in children aged 0–12 months between 2015/16 and 2018/19. Rotarix was detected in 10% of those eligible for the vaccine and was not found in those aged >7 months. Rotavirus typically peaks in March–May, but following vaccination, the seasonality became less defined. In 2015–16, G1P[8] was the most common genotype circulating; however, in 2019 G2P[4] was detected more often. Following the introduction of Rotarix, a reduction in numbers of rotavirus infections occurred, coinciding with an increase in genotype diversity, along with the first recorded detection of an equine-like G3 strain in Ireland.

**Keywords:** gastroenteritis; rotavirus; Rotarix; pediatric; diagnostics; molecular epidemiology; G3P[8]; equine-like

## 1. Introduction

Rotavirus is a leading cause of pediatric acute gastroenteritis, causing fever, vomiting, and diarrhoea. Mortality rates are highest in low income developing countries, where it causes approximately 128,000 fatal cases per year in those under five years old [1,2]. With the availability of rotavirus vaccines, the rate of global hospitalisations due to rotavirus or acute gastroenteritis, as well as deaths due to acute gastroenteritis, has decreased [3]. In Europe, pediatric rotavirus infection results in approximately 75,000–150,000 hospitalisations annually, with 2–4 times more children seeking out-patient medical care [4]. In Ireland, average crude incidence rates were 55 per 100,000 population in the 2007–2015 period [5], with hospitalisation rates of approximately 1190 per 100,000 [6], compared to the majority of EU member states, which report rates of 300–600 per 100,000 [4].

In 2009, the World Health Organisation (WHO) recommended global rotavirus vaccination [7] and, in Europe, 13 countries include it in their universal immunisation programmes, with a further five offering the vaccine for certain risk groups, specific regions, or requiring partial payment [8].

Two licensed live-attenuated vaccines are available in Europe; the pentavalent bovine-human reassortment rotavirus vaccine, RotaTeq (Merck & Co., West Point, PA, USA), and the human monovalent vaccine, Rotarix (GlaxoSmithKline, Rixensart, Belgium). In December 2016, Rotarix was introduced into the Irish national immunisation programme, with the vaccine administered in two doses at 2 and 4 months of age. Most recent figures (Q3, 2019) show the national uptake of the vaccine is 89% [9]. Rotavirus is a notifiable disease in Ireland, and laboratory confirmed cases are reported to the Health Protection Surveillance Centre. Effectiveness of both RotaTeq and Rotarix has been well documented, with the UK, Germany, and Belgium reporting an approximate 85% reduction in the presentation of severe rotavirus disease following vaccination [10–12].

Rotaviruses are double stranded RNA viruses containing 11 genome segments. There are 10 groups, A–J, defined by the middle VP6 capsid antigen, [13] two of which (I and J) were recently discovered in dogs and bats, respectively [14,15]. However, in humans, the majority of infections are caused by Group A rotavirus. Classification is a binary system depending on the expression of two outer proteins; the G and P-type, encoded by VP7 and VP4, respectively. Full genome analysis (where the VP7-VP4-VP6-VP1-VP2-VP3-NSP1-NSP2-NSP3-NSP4-NSP5/6 genes of rotavirus (RV) strains are described using the abbreviations Gx-P[x]-Ix-Rx-Cx-Mx-Ax-Nx-Tx-Ex-Hx), is required to monitor the evolution of the virus and detect reassortment [16].

Despite the theoretical possibility for numerous rotavirus G/P constellations, six account for 80–90% of circulating genotypes, namely G1P[8], G2P[4], G3P[8], G4P[8], G9P[8] and G12P[8]. Distribution of these commonly detected genotypes can vary by year, country, and age [17]. Despite the natural fluctuation of genotype diversity, increasing data suggest that the changes may be due to the impact of strain-specific vaccines [18]. Both in Belgium and the UK, before immunisation, G1P[8] was the most common circulating genotype; however, following vaccination, G2P[4] has been more frequently detected [19,20]. In Finland, following the introduction of RotaTeq, G9P[8] and G12P[8] have now become the main genotypes, where, previously, G1P[8] dominated [21]. However, changes in genotype distribution also occurs in countries with no immunisation [22,23], so whether the vaccine directly leads to a change in genotype diversity remains unclear [24,25].

Surveillance of rotavirus genotypes has been recommended by the WHO in countries with immunisation programmes to detect and monitor strain variation and ensure vaccine effectiveness is maintained [26]. The surveillance network, EuroRotaNet, has been monitoring rotavirus diversity in 12 European countries and has reported an increase in diversity since vaccination [17,27]. As Ireland is not currently part of any European or global surveillance network, we aim to fill that current gap of knowledge.

The purpose of this study is two-fold; firstly, to report on the viruses causing gastroenteritis, including rotavirus, 2 years prior and 3 years post implementation of the Rotarix immunisation programme, and, secondly, to describe the diversity of rotavirus genotypes in Ireland.

## 2. Results

### 2.1. Sample Demographics

Ireland has a population of 4.8 million with 36% of people living in the eastern health region, which includes Dublin, the surrounding areas, and the country's largest children's hospitals [28]. The National Virus Reference Laboratory (NVRL), Dublin, provides a diagnostic and reference service for all health care regions, though testing is also provided in regional hospitals.

This study analyzed the results from pediatric (≤5 years) patient samples received at the NVRL between 1 January 2015 and 31 December 2019 for the investigation of viral gastroenteritis. In total, 11,800 faecal samples were included in the analysis, 5267 (45%) from females, 6511 (55%) from males, and 22 (0.2%) for which details were not provided. Samples tested were predominantly from the eastern health region 10,644/11,800 (90%), and of these 10,180/10,644 (96%) were from a children's hospital. Other samples were from the northern 672/11,800 (6%), western 204/11,800 (2%), midlands 139/11,800

(1%), and southern health regions 141/11,800 (1%). As vaccine history was not available for each patient, cohorts are described as vaccine-eligible, using age as a proxy for vaccination status.

During 2015 to 2019, there were 312,013 births recorded in Ireland; 159,821 males (51.2%) and 152,192 females (48.8%). To establish how representative the samples tested were, the percentage of the annual birth cohort investigated for the detection of viruses causing gastroenteritis was calculated for those aged 0–12 months in each year. In 2015, 2280/65,536 (3.5%) were tested, in 2016 2065/63,841 (3.3%) were tested, in 2017 760/61,824 (1.2%) were tested, in 2018 587/61,016 (1%) were tested, and in 2019 608/59,796 (1%) were tested.

## 2.2. Detection of Viral Pathogens

The most frequently detected viral pathogen in 2015 and 2016 was rotavirus, followed by norovirus. Norovirus has been detected in approximately 12% of samples each year, whereas enteric adenovirus (adenovirus subgenus F), sapovirus, and astrovirus were detected in 2.8–6.3% of samples from 2015–2019 (Table 1). The number of samples with no virus detected ranged from 51.4% to 65.0%, depending on the year.

**Table 1.** Laboratory results for the investigation of viral gastroenteritis in 11,800 samples tested at the National Virus Reference Laboratory (NVRL), aged 0–5 years in 2015–2019.

| Virus Detected | Results (%) by Year | | | | | Total |
| --- | --- | --- | --- | --- | --- | --- |
| | 2015 | 2016 | 2017 | 2018 | 2019 | |
| Rotavirus-wild-type | 662 (15.03) | 519 (13.09) | 250 (15.49) | 53 (4.42) | 70 (5.93) | 1554 |
| Rotavirus-Rotarix | 0 (0.00) | 1 (0.03) | 61 (3.78) | 49 (4.08) | 69 (5.84) | 180 |
| Norovirus | 482 (10.94) | 492 (12.41) | 210 (13.01) | 158 (13.17) | 141 (11.94) | 1483 |
| Adenovirus F | 156 (3.54) | 155 (3.91) | 101 (6.26) | 64 (5.33) | 47 (3.98) | 523 |
| Sapovirus | 202 (4.59) | 167 (4.21) | 85 (5.27) | 72 (6.00) | 33 (2.79) | 559 |
| Astrovirus | 197 (4.47) | 121 (3.05) | 77 (4.77) | 68 (5.67) | 53 (4.49) | 516 |
| No virus detected | 2705 (61.42) | 2511 (63.31) | 830 (51.43) | 736 (61.33) | 768 (65.03) | 7550 |
| Total samples tested | 4199 | 3787 | 1499 | 1159 | 1156 | |
| Total results | 4404 [a] | 3966 [b] | 1614 [c] | 1200 [d] | 1181 [e] | |

[a] 185 dual infections, 10 triple infections [b] 154 dual infections, 11 triple infections, 1 quadruple infection, [c] 93 dual infections, 8 triple infections, 2 quadruple infections [d] 41 dual infections [e] 25 dual infections. Additional viruses detected in Rotarix samples, 2017: norovirus n = 3, adenovirus F n = 1, astrovirus n = 2; 2018: norovirus n = 8, adenovirus F n = 1; 2019: norovirus n = 3, sapovirus n = 1, astrovirus n = 1.

There were 1753 samples tested from vaccine-eligible children in 2017–2019, and of these 43 (2.5%) had wild-type rotavirus, 179 (10.2%) had Rotarix, 257 (14.7%) had norovirus, 113 (6.4%) had adenovirus F, 97 (5.5%) had sapovirus, and 95 (5.4%) had astrovirus detected. In this group, there were 70 dual infections and 1039 (59.3%) samples had no detectable virus.

## 2.3. Detection of Wild-Type Rotavirus

The median age of those testing positive for rotavirus in the pre-vaccine era, 2015–2016 (n = 1181), was significantly lower at 1.19 years (interquartile range (IQR) 0.64–1.85), compared to the median in the entire 3 years post-vaccine, 2017–2019 (n = 373) at 1.85 years (IQR 1.12–2.84) $p < 0.0001$ (Table 2).

In the 2015/16 pre-vaccine era, a total of 485/4345 (11.2%) children aged 0–1 year had detectable wild-type rotavirus. This compares with 12/1195 (1.0%) in the post-vaccine 2018 and 2019 era, representing a 91.1% relative decrease in the number of wild-type rotavirus detected in this age range. The 1–2-year age group showed a relative reduction of 79.1% when 2015/16 was compared with 2018/19; 444/1691 (26.3%) compared to 28/505 (5.5%), respectively. This contrasts with the 5–6-year age group, which showed an increase in the detection of rotavirus from 20/324 (6.2%) to 12/96 (12.5%).

**Table 2.** Number of wild-type rotavirus positive cases by age group in the pre-vaccine years (2015–2016) compared to the post-vaccine years (2017–2019).

|  | Year | Number of Wild-Type Rotavirus Positive Samples/Total Number of Samples Tested (%) | | | | | | | Median Age (IQR) |
|---|---|---|---|---|---|---|---|---|---|
|  |  | 0–1 Year | 1–2 Years | 2–3 Years | 3–4 Years | 4–5 Years | 5–6 Years | Total |  |
| Pre-vaccine | 2015 | 285/2280 (12.5) | 227/899 (25.3) | 90/413 (21.8) | 35/213 (16.4) | 17/213 (8.0) | 8/181 (4.4) | 662/4199 (15.8) | 1.17 (0.5-1.9) |
|  | 2016 | 200/2065 (9.7) | 217/792 (27.4) | 55/427 (12.9) | 24/224 (10.7) | 11/136 (8.1) | 12/143 (8.4) | 519/3787 (13.7) | 1.22 (0.8-1.8) |
| Post-vaccine | 2017 | 57/760 (7.5) | 110/374 (29.4) | 49/144 (34.0) | 19/105 (18.1) | 6/55 (10.9) | 9/61 (14.8) | 250/1499 (16.7) | 1.59 (1.0–2.4) |
|  | 2018 | 8/587 (1.4) | 12/272 (4.4) | 23/125 (18.4) | 2/62 (3.2) | 3/59 (5.1) | 5/54 (9.2) | 53/1159 (4.6) | 2.24 (1.6–2.9) |
|  | 2019 | 4/608 (0.7) | 16/233 (6.9) | 16/129 (12.4) | 21/86 (24.4) | 6/58 (10.3) | 7/42 (16.7) | 70/1156 (6.1) | 2.90 (1.9–3.5) |

Interquartile range (IQR).

## 2.4. Seasonal Variation of Wild-Type Rotavirus

Prior to vaccination, rotavirus was a seasonal infection. In 2015, the season ran from weeks 1–29, peaking in week 11; in 2016 from weeks 11–27, peaking in week 19; and in 2017 from weeks 2–30, peaking in week 11. However, in 2018 and 2019, there was no clear seasonal onset and end, and rotavirus was most frequently detected in weeks 14 and 22, respectively (Figure 1).

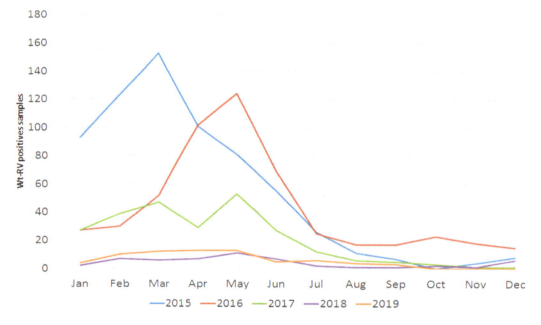

**Figure 1.** Number of wild-type rotavirus (Wt-RV) cases detected by month, 2015–2019.

## 2.5. Detection of Vaccine-Derived Rotavirus (Rotarix)

Of all 3814 samples tested in 2017–2019, 1753 (46.0%) were eligible for the vaccine, and Rotarix was detected in 179/1753 (10.2%) of these (Table 1). In addition, one sample from a vaccine eligible patient was received and tested in December 2016 and found to be positive for Rotarix. In 20/180 (11.1%) of Rotarix-positive samples, another virus was detected, most commonly norovirus.

The age at which Rotarix was most frequently detected was 2 months (Table 3). Rotarix was not detected in any samples from patients older than 7 months of age.

**Table 3.** Detection of Rotarix by age.

|  | Age | | | | | |
|---|---|---|---|---|---|---|
|  | 2 mts | 3 mts | 4 mts | 5 mts | 6 mts | 7 mts |
| Rotarix detected/total number Rotarix detected (%) | 99/180 (55.0) | 41/180 (22.8) | 26/180 (14.4) | 11/180 (6.1) | 2/180 (1.1) | 1/180 (0.6) |

## 2.6. Distribution of Genotypes in Ireland

In total, 786/1554 (51%) samples with detectable wild-type rotavirus were genotyped. Of these, 728 (93%) were from the eastern health board, 33 (4%) northern, 14 (2%) western, 8 (1%) southern, and 3 (0.4%) from the midlands. No significant correlation was observed between genotype and region or age (data not shown).

As the total numbers of rotavirus cases decreased following the introduction of immunization in December 2016, the proportion of samples genotyped was increased to reliably detect significant changes. In 2015, 293/662 (44%), and in 2016, 242/519 (47%) positive samples were genotyped, while in 2017, 135/250 (54%), in 2018, 48/53 (91%), and in 2019, 68/70 (97%) were genotyped.

## 2.7. Comparison of the Genotype Diversity Pre- and Post-Vaccine

G1P[8] was the most common genotype detected in 2015, 2016, and 2017 (Table 4). Conversely, G2P[4] was the most frequently detected genotype in 2019 (Figure 2). G3P[4], G8P[8], G9P[4], G12P[6], and G2P[8] remain uncommon genotypes in Ireland, detected in five, two, four, two, and one samples, respectively, over the 5-year period.

**Table 4.** Comparison of genotype diversity between the pre-vaccine (2015–2016) and post-vaccine (2017–2019) eras. Confidence interval (CI) significance 0.95. Comparison of the genotype proportion between pre- and post-vaccine year groups by Chi-square $p < 0.05$.

| Genotype | Pre-Vaccinen (%) 2015 | 2016 | Post-Vaccinen (%) 2017 | 2018 | 2019 | Pre-Vaccine Data Combined n (%) | CI 95% | Post-Vaccine Data Combined n (%) | CI 95% | Pre vs. Post $p =$ |
|---|---|---|---|---|---|---|---|---|---|---|
| G1P[8] | 125 (42.7) | 172 (71.1) | 70 (51.9) | 7 (14.6) | 3 (4.4) | 297 (55.5) | 51.3–59.7 | 80 (31.9) | 26.4–37.9 | <0.0001 |
| G2P[4] | 6 (2.0) | 16 (6.6) | 15 (11.1) | 7 (14.6) | 27 (39.7) | 22 (4.1) | 2.7–6.2 | 49 (19.5) | 15.1–24.9 | <0.0001 |
| G3P[8] | 10 (3.4) | 9 (3.7) | 17 (12.6) | 7 (14.6) | 16 (23.5) | 19 (3.6) | 2.3–5.5 | 40 (15.9) | 11.9–21.0 | <0.0001 |
| G4P[8] | 64 (21.8) | 0 (0.0) | 6 (4.4) | 11 (23.0) | 0 (0.0) | 64 (12.0) | 9.5–15.0 | 17 (6.8) | 4.3–10.6 | 0.0257 |
| G9P[8] | 69 (23.5) | 34 (14.1) | 20 (14.8) | 10 (20.9) | 4 (5.9) | 103 (19.3) | 16.1–22.8 | 34 (13.6) | 9.9–18.3 | 0.0493 |
| G12P[8] | 3 (1.0) | 4 (1.7) | 0 (0.0) | 1 (2.1) | 5 (7.4) | 7 (1.3) | 0.1–2.7 | 6 (2.4) | 1.1–5.1 | 0.2675 |
| Mixed | 7 (2.4) | 3 (1.2) | 1 (0.7) | 1 (2.1) | 4 (5.9) | 10 (1.9) | 1–3.4 | 6 (2.4) | 1.1–5.1 | 0.0014 |
| Uncommon | 2 (0.7) | 2 (0.8) | 1 (0.7) | 1 (2.1) | 8 (11.8) | 4 (0.8) | 0.03–1.9 | 10 (4.0) | 2.2–7.2 | 0.6295 |
| Untypable | 7 (2.4) | 2 (0.8) | 5 (3.7) | 3 (6.3) | 1 (1.5) | 9 (1.7) | 0.9–3.2 | 9 (3.6) | 1.9–6.7 | n/a |
| Total | 293 (100) | 242 (100) | 135 (100) | 48 (100) | 68 (100) | 535 (100) | n/a | 251 (100) | n/a | n/a |

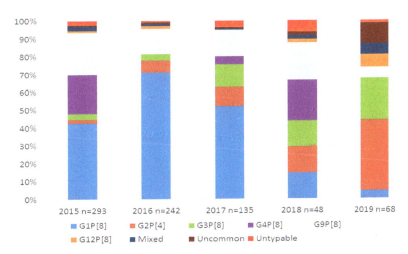

**Figure 2.** Genotype diversity in Ireland 2015–2019. Data are presented as the proportion (%) of a specific genotype compared to the total genotype results. Uncommon genotypes: <1% of total results, 2015: G9P[4] n = 2; 2016: G12P[6] n = 2; 2017: G8P[8] n = 1. 2018; G3P[4] n = 1; 2019 G2P[8] n = 1, G3P[4] n = 4, G8P[8] n = 1, G9P[4] n = 2. Mixed genotypes: those with >1 G or P-type, 2015: G1/4P[8] n = 7; 2016: G8/12P[8] n = 1, G2/3P[8] n = 1, G2/9 P[4/8] n = 1; 2017: G1/3P[8] n = 1; 2018: G1/3P[8] n = 1; 2019: G8/12P[8] n = 2, G3/12P[8] n = 1, G8P[8] n = 1, G9/12P[8] n = 1. Untypable results are those where either the G or P type was untypable.

## 2.8. Detection of Human and Equine-Like Rotavirus G3

G3P[8] was detected in 19/535 (4%) of genotyped samples in 2015–2016, compared to 40/251 (16%) in 2017–2019, a significant increase (p < 0.0001), whilst the uncommon G3P[4] was only detected in the post-vaccine era. Four G3 strains were detected as a mixed infection. Of the 68 G3 types (63 P[8] and 5 P[4]), 17 were selected for sequencing of the VP7 gene, which identified two G3P[8] samples from 2018, containing viruses that clustered within the equine-like G3 lineage and the remaining 15 G3 samples clustered within the human lineage (Figure 3).

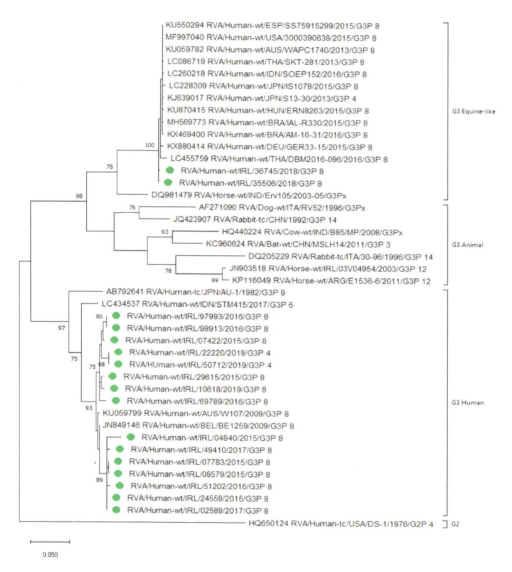

**Figure 3.** Phylogenetic tree of VP7 G3 rotavirus gene sequences. The tree was constructed by using the maximum likelihood method and the Tamura-Nei model [29]. Bootstrap values (1000 replicates) above 75% are shown. The tree is drawn to scale, with branch lengths measured in the number of substitutions per site. This analysis shows 46 nucleotide sequences; 17 from Irish strains identified in this study (colour coded with green circle) and 29 from reference strains in GenBank. Phylogenetic analyses were conducted in MEGA X [30].

## 2.9. Genotypes Detected in Rotavirus Positive Samples from Those of Vaccine-Eligible Age

There are six common genotypes circulating in Europe, namely, G1P[8], G2P[4], G3P[8], G4P[8], G9P[8], and G12P[8] [17], and all other genotypes are considered uncommon. Of the 43 samples with detectable wild-type rotavirus and of vaccine-eligible age, 37 were genotyped by RT-PCR (Table 5).

Of these, 30/37 (81.1%) had a common genotype, 4/37 (10.8%) had an uncommon genotype, 2/37 (5.4%) had a mixed infection, and one sample (2.7%) could not be fully genotyped. Ten of the 37 samples (27.0%) had G3 genotype detected (seven P[8] and three P[4]).

Table 5. Wild-type rotavirus genotypes detected in the age group eligible for the vaccine. Six additional samples had detectable wild-type rotavirus but were unavailable for genotyping.

| Genotype | Classification of Genotype | Number of Samples (%) |
|---|---|---|
| G1P[8] | Common | 5 (13.5) |
| G2P[4] | Common | 11 (29.7) |
| G3P[8] | Common | 6 (16.2) |
| G4P[8] | Common | 1 (2.7) |
| G9P[8] | Common | 4 (10.8) |
| G12P[8] | Common | 3 (8.1) |
| G3P[4] | Uncommon | 3 (8.1) |
| G9P[4] | Uncommon | 1 (2.7) |
| G1/3 P[8] | Mixed | 1 (2.7) |
| G9/12 P[8] | Mixed | 1 (2.7) |
| G9 P untypable | Untypable | 1 (2.7) |
| Total |  | 37 (100) |

## 3. Discussion

This study describes the reduction in rotavirus detection following implementation of a national immunization program for all children in Ireland, as well as previously unknown data regarding the extent of genotype diversity during 2015–2019. Our study shows that the largest reduction in the detection of rotavirus occurred in those aged 0–12 months, where a relative decrease of 91% was achieved between 2015/16 and 2018/19. Although the vaccine status was unknown in detail, the effectiveness of the vaccination program has been clearly shown. Our results support the national data collated by the Health Protection Surveillance Centre (HPSC), where a crude incidence rate (CIR) of rotavirus for all age groups was 13.3 per 100,000 population in 2018, representing a decrease of 76%, compared to the mean CIR during 2008–2017 of 55.5 per 100,000 [5]. In addition, since the introduction of the vaccine, there was a reduction in visits to three large pediatric emergency departments with acute gastroenteritis, where median weekly presentations in 2017–2018 (126; interquartile range (IQR), 103–165) were lower than in 2012–2016 (160; IQR 128–214) ($p < 0.001$) [31]. Furthermore, an 86% (95% CI 79.3–90.2%) decrease in hospitalizations due to rotavirus has been reported nationally in those aged <1 year [32]. In our study, we found that the median age of wild-type rotavirus infection significantly increased in the years following vaccination, from 1.2 years in 2015 to 2.9 years in 2019 ($p < 0.0001$). This is consistent with the findings of other researchers, who also noted the later age of infection in the post-vaccine era [11,33]. In Ireland, vaccination uptake is recorded by individual General Practitioners and health care professionals which are submitted to the HPSC on a quarterly basis. Vaccine uptake data from Q1 2017 to Q3 2017 was unavailable, but the evidence suggests that this must have been suboptimal as there was little change in rotavirus detection in those aged 0–1 year in 2016 compared to 2017 (9.7% versus 7.5%, respectively). The substantial increase in rotavirus infection in the post-vaccine years in the 5–6-year age group who would not be eligible for the vaccine was also somewhat surprising. Although the number of children tested in this age group were lower in the post-vaccine compared to pre-vaccine years, the proportion of positives was almost double (6.2% versus 12.5%). The short timeframe is a limitation of this study; however, collection of data is ongoing, and it will be of interest to follow up on the impact of vaccination on rotavirus detection in all age groups in the post-vaccine era. A further finding in our data is a diminution of the characteristic rotavirus seasonal pattern, a phenomenon that has been noted by others following introduction of the rotavirus vaccine [17,34].

The live-attenuated vaccine Rotarix replicates in the gut of the recipient and is excreted, albeit at lower amounts compared to a wild-type infection [35]. We detected Rotarix in 10% of patients who were of vaccine-eligible age and, as rotavirus is notifiable in Ireland, this highlights the importance of differentiating between wild-type and vaccine-derived viruses, particularly when screening with a sensitive method, such as RT-PCR. By not excluding vaccine-derived rotavirus from diagnostic tests, there may be an over-estimation of rotavirus disease burden and unnecessary clinical intervention [36–38]. We identified 180 samples with detectable Rotarix, 20 (11%) of which had another virus detected, the most common being norovirus. We found norovirus to be the second most common pathogen detected after rotavirus in 2015/16, which then became the most common cause of viral gastroenteritis in our study group in the post-vaccine era. Our results are consistent with that observed in earlier studies, where norovirus is now the leading cause of viral gastroenteritis in those vaccinated for rotavirus [39–41]. Of note, sapovirus, astrovirus, and enteric adenovirus were detected in similar proportions over the 5-year time period and demonstrated no increase or decrease in detection rates following Rotarix introduction. Depending on the year, we report that 51–65% had no detectable viral pathogen. This apparent diagnostic gap highlights a further limitation of this study, in that it is quite possible that parallel samples were sent for the investigation of bacterial or parasitic pathogens, which are common causes of gastroenteritis [42,43]. Unfortunately, we did not have access to these results. In addition, other viruses, such as bocavirus, enterovirus, and parechoviruses, which may cause gastroenteritis, would not have been detected by our routine screening test.

Prior to the introduction of Rotarix, we found the circulating genotypes in Ireland were comparable to other European countries, with G1P[8] being the most commonly detected. The findings of the current study are consistent with those observed in several earlier reports from samples tested in Ireland from 1995 to 2009, where it was reported that the most commonly detected genotype was G1P[8], with fluctuating levels of G2P[4], G3P[8], G4P[8], and G9P[8] [44–49]. The current study matches those findings. However, we can report that the diversity of genotypes increased in the years following the introduction of a vaccine and that, in 2018/19, G1P[8] was no longer the most common genotype. Furthermore, genotypes detected in children eligible for the vaccine was more varied than those detected in the vaccine-ineligible cohort. With regards to wild-type and vaccine rotavirus strains, they can be described in terms of being homotypic, partly heterotypic, and fully heterotypic based on the G and P proteins. For instance, the monovalent G1P[8] Rotarix vaccine is homotypic to other circulating G1P[8] strains (both proteins are the same), G12P[8] is partly heterotypic (one protein different), and G2P[4] is fully heterotypic (both G and P proteins are different) [50]. Rotarix provides exposure to G1P[8] rotavirus among infants, with protection that is likely to be higher against homotypic strains than heterotypic strains, such as G2P[4]. This suggests that natural infection leading to disease is more likely to be caused by such heterotypic strains [19,51] and that a vaccinated population could possibly drive selective pressure, increasing the likelihood of these genotypes to circulate in the community [52,53]. That being said, the monovalent vaccine Rotarix provides significant protection from G1, G2, G3, G4, and G9, and efficacy against severe G2 rotavirus gastroenteritis was as high as for other rotavirus types [54]. Clearly, the immune response to rotavirus infection is a complex issue, with a previous report suggesting that type-specific neutralizing antibodies induced by the vaccine against VP7/VP4 epitopes are not solely responsible for a protective effect [55]. The report proposes that, as there are a limited number of diverse circulating strains worldwide, these antibodies are not driving long-term selective pressure, which itself would favor antigenic drift or the emergence of novel genotypes.

Interestingly, the genotype G12P[8] was not circulating widely at the time of Rotarix and RotaTeq vaccine development; however, it has now become established as an increasingly common genotype [17]. A large study in the USA found G12P[8] more frequently than any other rotavirus genotype in fully vaccinated children [56]. Another example of an uncommon genotype becoming more prevalent is the recently emerged equine-like G3 strain, first identified in Japan in 2013 [57] but now detected world-wide [58–60]. We identified, for the first time in Ireland, two samples from 2018 that clustered within the equine-like G3 lineage. A further 15 G3 samples were sequenced and all clustered in the human lineage, suggesting that the equine-like lineage has not yet become established in Ireland compared to other countries [59,61]. Of note, five of the uncommon human G3P[4] strains were also identified in our study in 2018–2019, and this strain has been detected before in Ireland in 2006/07 [48]. The detection of uncommon genotypes, along with the additional potential for zoonotic reassortment [62,63], reinforces the WHO recommendation for surveillance, emphasising the need for continued monitoring of rotavirus vaccine efficacy against emerging rotavirus.

Several important limitations need to be considered for our study group. Firstly, the results are somewhat biased due to the observational nature of the study and samples tested would have been from those with moderate to severe gastroenteritis that warranted clinical investigation. In addition, there was no denominator for the population not suffering from symptoms of viral gastroenteritis, so we are unable to calculate incidence and prevalence of rotavirus infection. Furthermore, with no access to vaccination data, it was not possible to determine vaccine effectiveness rates or describe definitive vaccine failures. However, due to the large data set (n = 11,800), we can show relative reductions in the detection of rotavirus and the changes in the diversity of circulating genotypes. The geographical distribution of samples is nationwide, although the data are skewed to some extent due to the density of the population in Dublin and the location of the main children's hospitals, and therefore samples were predominantly from the eastern health region. It should also be noted that the number of samples tested has decreased year on year. The reason for this may be the decrease in symptomatic children or the increase in localized testing and possible availability of point of care assays. Finally, it was not possible to categorize samples as the community or hospital acquired and we could not identify samples belonging to outbreaks.

We have shown that rotavirus continues to circulate in the pediatric population, albeit in low numbers, and this is expected to decrease further with the increasing cohort of vaccinated children. Binary genotypic classification is useful to establish circulating genotypes and can be used for reassortment studies of the VP7 and VP4 encoding genes; however, whole genome genotyping is required for a more detailed analysis of the virus. Indeed, a future aim from this ongoing study is to perform whole genome sequencing from samples in this dataset to allow identification of possible reassortment of non VP7/VP4 genes or mutation events. In addition, all samples identified as G3 will be categorized as either equine-like or of human lineage. By collaborating with clinicians at the children's hospitals, it is hoped that any sample from a child with rotavirus with a full or partial vaccine history will be referred to the NVRL for whole genome sequencing to establish definitive strains circulating in this group of children.

In conclusion, we describe the detection and characterization of rotavirus in pediatric samples circulating in Ireland over a 5-year time period. We show that, following the introduction of Rotarix, there is a relative reduction in the number of rotavirus infections diagnosed, coinciding with an increase in genotype diversity, along with the first recorded detection of an equine-like G3 strain in Ireland.

## 4. Materials and Methods

### 4.1. Study Design

This opportunistic study presents the results of faecal samples from pediatric samples (≤5 years) investigated for viral gastroenteritis at the National Virus Reference Laboratory (NVRL), Dublin, Ireland. Test results for wild-type rotavirus, vaccine-derived rotavirus (Rotarix), norovirus, sapovirus, astrovirus, and enteric adenovirus subgenus F were obtained with genotype and sequence results, if available. Samples dated 1 January 2015 to 31 December 2019 were included in the study. Samples dated 1 January 2015 to 31 December 2016 were designated as "pre-vaccine". The first doses of Rotarix were given for those aged 2 months from the 1 December 2016. Only one sample was received from a 2-month old in December 2016, and this patient had detectable Rotarix. Samples dated 1 January 2017 to 31 December 2019 were designated as "post-vaccine". Routine testing for Rotarix was introduced into the NVRL from 11 December 2017. Rotavirus-positive samples received from 1 December 2016 to 10 December 2017 were tested for Rotarix, retrospectively.

*4.2. Annual Birth Cohort in Ireland*

The Central Office of Statistics provides the annual number of births in Ireland [64]. The number of annual births by year are: 2015: 65,536 (33,480 males, 32,056 females); 2016: 63,841 (32,709 males, 31,132 females); 2017: 61,824 (31,779 males, 30,045 females); 2018: 61,016 (31,298 males, 29,718 females); 2019: 59,796 (30,555 males, 29,241 females,). Data for 2018 and 2019 are provisional. The overall male: female ratio for 2015–2019 was 1.1: 1 (51.2% versus 48.8%).

*4.3. Data Analysis*

Data were extracted from the NVRL Laboratory Information Management System and analyzed in Excel. All samples were assumed to be from symptomatic patients. Samples with no date of birth recorded or duplicate samples were excluded from the study. Patients were de-identified, and the variables recorded in the database were patients' age at sample collection, sex, sample date, geographical region, and test result(s). Geographical regions were categorized as eastern (which includes Dublin), western, southern (south and south-east), northern (north-west and north-east), and midlands (midlands and mid-west), as defined by the Health Service Executive areas used by the Health Protection Surveillance Centre [5].

*4.4. Sampling Strategy for Genotyping and Sequencing of Samples*

To determine the sample size required to reliably detect a change in genotype frequency, a sample size calculator was used (CL95%, www.openepi.com), and then a random selection of wild-type rotavirus samples was selected for genotyping. In addition, all uncommon genotypes and a random subset of genotyped samples was selected for sequencing of VP7 and VP4 genes. A subset of those identified as G3 and were sequenced and analyzed to determine a human or equine-like lineage.

*4.5. Seasonality*

Seasonal onset, peak, and end were calculated: Onset: First of 2 consecutive weeks, where the median percentage of positive results was >10%. Peak: Week with the highest proportion of positive samples. End: Last of two consecutive weeks, where the median percentage was <10%. Denominator: total samples tested; numerator: the number of positive samples.

*4.6. Vaccine Eligibility*

The vaccine status was unknown, and patients were categorised by vaccine eligibility. Vaccine-eligible samples were those born after 1 October 2016 and were ≥2 months of age. Vaccine-ineligible samples were those born after 1 October 2016 and were <2 months of age or were born prior to 1 October 2016 and were aged 0–5 years of age.

*4.7. Laboratory Methods*

Upon receipt into the laboratory, approximately 20% $w/v$ suspension of the fecal sample was prepared in 400 µL Stool Transport and Recovery Buffer (Roche) and 400 µL external lysis buffer (Roche). A total of 450 µL of the suspension was extracted by Roche MagNAPure 96 and eluted into 100 µL. During extraction, Brome Mosaic Virus RNA (University of Indiana) was added as an internal control (IC) at 1 pg/µL to the sample prior to extraction. The eluates were tested in five one-step RT-PCR assays, as previously described [65–70]. Briefly, eluates were tested in a 25 µL or 10 µL reaction mixture (depending on the 96- or 384-well format, respectively), containing 2× Superscript™ III Platinum One-Step qRT-PCR mix (Invitrogen), as per product insert. Final concentrations of primers and probes ranged from 80 nM to 400 nM, depending on the target. Each sample eluate was tested by five (RT-)PCR reactions, namely: (i) norovirus G1/G2/IC; (ii) adenovirus F/pan-rotavirus/IC; (iii) Rotarix; iv) astrovirus/IC; v) sapovirus/IC. Amplification was performed on the ABI 7500 Fast (96-well format) or the ABI Viia7 (384-well format) instrument under the following conditions: 15 mins 50 °C, 2 mins 95 °C,

38 cycles of 15 secs 95 and 30 secs 60 °C (56 °C for norovirus). Amplification data was collected and analyzed with Sequence Detection Software version 2.3 or the Viia7 software version 1.2.1 (both from Applied Biosystems).

Genotyping was either by a multiplex RT-PCR [71,72] or by hemi-nested RT-PCR, as described previously [73], with fragment visualization and size determination performed on the TapeStation (Agilent software, version 2200). Samples with an indeterminate G or P type were tested by both methods before being categorized as untypable. A selection of genotypes were confirmed by Sanger sequencing of the VP7 and VP4 genes, using previously described methods [73] on the ABI 3500Dx genetic analyzer (Applied Biosystems) and typed using the RotaC typing tool [74] or by the Basic Local Alignment and Search Tool, BLAST (http://www.ncbi.nlm.nih.gov/blast/Blast.cgi). G3 VP7 sequences (450 nucleotides) were aligned with appropriate reference sequences using ClustalW. Phylogenetic analyses were conducted in MEGA X [30] using the maximum likelihood method, with 1000 bootstrap replicates, based on the Tamura-Nei model [29]. This model was selected as it generated the lowest Bayesian information criterion (BIC) score in MEGA X.

*4.8. GenBank Accession Numbers*

Partial VP7 fragments of the equine-like G3 strains identified in this study were deposited in GenBank under the following accession numbers: strains; MT475885 and MT4758866, whereas the human-lineage G3 VP7 fragments were MT537569-537583.

*4.9. Statistical Analysis*

The study was observational and therefore most data presented was descriptive. The median age of rotavirus infection in the pre- and post-vaccination groups was compared using Mann–Whitney $U$ test. The Chi-square test for proportions was used to compare genotypes in the pre- and post-vaccination groups. $P$ values for both tests of ≤0.05 were considered statistically significant. Confidence intervals (95%) were calculated using the Wilson method for a proportion of the genotypes detected. Statistical analysis was performed using SPSS 26 (IBM Corp; Armonk, NY, USA) software or www.openepi.com.

*4.10. Ethical Statement*

All procedures performed in studies involving human participants were in accordance with the ethical standards of the institutional and/or research committee and with the 1964 Helsinki declaration and its later amendments or comparable standards. This study was approved for ethical exemption by University College, Dublin LS-E-17-09.

**Author Contributions:** Conceptualization, Z.Y., S.C., and C.F.D.G.; data curation, S.C.; formal analysis, Z.Y.; investigation, Z.Y. and S.C.; methodology, Z.Y., S.C., and C.F.D.G.; project administration, Z.Y. and S.C.; resources, Z.Y., G.T., A.C., and C.F.D.G.; supervision, S.C. and C.F.D.G.; validation, Z.Y., S.C., and C.F.D.G.; visualization, Z.Y., S.C., and C.F.D.G.; writing—original draft, Z.Y.; Writing—review and editing, Z.Y., S.C., J.D., G.T., and C.F.D.G. All authors have read and agreed to the published version of the manuscript.

**Acknowledgments:** The authors would like to thank all clinicians and general practitioners for referring samples to the National Virus Reference Laboratory, Dublin, and to acknowledge the hard work of all the laboratory staff for processing and testing samples for the gastroenteritis screen.

**References**

1. Hungerford, D.; Smith, K.; Tucker, A.; Iturriza-Gomara, M.; Vivancos, R.; McLeonard, C.; N, A.C.; French, N. Population effectiveness of the pentavalent and monovalent rotavirus vaccines: A systematic review and meta-analysis of observational studies. *BMC Infect. Dis.* **2017**, *17*, 569. [CrossRef] [PubMed]
2. Troeger, C.; Blacker, B.; Khalil, I. Estimates of the global, regional, and national morbidity, mortality, and aetiologies of diarrhoea in 195 countries: A systematic analysis for the Global Burden of Disease Study 2016. *Lancet. Infect. Dis.* **2018**, *18*, 1211–1228. [CrossRef]

3. Burnett, E.; Parashar, U.D.; Tate, J.E. Global impact of rotavirus vaccination on diarrhea hospitalizations and deaths among children < 5 years old: 2006–2019. *J. Infect. Dis.* **2020**. [CrossRef] [PubMed]
4. European Centre for Disease Prevention and Control. *ECDC Report: Expert Opinion on Rotavirus Vaccination in Infancy*; ECDC: Stockholm, Sweden, 2017.
5. HSE Health Protection Surveillance Centre. *Rotavirus 2018 Annual Epidemiological Report*; HSE HPSC: Dublin, Ireland, 2019.
6. Lynch, M.; O'Halloran, F.; Whyte, D.; Fanning, S.; Cryan, B.; Glass, R.I. Rotavirus in Ireland: National estimates of disease burden, 1997 to 1998. *Pediatric Infect. Dis. J.* **2001**, *20*, 693–698. [CrossRef]
7. World Health Organization. Global Advisory Committee on Vaccine Safety, report of meeting held 17–18 June 2009. *Wkly. Epidemiol. Rec.* **2009**, *84*, 213–236.
8. Poelaert, D.; Pereira, P.; Gardner, R.; Standaert, B.; Benninghoff, B. A review of recommendations for rotavirus vaccination in Europe: Arguments for change. *Vaccine* **2018**, *36*, 2243–2253. [CrossRef]
9. Health Protection Surveillance Centre. Available online: https://www.hpsc.ie/az/vaccinepreventable/vaccination/immunisationuptakestatistics/immunisationuptakestatisticsat12and24monthsofage/ (accessed on 10 March 2020).
10. Walker, J.L.; Andrews, N.J.; Atchison, C.J.; Collins, S.; Allen, D.J.; Ramsay, M.E.; Ladhani, S.N.; Thomas, S.L. Effectiveness of oral rotavirus vaccination in England against rotavirus-confirmed and all-cause acute gastroenteritis. *Vaccine: X* **2019**, *1*, 100005. [CrossRef]
11. Pietsch, C.; Liebert, U.G. Rotavirus vaccine effectiveness in preventing hospitalizations due to gastroenteritis: A descriptive epidemiological study from Germany. *Clin. Microbiol. Infect.* **2019**, *25*, 102–106. [CrossRef]
12. Braeckman, T.; Van Herck, K.; Meyer, N.; Pircon, J.Y.; Soriano-Gabarro, M.; Heylen, E.; Zeller, M.; Azou, M.; Capiau, H.; De Koster, J.; et al. Effectiveness of rotavirus vaccination in prevention of hospital admissions for rotavirus gastroenteritis among young children in Belgium: Case-control study. *BMJ* **2012**, *345*, e4752. [CrossRef]
13. Matthijnssens, J.; Otto, P.H.; Ciarlet, M.; Desselberger, U.; Van Ranst, M.; Johne, R. VP6-sequence-based cutoff values as a criterion for rotavirus species demarcation. *Arch. Virol.* **2012**, *157*, 1177–1182. [CrossRef]
14. Mihalov-Kovács, E.; Gellért, Á.; Marton, S.; Farkas, S.L.; Fehér, E.; Oldal, M.; Jakab, F.; Martella, V.; Bányai, K. Candidate new rotavirus species in sheltered dogs, Hungary. *Emerg. Infect. Dis.* **2015**, *21*, 660–663. [CrossRef] [PubMed]
15. Bányai, K.; Kemenesi, G.; Budinski, I.; Földes, F.; Zana, B.; Marton, S.; Varga-Kugler, R.; Oldal, M.; Kurucz, K.; Jakab, F. Candidate new rotavirus species in Schreiber's bats, Serbia. *Infect. Genet. Evol.* **2017**, *48*, 19–26. [CrossRef] [PubMed]
16. Matthijnssens, J.; Ciarlet, M.; Heiman, E.; Arijs, I.; Delbeke, T.; McDonald, S.M. Full genome-based classification of rotaviruses reveals a common origin between human Wa-Like and porcine rotavirus strains and human DS-1-like and bovine rotavirus strains. *J. Virol.* **2008**, *82*. [CrossRef] [PubMed]
17. Hungerford, D.; Vivancos, R.; EuroRotaNet Network Members. In-season and out-of-season variation of rotavirus genotype distribution and age of infection across 12 European countries before the introduction of routine vaccination, 2007/08 to 2012/13. *Eurosurveillance* **2016**, *21*. [CrossRef] [PubMed]
18. Roczo-Farkas, S.; Kirkwood, C.D.; Cowley, D.; Barnes, G.L.; Bishop, R.F.; Bogdanovic-Sakran, N.; Boniface, K.; Donato, C.M.; Bines, J.E. The Impact of Rotavirus Vaccines on Genotype Diversity: A Comprehensive Analysis of 2 Decades of Australian Surveillance Data. *J. Infect. Dis.* **2018**, *218*, 546–554. [CrossRef] [PubMed]
19. Hungerford, D.; Allen, D.J.; Nawaz, S.; Collins, S.; Ladhani, S.; Vivancos, R.; Iturriza-Gomara, M. Impact of rotavirus vaccination on rotavirus genotype distribution and diversity in England, September 2006 to August 2016. *Eurosurveillance* **2019**, *24*, 1700774. [CrossRef]
20. Zeller, M.; Rahman, M.; Heylen, E.; De Coster, S.; De Vos, S.; Arijs, I.; Novo, L.; Verstappen, N.; Van Ranst, M.; Matthijnssens, J. Rotavirus incidence and genotype distribution before and after national rotavirus vaccine introduction in Belgium. *Vaccine* **2010**, *28*, 7507–7513. [CrossRef]
21. Markkula, J.; Hemming-Harlo, M.; Salminen, M.T.; Savolainen-Kopra, C.; Pirhonen, J.; Al-Hello, H.; Vesikari, T. Rotavirus epidemiology 5–6 years after universal rotavirus vaccination: Persistent rotavirus activity in older children and elderly. *Infect. Dis.* **2017**, *49*, 388–395. [CrossRef]
22. Kaplon, J.; Grangier, N.; Pillet, S.; Minoui-Tran, A.; Vabret, A.; Wilhelm, N.; Prieur, N.; Lazrek, M.; Alain, S.; Mekki, Y.; et al. Predominance of G9P[8] rotavirus strains throughout France, 2014–2017. *Clin. Microbiol. Infect.* **2018**, *24*, 660.e661–660.e664. [CrossRef]

23. Verberk, J.D.M.; Bruijning-Verhagen, P.; Melker, H.E. Rotavirus in the Netherlands: Background information for the Health Council. *RIVM* 2017. [CrossRef]
24. Matthijnssens, J.; Nakagomi, O.; Kirkwood, C.D.; Ciarlet, M.; Desselberger, U.; Ranst, M.V. Group A rotavirus universal mass vaccination: How and to what extent will selective pressure influence prevalence of rotavirus genotypes? *Expert Rev. Vaccines* 2012, *11*, 1347–1354. [CrossRef] [PubMed]
25. Matthijnssens, J.; Bilcke, J.; Ciarlet, M.; Martella, V.; Bányai, K.; Rahman, M.; Zeller, M.; Beutels, P.; Van Damme, P.; Van Ranst, M. Rotavirus disease and vaccination: Impact on genotype diversity. *Future Microbiol.* 2009, *4*, 1303–1316. [CrossRef] [PubMed]
26. World Health Organization. Available online: https://www.who.int/immunization/monitoring_surveillance/burden/estimates/rotavirus/Rota_virus_Q5_mortality_estimates_external_review_report_2006_may.pdf?ua=1 (accessed on 20 January 2020).
27. Iturriza-Gomara, M.; Dallman, T.; Banyai, K.; Bottiger, B.; Buesa, J.; Diedrich, S.; Fiore, L.; Johansen, K.; Koopmans, M.; Korsun, N.; et al. Rotavirus genotypes co-circulating in Europe between 2006 and 2009 as determined by EuroRotaNet, a pan-European collaborative strain surveillance network. *Epidemiol. Infect.* 2011, *139*, 895–909. [CrossRef] [PubMed]
28. Central Statistics Office. Available online: https://www.cso.ie/en/statistics/population (accessed on 8 May 2020).
29. Tamura, K.; Nei, M. Estimation of the number of nucleotide substitutions in the control region of mitochondrial DNA in humans and chimpanzees. *Mol. Biol. Evol.* 1993, *10*, 512–526. [CrossRef]
30. Kumar, S.; Stecher, G.; Li, M.; Knyaz, C.; Tamura, K. MEGA X: Molecular Evolutionary Genetics Analysis across Computing Platforms. *Mol. Biol. Evol.* 2018, *35*, 1547–1549. [CrossRef]
31. Coveney, J.; Barrett, M.; Fitzpatrick, P.; Kandamany, N.; McNamara, R.; Koe, S.; Okafor, I. National rotavirus vaccination programme implementation and gastroenteritis presentations: The paediatric emergency medicine perspective. *Ir. J. Med Sci.* 2019, *189*, 327–332. [CrossRef]
32. Burns, H.E.; Collins, A.M.; Fallon, U.B.; Marsden, P.V.; Ni Shuilleabhain, C.M. Rotavirus vaccination impact, Ireland, implications for vaccine confidence and screening. *Eur. J. Public Health* 2020, 281–285. [CrossRef]
33. Shim, J.O.; Chang, J.Y.; Shin, S.; Moon, J.S.; Ko, J.S. Changing distribution of age, clinical severity, and genotypes of rotavirus gastroenteritis in hospitalized children after the introduction of vaccination: A single center study in Seoul between 2011 and 2014. *BMC Infect. Dis.* 2016, *16*, 287. [CrossRef]
34. Tate, J.E.; Panozzo, C.A.; Payne, D.C.; Patel, M.M.; Cortese, M.M.; Fowlkes, A.L.; Parashar, U.D. Decline and change in seasonality of US rotavirus activity after the introduction of rotavirus vaccine. *Pediatrics* 2009, *124*, 465–471. [CrossRef]
35. Yandle, Z.; Coughlan, S.; Drew, R.J.; Cleary, J.; De Gascun, C. Diagnosis of rotavirus infection in a vaccinated population: Is a less sensitive immunochromatographic method more suitable for detecting wild-type rotavirus than real-time RT-PCR? *J. Clin. Virol.* 2018, *109*, 19–21. [CrossRef]
36. Gower, C.M.; Dunning, J.; Nawaz, S.; Allen, D.; Ramsay, M.E.; Ladhani, S. Vaccine-derived rotavirus strains in infants in England. *Arch. Dis. Child.* 2019, *105*, 1–5. [CrossRef] [PubMed]
37. Whiley, D.M.; Ye, S.; Tozer, S.; Clark, J.E.; Bletchly, C.; Lambert, S.B.; Grimwood, K.; Nimmo, G.R. Over-diagnosis of rotavirus infection in infants due to detection of vaccine virus. *Clin. Infect. Dis.* 2019, ciz1196. [CrossRef] [PubMed]
38. McAuliffe, G.N.; Taylor, S.L.; Moore, S.; Hewitt, J.; Upton, A.; Howe, A.S.; Best, E.J. Suboptimal performance of rotavirus testing in a vaccinated community population should prompt laboratories to review their rotavirus testing algorithms in response to changes in disease prevalence. *Diagn. Microbiol. Infect. Dis.* 2019, *93*, 203–207. [CrossRef] [PubMed]
39. Hemming, M.; Räsänen, S.; Huhti, L.; Paloniemi, M.; Salminen, M.; Vesikari, T. Major reduction of rotavirus, but not norovirus, gastroenteritis in children seen in hospital after the introduction of RotaTeq vaccine into the National Immunization Programme in Finland. *Eur. J. Pediatr.* 2013, *172*, 739–746. [CrossRef]
40. Bucardo, F.; Reyes, Y.; Svensson, L.; Nordgren, J. Predominance of norovirus and sapovirus in Nicaragua after implementation of universal rotavirus vaccination. *PLoS ONE* 2014, *9*, e98201. [CrossRef]
41. Koo, H.L.; Neill, F.H.; Estes, M.K.; Munoz, F.M.; Cameron, A.; DuPont, H.L.; Atmar, R.L. Noroviruses: The Most Common Pediatric Viral Enteric Pathogen at a Large University Hospital After Introduction of Rotavirus Vaccination. *J. Pediatric Infect. Dis. Soc.* 2013, *2*, 57–60. [CrossRef]

42. Steyer, A.; Jevšnik, M.; Petrovec, M.; Pokorn, M.; Grosek, Š.; Fratnik Steyer, A.; Šoba, B.; Uršič, T.; Cerar Kišek, T.; Kolenc, M.; et al. Narrowing of the Diagnostic Gap of Acute Gastroenteritis in Children 0–6 Years of Age Using a Combination of Classical and Molecular Techniques, Delivers Challenges in Syndromic Approach Diagnostics. *Pediatric Infect. Dis. J.* **2016**, *35*, e262–e270. [CrossRef]
43. Donaldson, A.L.; Clough, H.E.; O'Brien, S.J.; Harris, J.P. Symptom profiling for infectious intestinal disease (IID): A secondary data analysis of the IID2 study. *Epidemiol. Infect.* **2019**, *147*, e229. [CrossRef]
44. O'Mahony, J.; Foley, B.; Morgan, S.; Morgan, J.G.; Hill, C. VP4 and VP7 genotyping of rotavirus samples recovered from infected children in Ireland over a 3-year period. *J. Clin. Microbiol.* **1999**, *37*, 1699–1703. [CrossRef]
45. O'Halloran, F.; Lynch, M.; Cryan, B.; O'Shea, H.; Fanning, S. Molecular characterization of rotavirus in Ireland: Detection of novel strains circulating in the population. *J. Clin. Microbiol.* **2000**, *38*, 3370–3374. [CrossRef]
46. Reidy, N.; O'Halloran, F.; Fanning, S.; Cryan, B.; O'Shea, H. Emergence of G3 and G9 rotavirus and increased incidence of mixed infections in the southern region of Ireland 2001–2004. *J. Med Virol.* **2005**, *77*, 571–578. [CrossRef] [PubMed]
47. Lennon, G.; Reidy, N.; Cryan, B.; Fanning, S.; O'Shea, H. Changing profile of rotavirus in Ireland: Predominance of P[8] and emergence of P[6] and P[9] in mixed infections. *J. Med Virol.* **2008**, *80*, 524–530. [CrossRef] [PubMed]
48. Collins, P.J.; Mulherin, E.; O'Shea, H.; Cashman, O.; Lennon, G.; Pidgeon, E.; Coughlan, S.; Hall, W.; Fanning, S. Changing patterns of rotavirus strains circulating in Ireland: Re-emergence of G2P[4] and identification of novel genotypes in Ireland. *J. Med Virol.* **2015**, *87*, 764–773. [CrossRef] [PubMed]
49. Cashman, O.; Collins, P.J.; Lennon, G.; Cryan, B.; Martella, V.; Fanning, S.; Staines, A.; O'Shea, H. Molecular characterization of group A rotaviruses detected in children with gastroenteritis in Ireland in 2006-2009. *Epidemiol. Infect.* **2012**, *140*, 247–259. [CrossRef]
50. Bernstein, D.I. Rotavirus Vaccines: Mind Your Ps and Gs. *J. Infect. Dis.* **2018**, *218*, 519–521. [CrossRef]
51. Matthijnssens, J.; Zeller, M.; Heylen, E.; De Coster, S.; Vercauteren, J.; Braeckman, T.; Van Herck, K.; Meyer, N.; Pirçon, J.Y.; Soriano-Gabarro, M.; et al. Higher proportion of G2P[4] rotaviruses in vaccinated hospitalized cases compared with unvaccinated hospitalized cases, despite high vaccine effectiveness against heterotypic G2P[4] rotaviruses. *Clin. Microbiol. Infect.* **2014**, *20*, O702–O710. [CrossRef]
52. Pitzer, V.E.; Bilcke, J.; Heylen, E.; Crawford, F.W.; Callens, M.; De Smet, F.; Van Ranst, M.; Zeller, M.; Matthijnssens, J. Did Large-Scale Vaccination Drive Changes in the Circulating Rotavirus Population in Belgium? *Sci. Rep.* **2015**, *5*, 18585. [CrossRef]
53. Zeller, M.; Donato, C.; Trovão, N.S.; Cowley, D.; Heylen, E.; Donker, N.C.; McAllen, J.K.; Akopov, A.; Kirkness, E.F.; Lemey, P.; et al. Genome-Wide Evolutionary Analyses of G1P[8] Strains Isolated Before and After Rotavirus Vaccine Introduction. *Genome Biol. Evol.* **2015**, *7*, 2473–2483. [CrossRef]
54. Vesikari, T.; Karvonen, A.; Prymula, R.; Schuster, V.; Tejedor, J.C.; Cohen, R.; Meurice, F.; Han, H.H.; Damaso, S.; Bouckenooghe, A. Efficacy of human rotavirus vaccine against rotavirus gastroenteritis during the first 2 years of life in European infants: Randomised, double-blind controlled study. *Lancet* **2007**, *370*, 1757–1763. [CrossRef]
55. Clarke, E.; Desselberger, U. Correlates of protection against human rotavirus disease and the factors influencing protection in low-income settings. *Mucosal Immunol.* **2015**, *8*, 1–17. [CrossRef]
56. Ogden, K.M.; Tan, Y.; Akopov, A.; Stewart, L.S.; McHenry, R.; Fonnesbeck, C.J.; Piya, B.; Carter, M.H.; Fedorova, N.B.; Halpin, R.A.; et al. Multiple introductions and antigenic mismatch with vaccines may contribute to increased predominance of G12P[8] rotaviruses in the United States. *J. Virol.* **2018**. [CrossRef] [PubMed]
57. Malasao, R.; Saito, M.; Suzuki, A.; Imagawa, T.; Nukiwa-Soma, N.; Tohma, K.; Liu, X.; Okamoto, M.; Chaimongkol, N.; Dapat, C.; et al. Human G3P[4] rotavirus obtained in Japan, 2013, possibly emerged through a human-equine rotavirus reassortment event. *Virus Genes* **2015**, *50*, 129–133. [CrossRef] [PubMed]
58. Esposito, S.; Camilloni, B.; Bianchini, S.; Ianiro, G.; Polinori, I.; Farinelli, E.; Monini, M.; Principi, N. First detection of a reassortant G3P[8] rotavirus A strain in Italy: A case report in an 8-year-old child. *Virol. J.* **2019**, *16*, 64. [CrossRef] [PubMed]
59. Tacharoenmuang, R.; Komoto, S.; Guntapong, R.; Upachai, S.; Singchai, P.; Ide, T.; Fukuda, S.; Ruchusatsawast, K.; Sriwantana, B.; Tatsumi, M.; et al. High prevalence of equine-like G3P[8] rotavirus in children and adults with acute gastroenteritis in Thailand. *J. Med Virol.* **2020**, *92*, 174–186. [CrossRef]

60. Pietsch, C.; Liebert, U.G. Molecular characterization of different equine-like G3 rotavirus strains from Germany. *Infect. Genet. Evol.* **2018**, *57*, 46–50. [CrossRef]
61. Cowley, D.; Donato, C.M.; Roczo-Farkas, S.; Kirkwood, C.D. Emergence of a novel equine-like G3P[8] inter-genogroup reassortant rotavirus strain associated with gastroenteritis in Australian children. *J. Gen. Virol.* **2016**, *97*, 403–410. [CrossRef]
62. Kumar, N.; Malik, Y.S.; Sharma, K.; Dhama, K.; Ghosh, S.; Banyai, K.; Kobayashi, N.; Singh, R.K. Molecular characterization of unusual bovine rotavirus A strains having high genetic relatedness with human rotavirus: Evidence for zooanthroponotic transmission. *Zoonoses Public Health* **2018**, *65*, 431–442. [CrossRef]
63. Tamim, S.; Matthijnssens, J.; Heylen, E.; Zeller, M.; Van Ranst, M.; Salman, M.; Hasan, F. Evidence of zoonotic transmission of VP6 and NSP4 genes into human species A rotaviruses isolated in Pakistan in 2010. *Arch. Virol.* **2019**, *164*, 1781–1791. [CrossRef]
64. Central Statistics Office. Available online: https://www.cso.ie/en/statistics/birthsdeathsandmarriages (accessed on 30 May 2020).
65. Gautam, R.; Esona, M.D.; Mijatovic-Rustempasic, S.; Ian Tam, K.; Gentsch, J.R.; Bowen, M.D. Real-time RT-PCR assays to differentiate wild-type group A rotavirus strains from Rotarix(®) and RotaTeq(®) vaccine strains in stool samples. *Hum. Vaccines Immunother.* **2014**, *10*, 767–777. [CrossRef]
66. Kageyama, T.; Kojima, S.; Shinohara, M.; Uchida, K.; Fukushi, S.; Hoshino, F.B.; Takeda, N.; Katayama, K. Broadly reactive and highly sensitive assay for Norwalk-like viruses based on real-time quantitative reverse transcription-PCR. *J. Clin. Microbiol.* **2003**, *41*, 1548–1557. [CrossRef]
67. Tiemessen, C.T.; Nel, M.J. Detection and typing of subgroup F adenoviruses using the polymerase chain reaction. *J. Virol. Methods* **1996**, *59*, 73–82. [CrossRef]
68. Oka, T.; Katayama, K.; Hansman, G.S.; Kageyama, T.; Ogawa, S.; Wu, F.T.; White, P.A.; Takeda, N. Detection of human sapovirus by real-time reverse transcription-polymerase chain reaction. *J. Med. Virol.* **2006**, *78*, 1347–1353. [CrossRef] [PubMed]
69. Logan, C.; O'Leary, J.J.; O'Sullivan, N. Real-time reverse transcription PCR detection of norovirus, sapovirus and astrovirus as causative agents of acute viral gastroenteritis. *J. Virol. Methods* **2007**, *146*, 36–44. [CrossRef] [PubMed]
70. Freeman, M.M.; Kerin, T.; Hull, J.; McCaustland, K.; Gentsch, J. Enhancement of detection and quantification of rotavirus in stool using a modified real-time RT-PCR assay. *J. Med Virol.* **2008**, *80*, 1489–1496. [CrossRef] [PubMed]
71. Gautam, R.; Mijatovic-Rustempasic, S.; Esona, M.D.; Tam, K.I.; Quaye, O.; Bowen, M.D. One-step multiplex real-time RT-PCR assay for detecting and genotyping wild-type group A rotavirus strains and vaccine strains (Rotarix(R) and RotaTeq(R)) in stool samples. *PeerJ* **2016**, *4*, e1560. [CrossRef] [PubMed]
72. Andersson, M.; Lindh, M. Rotavirus genotype shifts among Swedish children and adults-Application of a real-time PCR genotyping. *J. Clin. Virol.* **2017**, *96*, 1–6. [CrossRef]
73. World Health Organization. Method 16: G and P genotyping. In *Manual of Rotavirus Detection and Characterization Methods*; WHO/IVB/08.17; WHO: Geneva, Switzerland, 2009; pp. 91–98.
74. Maes, P.; Matthijnssens, J.; Rahman, M.; Van Ranst, M. RotaC. A web based tool for the complete genome classification of group A rotaviruses. *BMC Microbiol.* **2009**, *9*, 238. [CrossRef]

# Molecular Characterisation of a Rare Reassortant Porcine-Like G5P[6] Rotavirus Strain Detected in an Unvaccinated Child in Kasama, Zambia

Wairimu M. Maringa [1], Peter N. Mwangi [1], Julia Simwaka [2], Evans M. Mpabalwani [3], Jason M. Mwenda [4], Ina Peenze [5], Mathew D. Esona [5], M. Jeffrey Mphahlele [5,6], Mapaseka L. Seheri [5] and Martin M. Nyaga [1,*]

[1] Next Generation Sequencing Unit, Division of Virology, Faculty of Health Sciences, University of the Free State, Bloemfontein 9300, South Africa; makena96wairimu@gmail.com (W.M.M.); nthigapete@gmail.com (P.N.M.)
[2] Virology Laboratory, Department of Pathology & Microbiology, University Teaching Hospital, Adult and Emergency Hospital, Lusaka 10101, Zambia; juliachibumbya@gmail.com
[3] Department of Paediatrics & Child Health, School of Medicine, University of Zambia, Ridgeway, Lusaka RW50000, Zambia; evans.mpabalwani@unza.zm
[4] World Health Organization, Regional Office for Africa, Brazzaville P.O. Box 06, Congo; mwendaj@who.int
[5] Diarrhoeal Pathogens Research Unit, Faculty of Health Sciences, Sefako Makgatho Health Sciences University, Medunsa, Pretoria 0204, South Africa; ina.peenze@smu.ac.za (I.P.); mathew.esona@gmail.com (M.D.E.); Jeffrey.Mphahlele@mrc.ac.za (M.J.M.); mapaseka.seheri@smu.ac.za (M.L.S.)
[6] South African Medical Research Council, 1 Soutpansberg Road, Pretoria 0001, South Africa
* Correspondence: NyagaMM@ufs.ac.za;

**Abstract:** A human-porcine reassortant strain, RVA/Human-wt/ZMB/UFS-NGS-MRC-DPRU4723/2014/G5P[6], was identified in a sample collected in 2014 from an unvaccinated 12 month old male hospitalised for gastroenteritis in Zambia. We sequenced and characterised the complete genome of this strain which presented the constellation: G5-P[6]-I1-R1-C1-M1-A8-N1-T1-E1-H1. The genotype A8 is often observed in porcine strains. Phylogenetic analyses showed that VP6, VP7, NSP2, NSP4, and NSP5 genes were closely related to cognate gene sequences of porcine strains (e.g., RVA/Pig-wt/CHN/DZ-2/2013/G5P[X] for VP7) from the NCBI database, while VP1, VP3, VP4, and NSP3 were closely related to porcine-like human strains (e.g., RVA/Human-wt/CHN/E931/2008/G4P[6] for VP1, and VP3). On the other hand, the origin of the VP2 was not clear from our analyses, as it was not only close to both porcine (e.g., RVA/Pig-tc/CHN/SWU-1C/2018/G9P[13]) and porcine-like human strains (e.g., RVA/Human-wt/LKA/R1207/2009/G4P[6]) but also to three human strains (e.g., RVA/Human-wt/USA/1476/1974/G1P[8]). The VP7 gene was located in lineage II that comprised only porcine strains, which suggests the occurrence of independent porcine-to-human reassortment events. The study strain may have collectively been derived through interspecies transmission, or through reassortment event(s) involving strains of porcine and porcine-like human origin. The results of this study underline the importance of whole-genome characterisation of rotavirus strains and provide insights into interspecies transmissions from porcine to humans.

**Keywords:** whole-genome; genotype constellation; interspecies transmission; reassortment; porcine; porcine-like human

## 1. Introduction

Group A rotaviruses (RVA), of the family *Reoviridae*, are the number one viral pathogens causing severe diarrhoea in children below five years of age [1]. In 2016, an estimated 128,000 deaths in children below five years were due to RVA infections, 90% of which occurred in developing countries [2,3]. Similarly, RVA are the primary cause of acute gastroenteritis in new-born piglets [4].

Rotaviruses have a distinctive morphology which comprises a nonenveloped, three-layered icosahedral protein shell. The rotavirus genome within the protein shell comprises 11 segments of double-stranded (dsRNA) that encode six structural viral proteins (VP1 to VP4, VP6, and VP7) and five or six nonstructural proteins (NSP1 to NSP5/6) [1]. A binary classification system is used to distinguish RVA based on the antigenic properties of the outer shell proteins, VP7 and VP4, that determine the G-genotype and P-genotype, respectively [1]. Furthermore, RVA can be separated into two main genogroups and one minor genogroup according to a whole-genome classification system, whereby a specific genotype is assigned to the 11 gene segments. These genogroups represent the genotype constellations that are present in most human strains globally [5,6]. Genogroup 1 (Wa-like) bears the constellation I1-R1-C1-M1-A1-N1-T1-E1-H1 and is often associated with the G genotypes G1, G3, G4, G9, and G12 and P genotype P[8]. Genogroup 2 (DS-1-like) includes G2P[4] strains and bears the constellation I2-R2-C2-M2-A2-N2-T2-E2-H2. Lastly, the minor genogroup 3 (AU-1-like) bears the I3-R3-C3-M3-A3-N3-T3-E3-H3 constellation and includes G3P[9] strains [7]. As of 5th May 2020, the Rotavirus Classification Working Group had identified at least 36 G, 51 P, 26 I, 22 R, 20 C, 20 M, 31 A, 22 N, 22 T, 27 E, and 22 H genotypes [8]. The whole-genome classification system has made it possible to analyse and understand the origin of various strains, interspecies transmission, and animal–human reassortment events [9]. Human Wa-like strains and porcine rotavirus strains share a common origin, whereas DS-1-like and AU-1-like strains have a common origin with bovine and feline strains, respectively [5].

In humans, G1-G4, G9, and G12 along with P[4], P[6], and P[8] are the most frequently detected, globally [10–13]. On the contrary, in porcine, predominant genotypes are G3-G5, G9, and G11 along with P[6], P[7], and P[13] [4,14]. Porcine rotaviruses bear the constellation I5-R1-C1-M1-A8-N1-T1/T7-E1-H1 [5,15–20]. While human Wa-like RVA differ from porcine rotaviruses in some gene segments (VP4, VP6, VP7, and NSP1), they both appear to have genotype 1 in the VP1, VP2, VP3, NSP2, NSP3, NSP4, and NSP5 gene segments. Hence, the suggestion that human Wa-like and porcine RVAs have arisen from a common ancestor [5].

The findings that show animals can serve as potential reservoirs for genetically diverse rotavirus strains that can be passed on to humans have elicited a large amount of interest and topics for further research [21]. Several novel and rare animal-like or animal–human reassortant rotavirus strains have been identified globally [22–28]. The detection of animal strains in humans is presumed to be as a result of zoonotic transmission, along with reassortment, which contributes to the diversity of circulating RVA [4,29,30]. Inter and intragenogroup reassortment may occur when multiple RVA simultaneously infect a host. This is attributed to the segmented nature of the rotavirus genome [1,31]. It is, therefore, necessary to continuously carry out the monitoring of animal RVA and the role they play in contributing to the diversity of circulating RVA in humans.

The G5, one of the most common porcine genotypes, has sporadically been identified in human populations in Brazil (G5P[X]), Cameroon (G5P[7] and G5P[8]), Argentina (G5P[8]), and the United Kingdom(G5P[X]) [32–36]. The P[6] is presumed to be of porcine origin. They have also been identified in human populations [37–40]. The first human G5P[6] strain, LL36755, was detected in a child who had acute gastroenteritis in China in 2007 [41]. Other G5P[6] strains were detected in Vietnam, Taiwan, Bulgaria, Japan, and Thailand [37,42–45]. To date, the whole-genome of only two human G5P[6] strains—Bulgarian BG620 (nt sequences unavailable in the DDBJ, EMBL, and GenBank data libraries as of 13 August 2020) and Japanese Ryukyu-1120 (full open reading frame, available in GenBank)—have been analysed [45,46].

Diarrhoea is a burden for the Zambian healthcare system, with about 33% of the extreme cases being attributable to RVA [47–49]. In an attempt to generate disease burden attributable to rotavirus diarrhoea in children, the Zambian Ministry of Health, with support from WHO, launched rotavirus surveillance at the University Teaching Hospital (UTH) in 2006 [50,51]. Surveillance data generated provided evidence of the burden of rotavirus diarrhoea that supported the introduction of the rotavirus vaccine, Rotarix®, as a pilot project in Lusaka, Zambia in 2012, and was later rolled out nationwide in November 2013 [50]. According to the estimates reported by the World Health Organization (WHO) and the United Nations International Children's Emergency Fund (WHO/UNICEF), rotavirus vaccine coverage in Zambia has been consistently high for the last six years, increasing from 73% in 2014 to 90% in 2019 [52]. Over this period, a sustained and significant reduction in rotavirus-associated hospitalisations and mortality was observed in children under 5 years [51].

The African Rotavirus Surveillance Network, coordinated by the World Health Organization Regional Office for Africa (WHO/AFRO), is actively monitoring the diversity and distribution of RVA genotypes in children hospitalised with acute diarrhoea [53]. Initially, the network was established with four countries in 2006, and expanded to 29 countries by the end of 2016 [54,55]. The Diarrhoeal Pathogens Research Unit at Sefako Makgatho University in Pretoria (South Africa) and the Noguchi Memorial Institute for Medical Research in Accra (Ghana) are the two WHO Rotavirus Regional Reference Laboratories (RRLs) for the network that conducts monitoring of rotavirus epidemiology in Africa [55]. The WHO/AFRO is currently supporting the University of the Free State-Next Generation Sequencing (UFS-NGS) unit to undertake rotavirus surveillance of rotavirus strains that circulated in Zambia between 2013 and 2016 at the whole-genome level. A G5P[6] strain, UFS-NGS-MRC-DPRU4723, was identified among these strains and was analysed so as to elucidate its origin and evolution. The sample was collected in 2014 from an unvaccinated 12 month old male hospitalised for gastroenteritis at Arthur Davison Children's Hospital in Ndola, Zambia.

## 2. Results

### 2.1. Nucleotide Sequencing and Identity of the Strain

Illumina® MiSeq sequencing exhibited a phred score of Q30 and collectively yielded 98.8 Mbs of data for this specific sample. The whole genome of RVA/Human-wt/ ZMB/UFS-NGS-MRC-DPRU4723/2014/G5P[6] was 18272 bps in size. The length and ORF of the 11 gene segments as determined by nucleotide sequencing are shown in Table 1. A BLASTn search was performed, and it appeared to exhibit maximum sequence identities of 95.7%–98.0% with porcine and human porcine-like strains (Table 1). Based on the whole genome classification system, RVA/Human-wt/ZMB/UFS-NGS-MRC-DPRU4723/2014/G5P[6] exhibited a G5-P[6]-I1-R1-C1-M1-A8-N1-T1-E1-H1 genotype constellation (Table 2). The genetic constellation of the study strain was compared to those of other G5 and non-G5 strains retrieved from the GenBank (Table 2).

Table 1. The segment and ORF lengths of strain UFS-NGS-MRC-DPRU4723 and the highest sequence identities obtained using the Basic Local Alignment Search Tool (BLAST).

| GENOME SEGMENT Encoding | GenBank Accession no. | Segment Length | ORF Length | Results of Blast Search | | | Reference |
|---|---|---|---|---|---|---|---|
| | | | | Most Similar Strain | GenBank Accession no. | Similarity (%) | |
| VP1 | MT271025 | 3302 | 3267 | GX54 | KF041441 | 96.7 | [56] |
| VP2 | MT271026 | 2673 | 2673 | R1207 | LC389886 | 96.5 | [57] |
| VP3 | MT271027 | 2591 | 2508 | R946 | KF726060 | 95.7 | [58] |
| VP4 | MT271028 | 2359 | 2328 | KisB332 | KJ870903 | 98.0 | [59] |
| NSP1 | MT271029 | 1512 | 1482 | NT0042 | LC095894 | 98.1 | [60] |
| VP6 | MT271030 | 1356 | 1194 | KYE-14-A048 | KX988279 | 98.7 | [29] |
| NSP3 | MT271031 | 1076 | 942 | 12070-4 | KX363287 | 97.1 | [61] |
| NSP2 | MT271032 | 954 | 954 | YN | KJ466987 | 96.8 | [https://www.ncbi.nlm.nih.gov/nuccore/KJ466987] |
| VP7 | MT271033 | 1054 | 981 | JN-2 | KT820777 | 98.0 | [https://www.ncbi.nlm.nih.gov/nuccore/KT820777] |
| NSP4 | MT271034 | 751 | 528 | 14150-54 | KX363354 | 97.7 | [61] |
| NSP5 | MT271035 | 644 | 594 | R479 | GU189559 | 97.6 | [62] |

## 2.2. Sequence and Phylogenetic Analysis

To investigate the potential origin of RVA/Human-wt/ZMB/UFS-NGS-MRC-DPRU4723/2014/G5P[6], phylogenetic trees were constructed for each of the 11 gene segments along with cognate gene sequences of RVA strains obtained from the GenBank.

### 2.2.1. Sequence and Phylogenetic Analysis of the VP7 Gene

Phylogenetically, there are three known VP7 G5 lineages (I-III) [63]. The VP7 genes of RVA/Human-wt/ZMB/UFS-NGS-MRC-DPRU4723/2014/G5P[6] clustered into lineage II, which consisted only of porcine G5 strains from mainly Asia and the Americas (Figure 1). The VP7 gene showed the highest nucleotide (nt) and amino acid (aa) identities with the Chinese porcine strains RVA/Pig-wt/CHN/DZ-2/2013/ G5P[X] nt (aa), 98.6% (99.0%), and RVA/Pig-wt/CHN/JN-2/2014/G5P[X] 98.5% (99.0%) and was distantly related to the strains within lineage III with lower sequence identities (nt, 83.4%–86.5%; aa, 90.4%–94.5%) (Figure 1; Supplementary data 1). Overall, strains within lineage II exhibited sequence identities that were in the range nt, 89.6%–98.6%; aa, 92.4%–99.0% (Supplementary data 1).

The comparison of the amino acid sequence of RVA/Human-wt/ZMB/UFS-NGS-MRC-DPRU4723/2014/G5P[6] to reference G5 strains e.g., RVA/Pig-wt/THA/CMP-001-12/2012/G5P[13] (lineage I), RVA/Pig-wt/BRA/ROTA24/2013/G5P[6] (lineage II) and RVA/Human-wt/JPN/Ryukyu-1120/2011/G5P[6] (lineage III) within each of the three lineages revealed a high identity (range 90.0%–94.9% (Supplementary data 1; Supplementary data 2a). Numerous substitutions were identified in the nine VP7 variable regions, VR-1 to VR-9 [64]: VR-1 (I9V and I19V), VR-2 (V27T and V29T), VR-3 M/F39L, I40V, V41I, L/I43V, I/L/V47F, R49K, and A50T), VR-4 (K/A65T, V/M68A, M/A72T, and M/Q75T), VR-5/antigenic site A (N/S/D/T96A), VR-6 (I129V and D130E), VR-7/antigenic site B (N145D and A/V/E146G), VR-8/antigenic site C (L/S208T, A210T, T/V212I, S/A213I, I/M217T, V218I, and S220N), and VR-9/antigenic site F (A/M241T and S242N).

**Table 2.** Genotype natures of the 11 gene segments of Zambian strain UFS-NGS-MRC-DPRU4723 compared with those of selected human and porcine strains.

| Strain | Genotype | | | | | | | | | | |
|---|---|---|---|---|---|---|---|---|---|---|---|
| | VP7 | VP4 | VP6 | VP1 | VP2 | VP3 | NSP1 | NSP2 | NSP3 | NSP4 | NSP5 |
| RVA/Human-wt/ZMB/UFS-NGS-MRC-DPRU4723/2014/G5P[6] | G5 | P[6] | I1 | R1 | C1 | M1 | A8 | N1 | T1 | E1 | H1 |
| RVA/Human-wt/BGR/BG260/2008/G5P[6] * | G5 | P[6] | I1 | R1 | C1 | M1 | A8 | N1 | T1 | E1 | H1 |
| RVA/Human-wt/JPN/Ryukyu-1120/2011/G5P[6] | G5 | P[6] | I5 | R1 | C1 | M1 | A8 | N1 | T1 | E1 | H1 |
| RVA/Human-wt/CHN/LL3354/2000/G5P[6] | G5 | P[6] | I5 | - | - | - | - | - | - | E1 | - |
| RVA/Human-wt/CHN/LL4260/2001/G5P[6] | G5 | P[6] | - | - | - | - | - | - | - | E1 | - |
| RVA/Human-wt/CHN/LL36755/2003/G5P[6] | G5 | P[6] | - | - | - | - | - | - | - | E1 | - |
| RVA/Human-wt/VNM/KH210/2004/G5P[6] | G5 | P[6] | I5 | - | - | - | - | - | - | E1 | - |
| RVA/Human-wt/TWN/03-98P50/2009/G5P[6] * | G5 | P[6] | I5 | - | - | - | - | - | - | E1 | - |
| RVA/Human-wt/CMR/6784/ARN/2000/G5P[7] | G5 | P[7] | I5 | R1 | C1 | M1 | A1 | N1 | T1 | E1 | H1 |
| RVA/Human-tc/BRA/IAL28/1992/G5P[8] | G5 | P[8] | I5 | R1 | C1 | M1 | A1 | N1 | T1 | E1 | H1 |
| RVA/Pig-tc/USA/OSU/1975/G5P[7] | G5 | P[7] | I5 | R1 | C1 | M1 | A1 | N1 | T1 | E1 | H1 |
| RVA/Pig-wt/BEL/12R002/2012/G5P[7] | G5 | P[7] | I5 | R1 | C1 | M1 | A8 | N1 | T7 | E1 | H1 |
| RVA/Pig-wt/JPN/BU2/2014/G5P[7] | G5 | P[7] | I5 | R1 | C1 | M1 | A8 | N1 | T1 | E1 | H1 |
| RVA/Human-tc/USA/Wa/1974/G1P[8] | G1 | P[8] | I1 | R1 | C1 | M1 | A1 | N1 | T1 | E1 | H1 |
| RVA/Human-tc/USA/DS-1/1976/G2P[4] | G2 | P[4] | I2 | R2 | C2 | M2 | A2 | N2 | T2 | E2 | H2 |
| RVA/Human-tc/JPN/AU-1/1982/G3P[9] | G3 | P[9] | I3 | R3 | C3 | M3 | A3 | N3 | T3 | E3 | H3 |
| RVA/Pig-wt/BEL/12R006/2012/G3P[6] | G3 | P[6] | I5 | R1 | C1 | M1 | A8 | N1 | T1 | E1 | H1 |
| RVA/Human-tc/GBR/ST3/1974/G4P[6] | G4 | P[6] | I1 | R1 | C1 | M1 | A1 | N1 | T1 | E1 | H1 |
| RVA/Pig-tc/USA/Gottfried/1975/G4P[6] | G4 | P[6] | I1 | R1 | C1 | M1 | A8 | N1 | T1 | E1 | H1 |
| RVA/Human-tc/CHN/R479/2004/G4P[6] | G4 | P[6] | I5 | R1 | C1 | M1 | A1 | N1 | T1 | E1 | H1 |
| RVA/Human-wt/CHN/E931/2008/G4P[6] | G4 | P[6] | I1 | R1 | C1 | M1 | A8 | N1 | T1 | E1 | H1 |
| RVA/Human-wt/COD/KisB332/2008/G4P[6] | G4 | P[6] | I1 | R1 | C1 | M1 | A1 | N1 | T7 | E1 | H1 |
| RVA/Human-wt/CHN/GX54/2010/G4P[6] | G4 | P[6] | I1 | R1 | C1 | M1 | A8 | N1 | T1 | E1 | H1 |

Table 2. Cont.

| Strain | Genotype | | | | | | | | | | |
|---|---|---|---|---|---|---|---|---|---|---|---|
| | VP7 | VP4 | VP6 | VP1 | VP2 | VP3 | NSP1 | NSP2 | NSP3 | NSP4 | NSP5 |
| RVA/Pig-wt/BEL/12R005/2012/G4P[7] | G4 | P[7] | I5 | R1 | C1 | M1 | **A8** | N1 | T7 | E1 | H1 |
| RVA/Human-wt/BEL/BE2001/2009/G9P[6] | G9 | P[6] | I5 | R1 | C1 | M1 | **A8** | N1 | T7 | E1 | H1 |
| RVA/Human-tc/USA/WI61/1983/G9P[8] | G9 | P[8] | I1 | R1 | C1 | M1 | A1 | N1 | T1 | E1 | H1 |
| RVA/Human-wt/BEL/B3458/2003/G9P[8] | G9 | P[8] | I1 | R1 | C1 | M1 | A1 | N1 | T1 | E1 | H1 |
| RVA/Human-tc/IND/mani-97/2006/G9P[19] | G9 | P[19] | I5 | R1 | C1 | M1 | **A8** | N1 | T1 | E1 | H1 |
| RVA/Human-wt/BGD/Dhaka6/2001/G11P[25] | G11 | P[25] | I1 | R1 | C1 | M1 | A1 | N1 | T1 | E1 | H1 |
| RVA/Human-wt/VNM/30378/2009/G26P[19] | G26 | P[19] | I5 | R1 | C1 | M1 | **A8** | N1 | T1 | E1 | H1 |
| RVA/Human-wt/BRA/rj24598/2015/G26P[13] | G26 | P[19] | I5 | R1 | C1 | M1 | **A8** | N1 | T1 | E1 | H1 |

Blue shading indicates the gene segments with genotypes identical to those of UFS-NGS-MRC-DPRU4723. Bold font indicates genotypes associated with porcine strains. "—" indicates that no sequence data were available in GenBank/EMBL/DDBJ data banks. * Genotype assignment based on reports by [37] (strain 03-98sP50) and (strain BG260) [46]. To date, the nucleotide accession numbers for the 11 gene segments of strains 03-98sP50 and BG260 are not available in the GenBank, EMBL, or DDBJ data banks.

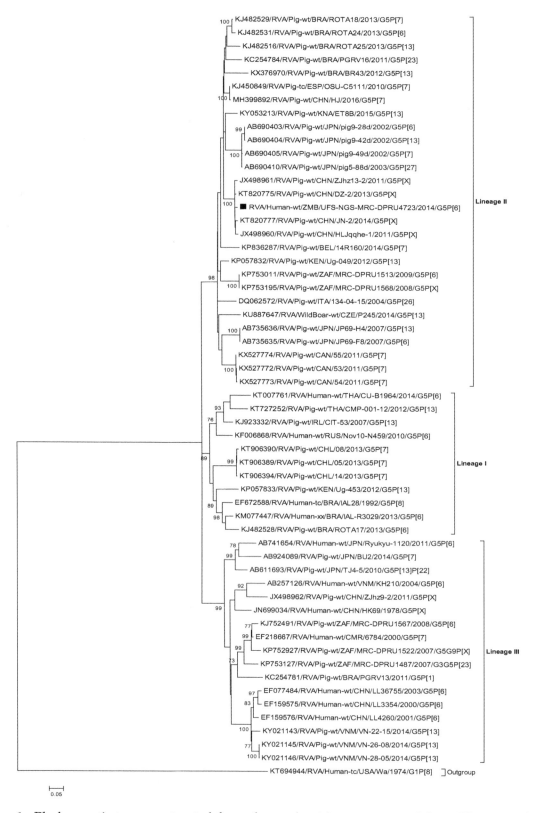

**Figure 1.** Phylogenetic tree constructed from the nucleotide sequences of the VP7 genes of strain RVA/Human-wt/ZMB/UFS-NGS-MRC-DPRU4723/2014/G5P[6] and representative strains. The position of strain RVA/Human-wt/ZMB/UFS-NGS-MRC-DPRU4723/2014/G5P[6] is shown by the black square (■). Reference strains obtained from GenBank are represented by accession number, strain name, country, and year of isolation. The three closest strains, as identified by BLASTn, are also included. Bootstrap values ≥70% are shown adjacent to each branch node. Scale bar: 0.05 substitutions per nucleotide.

## 2.2.2. Sequence and Phylogenetic Analysis of the VP4 Gene

The VP4 gene of RVA/Human-wt/ZMB/UFS-NGS-MRC-DPRU4723/2014/G5P[6] was phylogenetically compared to the already established five lineages (I-V) of genotype P[6] [65] (Figure 2). The P[6] gene of the study strain clustered into lineage V, which consisted of porcine and putative human porcine-like strains detected in parts of Europe and one African strain. A similarity analysis of the P[6] gene of the study strain with strains obtained from GenBank showed that the Zambian G5P[6] exhibited the highest sequence identity of 98.1% (98.3%) with a porcine-like human strain RVA/Human-wt/COD/KisB332/2008/G4P[6] from the Democratic Republic of Congo (Supplementary data 1). All the African strains clustered into a separate lineage, lineage I, with sequence identities of 85.7%–86.8% (92.5%–93.9%) (Supplementary data 1).

The deduced amino acid sequences of the VP4 gene of RVA/Human-wt/ZMB/UFS-NGS-MRC-DPRU4723/2014/G5P[6] along with the reference P[6] strain from each of the five lineages was compared (Supplementary data 2b). The reference strains shared high amino acid identities ranging from 91.0% to 98.3% (Supplementary data 1). Several amino acid changes were identified throughout the VP4 protein, and most of the substitutions were concentrated in the hypervariable region (amino acid 71-208) which houses the VR-3 (92–192) and includes a neutralization site at amino acid 135 [66,67]. Several amino acid substitutions were observed among the P[6] lineage I strains [65] at the VR-3 (L105I, V108I and T134S) and VR-8 (D602N) variable regions. Other amino acid substitutions were identified among the P[6] lineages at VR-1 (S30N), VR-2 (I61V), VR-3 (V112I, N114S, V130I, H182N and T189S), VR-4 (I280V), and VR-9 (E698K). The potential trypsin cleavage sites at residues 241 and 247 [68] were highly conserved in all the strains with three substitutions at positions 242 (I to V), 243 (A to T), and 244 (H to Y).

## 2.2.3. Phylogenetic Analysis of the VP6 Gene

The VP6 gene of RVA/Human-wt/ZMB/UFS-NGS-MRC-DPRU4723/2014/G5P[6] clustered closely with divergent African porcine strains from Uganda (RVA/Pig-wt/UGA/BUW-14-A003/2014/G3P[13], RVA/Pig-wt/UGA/KYE-14-A048/2014/G3P[13], and RVA/Pig-wt/UGA/KYE-14-A047/2014/G3P[13]) and a human porcine-like strain from the Democratic Republic of Congo (RVA/Human-wt/COD/KisB332/2008/G4P[6]) which displayed nt(aa) sequence identities ranging from 98.6% to 98.9% (98.9%–99.7%) (Figure 3, Supplementary data 1). Porcine-like Asian strains such as RVA/Human-wt/CHN/GX54/2010/G4P[6] and RVA/Human-wt/CHN/E931/2008/G4P[6] clustered separately, displaying identities of 88.7%–90.2% (97.5%–98.7%) (Supplementary data 1).

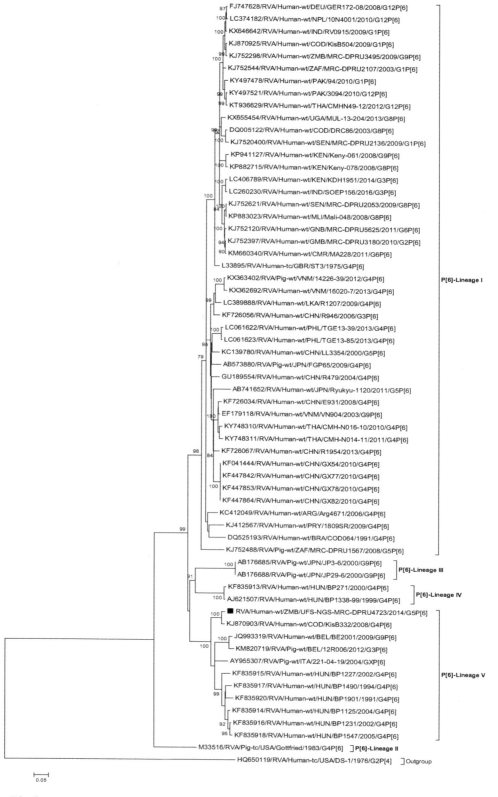

**Figure 2.** Phylogenetic tree constructed from the nucleotide sequences of the VP4 genes of strain RVA/Human-wt/ZMB/UFS-NGS-MRC-DPRU4723/2014/G5P[6] and representative strains. The position of strain RVA/Human-wt/ZMB/UFS-NGS-MRC-DPRU4723/2014/G5P[6] is shown by the black square (■). Reference strains obtained from GenBank are represented by accession number, strain name, country, and year of isolation. The three closest strains, as identified by BLASTn, are also included. Bootstrap values ≥70% are shown adjacent to each branch node. Scale bar: 0.05 substitutions per nucleotide.

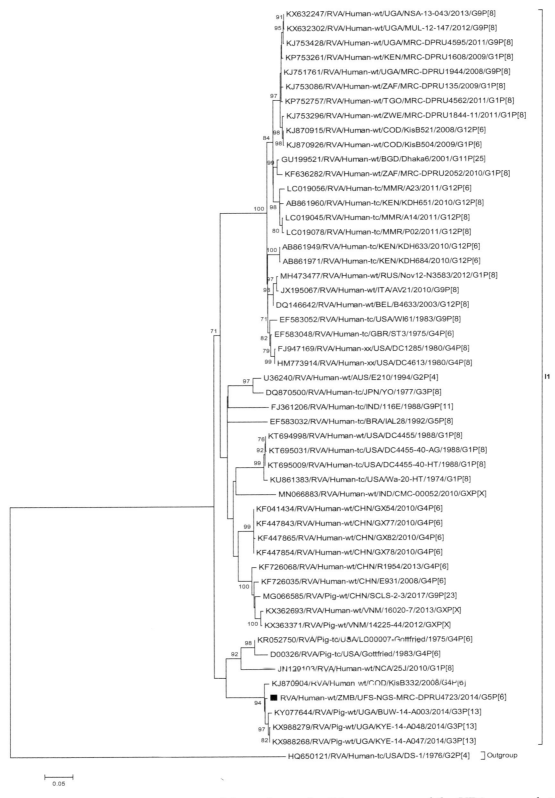

**Figure 3.** Phylogenetic tree constructed from the nucleotide sequences of the VP6 genes of strain RVA/Human-wt/ZMB/UFS-NGS-MRC-DPRU4723/2014/G5P[6] and representative strains. The position of strain RVA/Human-wt/ZMB/UFS-NGS-MRC-DPRU4723/2014/G5P[6] is shown by the black square (∎). Reference strains obtained from GenBank are represented by accession number, strain name, country, and year of isolation. The three closest strains, as identified by BLASTn, are also included. Bootstrap values ≥70% are shown adjacent to each branch node. Scale bar: 0.05 substitutions per nucleotide.

2.2.4. Phylogenetic Analysis of VP1 Gene

The VP1 gene of RVA/Human-wt/ZMB/UFS-NGS-MRC-DPRU4723/2014/G5P[6] clustered only with porcine and porcine-like human strains from Asia (China and Vietnam) (Supplementary data 3a). The VP1 gene exhibited a maximum nt (aa) sequence identity of 96.8% (98.9%) with the Chinese human porcine-like reassortant strains RVA/Human-wt/CHN/GX82/2010/G4P[6], RVA/Human-wt/CHN/GX78/2010/G4P[6], RVA/Human-wt/CHN/GX77/2010/G4P[6], and RVA/Human-wt/CHN/GX54/2010/G4P[6] (Supplementary data 1). Overall, the Asian strains within the cluster showed sequence identities of 94.1%–96.8% (97.9%–98.9%). Human non-porcine African strains clustered separately, with lower identities of 88.2%–88.8% (96.3%–97.3%) (Supplementary data 1).

2.2.5. Phylogenetic Analysis of VP2 Gene

The VP2 gene of strain RVA/Human-wt/ZMB/UFS-NGS-MRC-DPRU4723/2014/G5P[6] fell into a distinct cluster predominantly composed of porcine and porcine-like human strains from Asia (China, India, Vietnam, South Korea, and Sri Lanka) (Supplementary data 3b). The VP2 gene of the study strain showed a maximum nt (aa) sequence identity of 96.6% (90.9%) with a Sri Lankan porcine-like human strain RVA/Human-wt/LKA/R1207/2009/G4P[6] (Supplementary data 1).

2.2.6. Phylogenetic Analysis of VP3 Gene

The VP3 gene of strain RVA/Human-wt/ZMB/UFS-NGS-MRC-DPRU4723/2014/G5P[6] clustered in a lineage composed mainly of Asian (Asia and Thailand) porcine and porcine-like human strains (Supplementary data 3c), and exhibited the highest nt (aa) sequence identity with the Chinese porcine-like human strains—RVA/Human-wt/CHN/R946/2006/G3P[6], 95.8% (97.8%) and RVA/Human-wt/CHN/E931/2008/G4P[6], 95.7% (98.0%) (Supplementary data 1). The overall similarities of the Asian strains within the lineage ranged from 84.8% to 95.8% (92.7%–97.8%) (Supplementary data 1). Non-porcine African strains clustered separately and showed lower sequence identities of 84.1%–84.5% (92.1%–92.7%) (Supplementary data 1).

2.2.7. Phylogenetic Analysis of NSP1 Gene

The NSP1 gene of strain RVA/Human-wt/ZMB/UFS-NSG-MRC-DPRU4723/2014/G5P[6] was assigned to a porcine genotype A8 and clustered among Asian (Vietnam, China, and Bangladesh) porcine and porcine-like human strains and an African (Ghana) porcine strain (Supplementary data 3d). The NSP1 gene of the study strain was closest to strain RVA/Human-tc/VNM/NT0042/2007/G4P[6] displaying a nt(aa) sequence identity of 98.2% (97.9%) (Supplementary data 1). The porcine and porcine-like human strains from Europe and the Americas clustered separately showing sequence identities of 84.2%–85.9% (85.4%–88.2%) and 84.1%–85.9% (83.7%–88.3%), respectively (Supplementary data 1).

2.2.8. Phylogenetic Analysis of NSP2 Gene

The NSP2 gene of strain RVA/Human-wt/ZMB/UFS-NGS-MRC-DPRU4723/2014/G5P[6] clustered with Asian and European porcine and porcine-like human strains (Supplementary data 3e). The Nt(aa) similarity analysis showed that the NSP2 gene of the study strain was most similar to the Chinese porcine strains RVA/Pig-wt/CHN/YN/2012/GXP[X] and RVA/Pig-tc/CHN/SCMY-A3/2017/G9P[23]—96.8% (97.8%) (Supplementary data 1). Two African porcine strains, RVA/Pig-wt/ZAF/MRC-DPRU1487/2007/G3G5P[23] and RVA/Pig-wt/ZAF/MRC-DPRU1557/2008/G4G5P[23], were seen to cluster within the same lineage with sequence identities of 93.6%–93.7% (97.5%–97.8%) (Supplementary data 1).

2.2.9. Phylogenetic Analysis of NSP3 Gene

The NSP3 gene of strain RVA/Human-wt/ZMB/UFS-NGS-MRC-DPRU4723/2014/G5P[6] clustered closely with porcine and porcine-like human strains mainly from Asia (Thailand and

Vietnam) and exhibited a maximum nt(aa) sequence identities of 96.5%–97.0% (98.4%–98.7%) with the strains RVA/Human-wt/VNM/30378/2009/G26P[19], RVA/Pig-wt/VNM/12070-4/2012/GXP[X], RVA/Human-wt/VNM/NT0205/2007/G4P[6], and RVA/Human-wt/VNM/NT0621/2008/G4P[6] (Supplementary data 1; Supplementary data 3f).

### 2.2.10. Phylogenetic Analysis of NSP4 Gene

The NSP4 gene of strain RVA/Human-wt/ZMB/UFS-NGS-MRC-DPRU4723/2014/G5P[6] clustered with porcine and porcine-like human strains identified in Asia (China and Vietnam) and a porcine-like human strain from the Americas (Brazil) (Supplementary data 3g). In this cluster, the closest strains to UFS-NGS-MRC-DPRU4723 were the wild pig strains (RVA/WildBoar-wt/CZE/P828/2015/G9P[23] and RVA/WildBoar-wt/CZE/P830/2015/G9P[23]) from the Czech Republic, with nt(aa) sequence identities of 97.5% (98.3%) (Supplementary data 1). The Asian strains within the cluster showed nt(aa) similarities of 96.2%–97.3% (97.7%–98.9%). Porcine and porcine-like human strains from the Americas clustered separately and exhibited identities of 87.2%–96.4% (94.3%–98.9%) (Supplementary data 1).

### 2.2.11. Phylogenetic Analysis of the NSP5 Gene

The NSP5 gene of strain RVA/Human-wt/ZMB/UFS-NGS-MRC-DPRU4723/2014/G5P[6] clustered with porcine strains from Asia and showed the highest nt(aa) sequence identity of 98.6% (100%) with the porcine strains RVA/Pig-wt/CHN/TM-a/2009/G3P[8] and RVA/Pig-tc/CHN/TM-a-P20/2018/G9P[23] identified in China (Supplementary data 1; Supplementary data 3h). Overall, the porcine and porcine-like human strains from Asia and the Americas displayed nt(aa) identities of in the range 94.8%–98.6% (98.0%–100%) and 93.9%–96.1% (95.9%–99.0%), respectively (Supplementary data 1).

### 2.3. Reassortment Analysis

The concatenated whole genome alignment of RVA/Human-wt/ZMB/UFS-NGS-MRC-DPRU4723/2014/G5P[6], together with the Japanese G5P[6] strain and selected Chinese porcine-like human P[6] strains, was visualised (Figure 4). The whole genome of the Zambian G5P[6] strain demonstrated a relatively high degree of conservation with the Japanese G5P[6] strain and the two Chinese G4P[6] strains. With the exception of VP7 and VP4, the genome of the Chinese strain E931 exhibited the overall highest genomic conservation to the study strain. With the exception of VP7, VP3, and NSP1 genes, the Chinese strain GX54 shared a highly conserved genome with the study strain. The Japanese strain Ryukyu-1120 demonstrated a highly similar genome to the study strain for seven of the 11 genes, the exceptions being VP1, VP3, VP6, and VP7. The results of this analysis confirmed the genetic similarity between RVA/Human-wt/ZMB/UFS-NGS-MRC-DPRU4723/2014/G5P[6] and Asian (Chinese) porcine-like human strains, hence suggesting that the Zambian G5P[6] strain may have been derived via reassortment events.

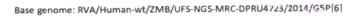
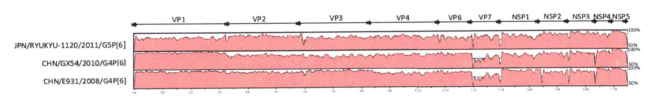

**Figure 4.** mVISTA whole genome nucleotide alignment comparing the Zambian G5P[6] strain (RVA/Human-wt/ZMB/UFS-NGS-MRC-DPRU4723/2014G5P[6]) with the G5P[6] strain from Japan (Ryukyu-1120), whose whole genome sequence had been determined, and with selected porcine-like human P[6] strains from China (GX54 and E931). Strain names are shown on the left, and the proteins VP1-VP4, VP6-VP7, and NSP1-NSP5 are indicated on the top. The bottom scale indicates distance in kb. Percentile values on the right indicate sequence-based similarity between the study strain and the respective reference strains. Shading indicates the level of conservation.

## 3. Discussion

The detection of genotype G5 in humans, which is typical for pigs, is possibly due to interspecies transmission [35,45]. In Zambia, as with many countries in Africa, humans and farm animals live in proximity. The interaction between humans and animals could be the primary cause for zoonotic transmission, which could result in genetic reassortments and perhaps other mechanisms of genetic diversity, ultimately leading to the introduction and spread of animal genotypes into human populations [69].

In this study, an analysis was conducted on a sample collected from a child admitted to a paediatric ward presenting with clinical symptoms (vomiting, diarrhoea, and fever) that are usually present during typical rotavirus infection. This raises the question whether such animal-derived strains are capable of mutating and effectively spreading within/across human populations as in the case of established typical Wa-like and DS-1-like genotype constellations, with the same magnitude of rotavirus disease severity. Furthermore, taking into consideration that the G5 and P[6] genotypes are not included in the currently available vaccines, the probability for such strains to have the potential to spread more swiftly from human to human may have implications for the effectiveness of current rotavirus vaccine candidates that are in use in African countries.

This study identified the complete genome of a reassortant porcine-like human strain, G5P[6], that showed the genotype constellation G5-P[6]-I1-R1-C1-M1-A8-N1-T1-E1-H1, which is commonly found in porcine and porcine-like human rotavirus strains [19]. RVA/Human-wt/ZMB/UFS-NGS-MRC-DPRU4723/2014/G5P[6] was found to share the same constellation (I1-R1-C1-M1-A8-N1-T1-E1-H1) with the archival porcine strain, Gottfried, and porcine-like human strains—BG260, E931, and GX54 [5,46,56,58]. In addition, porcine strains 12R002, 12R005, and 12R006, as well as porcine-like human strains Ryukyu-1120, mani-97, 30378, rj24598, and BE2001 shared the same constellation with strain RVA/Human-wt/ZMB/UFS-NGS-MRC-DPRU4723/2014/G5P[6] with the exception of VP6 (I5 instead of I1) and NSP3 (T7 instead of T1 gene segments) [20,25,26,45,70].

A phylogenetic analysis of RVA/Human-wt/ZMB/UFS-NGS-MRC-DPRU4723/2014/G5P[6] showed that this strain was a possible reassortant, as it was closely related to both porcine and porcine-like human strains, predominantly from Asia, than to typical human RVA strains. The VP6, VP7, NSP2, NSP4, and NSP5 segments of this strain showed a close similarity to porcine strains. Although the remaining gene segments (VP1, VP3, VP4, and NSP3) were closely related to human strains, all of these were porcine-like human strains [26,56,58–60,70]. With a genotype 1 (Wa-like) backbone, this finding is consistent with the hypothesis that human Wa-like strains and porcine strains have a common ancestor [5]. However, the origin of the VP2 gene of the study strain was not very definitive, as it was not only close to porcine and porcine-like human strains but also to three human strains (DC1476, DC582, and DC1127). Phylogenetically, the clusters of these three strains were shown to be distinctive from the genes of contemporary, wild-type human strains [71]. Notably, the VP7 gene of RVA/Human-wt/ZMB/UFS-NGS-MRC-DPRU4723/2014/G5P[6] was located in lineage II, which comprised only porcine strains, hence implying the possibility of porcine-to-human interspecies transmission [63]. Phylogenetic analysis of porcine and human P[6] strains indicated that both porcine and human P[6] strains were present in P[6] lineages I, III, and V, hence showing that human P[6] strains might have separately emerged from at least three porcine-to-human transmissions [65]. This finding supports the Zambian G5P[6] strain, as the VP4 gene clustered and shared high nucleotide and amino acid identities with lineage V of P[6] porcine and porcine-like human strains. The NSP1 gene was most similar to porcine-like human strains. However, it was revealed to have the porcine genotype A8. Taking this together, it is likely that RVA/Human-wt/ZMB/UFS-NGS-MRC-DPRU4723/2014/G5P[6] originated by zoonotic transmission, coupled with reassortment events.

Several amino acid changes were identified in the nine variable regions when the VP7 gene of the study strain was compared to other G5 strains within each of the three lineages [64]. Additionally, the previously described conserved N-glycosylation site at residues 69–71 within the variable region 4 (VR-4) was found to be conserved in all the G5 strains used in this analysis [64,72]. Four major antigenic regions have been described for the VP7 protein in rotaviruses (A, B, C and F) [73,74]. Marked differences in the antigenic regions of RVA/Human-wt/ZMB/UFS-NGS-MRC-DPRU4723/2014/G5P[6] were seen when it was compared to other globally circulating G5 strains. Usually, antigenic regions A and C are said to be conserved within serotypes [75]. However, multiple substitutions were observed in these regions when comparing the Zambian G5 strain to other G5 strains globally.

The amino acid sequence for the VP4 gene was 775 amino acids long and displayed amino acid identity values ranging from 91.0% to 98.3% with the reference P[6] strains. Considering it has been established that strains with amino acid identities greater than 89% belong to the same P genotype [76], our findings show that RVA/Human-wt/ZMB/UFS-NGS-MRC-DPRU4723/2014/G5P[6] belongs to the genotype P[6]. The analysis of the amino acid sequences showed that the hypervariable region (amino acid 71-208) which houses the variable region 3 (VR-3) contained most of the substitutions. Furthermore, the potential trypsin cleavage sites [68] were conserved in all the P[6] strains. Several amino acid substitutions were observed among the lineage I P[6] strains. The presence of several amino acid changes in the VP4 gene of this strain compared to other circulating P[6] strains globally is in agreement with the hypothesis that the P[6] gene has been introduced to humans via independent reassortment events [40,65,77].

Rotaviruses are genetically diverse in nature and are host-species specific, suggesting that host species barriers and restrictions exist. However, rotaviruses of animal origin may cross the host species barrier and may acquire human rotavirus gene segments, which enables the viruses to efficiently spread across human populations [4]. In this regard, G5 rotavirus strains have sporadically been documented in Latin America, Asia, Europe, and Africa [33–37,41,45,46]. Porcine P[6] strains seem to pose a lesser species barrier to humans [20]. Even though the relationship between porcine and human rotaviruses has already been established [5], whole genome analysis in this study presented the possible occurrence of interspecies transmission and reassortment between human and porcine rotaviruses.

## 4. Materials and Methods

### 4.1. Ethics Statement

This is a subset of a major project which involved the whole genome characterisation of 133 specimens collected in Zambia from 2013 through 2016 as part of the surveillance supported by the WHO/AFRO (reference 2017/757922-0) in collaboration with the University of the Free State (UFS-NGS). Ethical clearance for the main project was obtained under ethics number HSREC130/2016(UFS-HSD2016/1082) from the Health Science Research Ethics Committee (HSREC), University of the Free State, Bloemfontein, South Africa. Furthermore, this specific study was approved by the HSREC under ethics number UFS-HSD2020/0277/2104.

### 4.2. Sample Collection

The sample was collected in 2014 from an unvaccinated 12 month old male at Arthur Davidson Children's Hospital (ADCH) in Ndola, a rotavirus surveillance sentinel site. The child had travelled with parents from Kasama, a town in the Northern Province of Zambia which is approximately 760 km away from Ndola, Zambia. This child was admitted to a paediatric ward at ADCH, with gastroenteritis of four days duration and a history of fever. Frequency of vomiting and diarrhoea was three episodes and two episodes, respectively, in the previous 24 h. The level of dehydration was assessed as mild and the child received an oral rehydration solution and was discharged after a few days. The stool sample was screened using the enzyme immunoassay (EIA) technique for the presence of RVA antigen in the Virology laboratory in Lusaka. It was randomly picked and sent to the Diarrhoeal Pathogens Research Unit (DPRU), a World Health Organization Rotavirus Regional Reference Laboratory (WHO-RRL) in Pretoria, South Africa, as part of the WHO/AFRO annual rotavirus surveillance. Conventional genotyping was carried out at DPRU. Thereafter, the sample was shipped to the UFS-NGS unit for sequencing and whole-genome analysis.

*4.3. Viral dsRNA Extraction*

The viral double-stranded RNA (dsRNA) was extracted from human stool suspensions using a previously described method with modifications [78]. Approximately 100 mg stool was suspended in 200 µL phosphate-buffered saline (PBS) solution (Sigma-Aldrich®, St Louis, MO, United States). The faecal suspension was mixed with 900 µL TRI Reagent® LS (Molecular Research Centre, Cincinnati, OH, United States) and homogenized for five minutes. A 300 µL volume of chloroform (Sigma-Aldrich®, St Louis, MO, United States) was used to achieve phase separation, which was followed by centrifugation (Eppendorf microcentrifuge 5427 R, Germany) at 17,319× g for 20 min at 4 °C. The supernatant was precipitated using 700 µL ice-cold isopropanol (Sigma-Aldrich®, United States) and centrifuged (Eppendorf microcentrifuge 5427 R, Germany) at 17,319× g for 30 min at 4 °C. The supernatant was discarded, and the tubes were air-dried for 5 min, followed by the precipitation of single-stranded RNA (ssRNA) using 30 µL 8 M lithium chloride (Sigma, St Louis, MO, United States) at 4 °C for 16 h. The dsRNA was purified using the MinElute gel extraction kit (Qiagen, Hilden, Germany). RNA integrity was determined by electrophoresis on 1% TBE agarose gel stained with ethidium bromide (Sigma-Aldrich®, St Louis, MO, United States), which was visualised on a G: Box UV transilluminator (Syngene, Cambridge, United Kingdom).

*4.4. cDNA Synthesis and Purification*

cDNA synthesis was carried out using the Maxima H Minus Double-stranded cDNA kit (Thermo Fisher Scientific, Waltham, MA, United States) according to the manufacturer's instructions with minor modifications captured at the UFS-NGS SOP, whereby the dsRNA was denatured at 95 °C for 5 min. First strand synthesis was carried out for two hours at 50 °C. Random hexamer primer was employed for cDNA synthesis. The cDNA was purified using the MSB® Spin PCRapace purification kit (Stratec, Invitek Molecular, Berlin, Germany).

*4.5. DNA Library Preparation and Illumina® MiSeq Sequencing*

DNA libraries for Illumina® sequencing were prepared using the Nextera® XT DNA library preparation kit (Illumina, San Diego, CA, United States) according to the manufacturer's instructions. Briefly, DNA was tagmented at 55 °C for five minutes followed by ligation to Illumina® sequencing index 1 and index 2 adapters by PCR amplification. Size selection and clean-up of the DNA libraries was performed using Agencourt AMPure XP beads (Beckman Coulter, South Kraemer Boulevard Brea, CA, United States). The quantity of DNA was determined on the Qubit 2.0 fluorimeter (Invitrogen, Carlsbad, CA, United States), and a quality check of the libraries was performed on a Bioanalyzer 2100 (Agilent Technologies, Santa Clara, CA, United States). After this, sequencing was performed on an Illumina® MiSeq sequencer (Illumina, San Diego, CA, United States) using a MiSeq reagent kit v3 for 600 cycles (2 × 300 bp paired reads) with a 10% PhiX DNA control spike-in.

*4.6. Genome Assembly*

The raw reads obtained in FASTQ format were assembled using Geneious Prime® 2019.2.1 (https://www.geneious.com/; [79]). Briefly, the paired-end reads were merged into single reads and trimmed to remove low quality and short reads. The reads were mapped to reference sequences obtained from GenBank. Consensus sequences covering the complete open reading frame (ORF) were submitted to the National Centre for Biotechnology Information (NCBI) GenBank and assigned accession numbers MT271025–MT271035. The ORF lengths were 3267 (VP1), 2673 (VP2), 2508 (VP3), 2328 (VP4), 1194 (VP6), 981 (VP7), 1482 (NSP1), 954 (NSP2), 942 (NSP3), 528 (NSP4), and 594 (NSP5).

*4.7. Assignment of Genotypes*

The genotypes of each of the 11 rotavirus genome segments were determined using the online Virus Pathogen Resource (ViPR).

## 4.8. Phylogenetic Analysis

Gene-specific multiple sequence alignments were made using the MAFFT plugin implemented in Geneious Prime® 2019.2.1 and the MUSCLE algorithm embedded in MEGA 6.06 (for the VP2 and NSP1 segments) [80,81]. Once aligned, the DNA Model Test program in MEGA 6.06 was used to identify the optimal evolutionary model for each genome segment [82]. Using an Akaike information criterion (corrected) (AICc), the following models were found to best fit the data: HKY+G+I (VP1), GTR+G+I (VP2, VP3, and VP4), T92+G (VP6, NSP1, NSP2, NSP3, NSP4, and NSP5), and T92+G+I (VP7). Maximum likelihood trees were constructed using the optimal models in MEGA version 6.06 [82,83] with 1000 bootstrap replicates to estimate branch support [84]. The shared nucleotide and amino acid sequence identities among strains were calculated for each gene using the *p*-distance algorithm in MEGA 6.06. Analysis and visualization of the aligned concatenated whole genomes was performed on the mVISTA online platform [85].

## 5. Conclusions

In summary, RVA/Human-wt/ZMB/UFS-NGS-MRC-DPRU4723/2014/G5P[6] was a reassortant possessing gene segment of porcine and porcine-like human origin, and was closest to Asian strains. It is presumed that pigs play a crucial part as a source for new or newly-evolved emerging human rotaviruses. This highlights the need for continuous large-scale surveillance and whole genome analysis of circulating porcine and human rotaviruses. Furthermore, it was imperative to examine the prevalence of G5P[6] strains in Zambia. Eventually, this should result in a greater understanding of the genes that determine the transmission between hosts successfully as well as to gain insights on complex reassortment patterns between porcine and human rotaviruses.

**Author Contributions:** M.M.N., M.J.M., M.L.S., and J.M.M. conceptualised the main project. W.M.M., P.N.M., J.S., E.M.M., and M.M.N. performed the laboratory experiments. M.M.N., J.S., E.M.M., M.J.M., I.P., M.L.S., and J.M.M. facilitated the obtaining of the sample. Formal analysis was performed by W.M.M., M.D.E., and M.M.N. Data curation was performed by W.M.M., P.N.M., and M.M.N. Writing (original draft preparation) was performed by W.M.M. Review of the drafts was performed by all co-authors. Supervision, project administration, and funding acquisition was conducted by M.M.N. and J.M.M. All authors have read and agreed to the published version of the manuscript.

**Acknowledgments:** We greatly thank the Zambia team who assisted with sample collection and ELISA testing. We would like to thank Khutso Mothapo, Kebareng Rakau, and Nonkululeko Magagula at the WHO-RRL (Pretoria, South Africa) who assisted with the retrieval of samples. We would also like to thank Sebotsana Rasebotsa, Milton Mogotsi, Emmanuel Ayodeji, Teboho Mooko, and Gilmore Pambuka for their assistance with laboratory work. We are grateful to Stephanus Riekert for technical ICT support.

## References

1. Estes, M.K.; Greenberg, H.B. Rotaviruses. In *Fields Virology*, 6th ed.; Knipe, D.M., Howley, P.M., Eds.; Wolters Kluwer Health/Lippincott, Williams and Wilkins: Philadelphia, PA, USA, 2013; pp. 1347–1401.
2. Tate, J.E.; Burton, A.H.; Boschi-Pinto, C.; Parashar, U.D. World Health Organization—Coordinated Global Rotavirus Surveillance Network. Global, regional, and national estimates of rotavirus mortality in children <5 years of age, 2000–2013. *Clin. Infect. Dis.* **2016**, *62* (Suppl. 2), S96–S105. [CrossRef] [PubMed]
3. Troeger, C.; Khalil, I.A.; Rao, P.C.; Cao, S.; Blacker, B.F.; Ahmed, T.; Armah, G.; Bines, J.E.; Brewer, T.G.; Colombara, D.V.; et al. Rotavirus vaccination and the global burden of rotavirus diarrhoea among children younger than 5 years. *JAMA Pediatr.* **2018**, *172*, 958–965. [CrossRef] [PubMed]
4. Martella, V.; Bányai, K.; Matthijnssens, J.; Buonavoglia, C.; Ciarlet, M. Zoonotic aspects of rotaviruses. *Vet. Microbiol.* **2010**, *140*, 246–255. [CrossRef] [PubMed]
5. Matthijnssens, J.; Ciarlet, M.; Heiman, E.; Arijs, I.; Delbeke, T.; McDonald, S.M.; Palombo, E.A.; Iturriza-Gomara, M.; Maes, P.; Patton, J.T.; et al. Full genome-based classification of rotaviruses reveals a common origin between human Wa-like and porcine rotavirus strains and human DS-1-like and bovine rotavirus strains. *J. Virol.* **2008** *82*, 3204–3219. [CrossRef]

6. Matthijnssens, J.; Ciarlet, M.; McDonald, S.M.; Attoui, H.; Bányai, K.; Brister, J.R.; Buesa, J.; Esona, M.D.; Estes, M.K.; Gentsch, J.R.; et al. Uniformity of rotavirus strain nomenclature proposed by the Rotavirus Classification Working Group (RCWG). *Arch. Virol.* **2011**, *156*, 1397–1413. [CrossRef]
7. Matthijnssens, J.; Van Ranst, M. Genotype constellation and evolution of group A rotaviruses infecting humans. *Curr. Opin. Virol.* **2012**, *2*, 426–433. [CrossRef]
8. RCWG. Rotavirus Classification Working Group–Laboratory of Viral Metagenomics. 2018. Available online: https://rega.kuleuven.be/cev/viralmetagenomics/virus-classification/rcwg (accessed on 5 May 2020).
9. Ghosh, S.; Kobayashi, N. Whole-genomic analysis of rotavirus strains: Current status and future prospects. *Future Microbiol.* **2011**, *6*, 1049–1065. [CrossRef]
10. Iturriza-Gómara, M.; Dallman, T.; Bányai, K.; Böttiger, B.; Buesa, J.; Diedrich, S.; Fiore, L.; Johansen, K.; Koopmans, M.; Korsun, N.; et al. Rotavirus genotypes co-circulating in Europe between 2006 and 2009 as determined by EuroRotaNet, a pan-European collaborative strain surveillance network. *Epidemiol. Infect.* **2011**, *139*, 895–909. [CrossRef]
11. Matthijnssens, J.; Heylen, E.; Zeller, M.; Rahman, M.; Lemey, P.; Van Ranst, M. Phylodynamic analyses of rotavirus genotypes G9 and G12 underscore their potential for swift global spread. *Mol. Biol. Evol.* **2010**, *27*, 2431–2436. [CrossRef]
12. Patel, M.M.; Steele, D.; Gentsch, J.R.; Wecker, J.; Glass, R.I.; Parashar, U.D. Real-world impact of rotavirus vaccination. *Pediatr. Infect. Dis. J.* **2011**, *30*, 1–5. [CrossRef]
13. Rahman, M.; Matthijnssens, J.; Yang, X.; Delbeke, T.; Arijs, I.; Taniguchi, K.; Iturriza-Gomara, M.; Iftekharuddin, N.; Azim, T.; Van Ranst, M. Evolutionary history and global spread of the emerging G12 human rotaviruses. *J. Virol.* **2007**, *81*, 2382–2390. [CrossRef] [PubMed]
14. Papp, H.; László, B.; Jakab, F.; Ganesh, B.; De Grazia, S.; Matthijnssens, J.; Ciarlet, M.; Martella, V.; Bányai, K. Review of group A rotavirus strains reported in swine and cattle. *Vet. Microbiol.* **2013**, *165*, 190–199. [CrossRef] [PubMed]
15. Agbemabiese, C.A.; Nakagomi, T.; Gauchan, P.; Sherchand, J.B.; Pandey, B.D.; Cunliffe, N.A.; Nakagomi, O. Whole genome characterisation of a porcine-like human reassortant G26P[19] Rotavirus A strain detected in a child hospitalised for diarrhoea in Nepal, 2007. *Infect. Genet. Evol.* **2017**, *54*, 164–169. [CrossRef] [PubMed]
16. Kim, H.H.; Matthijnssens, J.; Kim, H.J.; Kwon, H.J.; Park, J.G.; Son, K.Y.; Ryu, E.H.; Kim, D.S.; Lee, W.S.; Kang, M.I.; et al. Full-length genomic analysis of porcine G9P[23] and G9P[7] rotavirus strains isolated from pigs with diarrhoea in South Korea. *Infect. Genet. Evol.* **2012**, *12*, 1427–1435. [CrossRef] [PubMed]
17. Martel-Paradis, O.; Laurin, M.A.; Martella, V.; Sohal, J.S.; L'Homme, Y. Full-length genome analysis of G2, G9 and G11 porcine group A rotaviruses. *Vet. Microbiol.* **2013**, *162*, 94–102. [CrossRef]
18. Monini, M.; Zaccaria, G.; Ianiro, G.; Lavazza, A.; Vaccari, G.; Ruggeri, F.M. Full-length genomic analysis of porcine rotavirus strains isolated from pigs with diarrhoea in Northern Italy. *Infect. Genet. Evol.* **2014**, *25*, 4–13. [CrossRef]
19. Silva, F.D.; Gregori, F.; McDonald, S.M. Distinguishing the genotype 1 genes and proteins of human Wa-like rotaviruses vs. porcine rotaviruses. *Infect. Genet. Evol.* **2016**, *43*, 6–14. [CrossRef]
20. Theuns, S.; Heylen, E.; Zeller, M.; Roukaerts, I.D.; Desmarets, L.M.; Van Ranst, M.; Nauwynck, H.J.; Matthijnssens, J. Complete genome characterisation of recent and ancient Belgian pig Group A rotaviruses and assessment of their evolutionary relationship with human rotaviruses. *J. Virol.* **2015**, *89*, 1043–1057. [CrossRef]
21. Doro, R.; Farkas, S.L.; Martella, V.; Banyai, K. Zoonotic transmission of rotavirus: Surveillance and control. *Expert Rev. Anti. Infect. Ther.* **2015**, *13*, 1337–1350. [CrossRef]
22. Cowley, D.; Donato, C.M.; Roczo-Farkas, S.; Kirkwood, C.D. Novel G10P[14] Rotavirus Strain, Northern Territory, Australia. *Emerg. Infect. Dis.* **2013**, *19*, 1324–1327. [CrossRef]
23. Komoto, S.; Tacharoenmuang, R.; Guntapong, R.; Ide, T.; Sinchai, P.; Upachai, S.; Fukuda, S.; Yoshikawa, T.; Tharmaphornpilas, P.; Sangkitporn, S.; et al. Identification and characterisation of a human G9P[23] rotavirus strain from a child with diarrhoea in Thailand: Evidence for porcine-to-human interspecies transmission. *J. Gen. Virol.* **2017** *98*, 532–538. [CrossRef] [PubMed]
24. Malasao, R.; Khamrin, P.; Kumthip, K.; Ushijima, H.; Maneekarn, N. Complete genome sequence analysis of rare G4P[6] rotavirus strains from human and pig reveals the evidence for interspecies transmission. *Infect. Genet. Evol.* **2018**, *65*, 357–368. [CrossRef] [PubMed]

25. Mukherjee, A.; Ghosh, S.; Bagchi, P.; Dutta, D.; Chattopadhyay, S.; Kobayashi, N.; Chawla-Sarkar, M. Full genomic analyses of human rotavirus G4P[4], G4P[6], G9P[19] and G10P[6] strains from north-eastern India: Evidence for interspecies transmission and complex reassortment events. *Clin. Microbiol. Infect.* **2011**, *17*, 1343–1346. [CrossRef] [PubMed]
26. My, P.V.; Rabaa, M.A.; Donato, C.; Cowley, D.; Phat, V.V.; Dung, T.T.; Anh, P.H.; Vinh, H.; Bryant, J.E.; Kellam, P.; et al. Novel porcine-like human G26P[19] rotavirus identified in hospitalised paediatric diarrhoea patients in Ho Chi Minh City, Vietnam. *J. Gen. Virol.* **2014**, *95*, 2727–2733. [CrossRef] [PubMed]
27. Quaye, O.; Roy, S.; Rungsrisuriyachai, K.; Esona, M.D.; Xu, Z.; Tam, K.I.; Banegas, D.J.; Rey-Benito, G.; Bowen, M.D. Characterisation of a rare, reassortant human G10P[14] rotavirus strain detected in Honduras. *Mem. Inst. Oswaldo Cruz.* **2018**, *113*, 9–16. [CrossRef] [PubMed]
28. Tacharoenmuang, R.; Komoto, S.; Guntapong, R.; Ide, T.; Singchai, P.; Upachai, S.; Fukuda, S.; Yoshida, Y.; Murata, T.; Yoshikawa, T.; et al. Characterisation of a G10P[14] rotavirus strain from a diarrhoeic child in Thailand: Evidence for bovine-to-human zoonotic transmission. *Infect. Genet. Evol.* **2018**, *63*, 43–57. [CrossRef]
29. Bwogi, J.; Jere, K.C.; Karamagi, C.; Byarugaba, D.K.; Namuwulya, P.; Baliraine, F.N.; Desselberger, U.; Iturriza-Gomara, M. Whole genome analysis of selected human and animal rotaviruses identified in Uganda from 2012 to 2014 reveals complex genome reassortment events between human, bovine, caprine and porcine strains. *PLoS ONE* **2017**, *12*, e0178855. [CrossRef]
30. Matthijnssens, J.; Bilcke, J.; Ciarlet, M.; Martella, V.; Bányai, K.; Rahman, M.; Zeller, M.; Beutels, P.; Van Damme, P.; Van Ranst, M. Rotavirus disease and vaccination: Impact on genotype diversity. *Future Microbiol.* **2009**, *4*, 1303–1316. [CrossRef]
31. Nyaga, M.M.; Jere, K.C.; Esona, M.D.; Seheri, M.L.; Stucker, K.M.; Halpin, R.A.; Akopov, A.; Stockwell, T.B.; Peenze, I.; Diop, A.; et al. Whole genome detection of rotavirus mixed infections in human, porcine and bovine samples co-infected with various rotavirus strains collected from sub-Saharan Africa. *Infect. Genet. Evol.* **2015**, *31*, 321–334. [CrossRef]
32. Beards, G.; Graham, C. Temporal distribution of rotavirus G-serotypes in the West Midlands region of the United Kingdom, 1983–1994. *J. Diarrhoeal Dis. Res.* **1995**, *13*, 235–237.
33. Bok, K.; Castagnaro, N.; Borsa, A.; Nates, S.; Espul, C.; Fay, O.; Fabri, A.; Grinstein, S.; Miceli, I.; Matson, D.O.; et al. Surveillance for rotavirus in Argentina. *J. Med. Virol.* **2001**, *65*, 190–198. [CrossRef] [PubMed]
34. Esona, M.D.; Armah, G.E.; Geyer, A.; Steele, A.D. Detection of an unusual human rotavirus strain with G5P[8] specificity in a Cameroonian child with diarrhoea. *J. Clin. Microbiol.* **2004**, *42*, 441–444. [CrossRef] [PubMed]
35. Esona, M.D.; Geyer, A.; Banyai, K.; Page, N.; Aminu, M.; Armah, G.E.; Hull, J.; Steele, D.A.; Glass, R.I.; Gentsch, J.R. Novel human rotavirus genotype G5P[7] from child with diarrhoea, Cameroon. *Emerg. Infect. Dis.* **2009**, *15*, 83–86. [CrossRef] [PubMed]
36. Gouvea, V.; de Castro, L.; Timenetsky Mdo, C.; Greenberg, H.; Santos, N. Rotavirus serotype G5 associated with diarrhoea in Brazilian children. *J. Clin. Microbiol.* **1994**, *32*, 1408–1409. Erratum appears in *J. Clin. Microbiol.* **1994**, *32*, 1834. [CrossRef] [PubMed]
37. Hwang, K.P.; Wu, F.T.; Bányai, K.; Wu, H.S.; Yang, D.C.; Huang, Y.C.; Lin, J.S.; Hsiung, C.A.; Huang, J.C.; Jiang, B.; et al. Identification of porcine rotavirus-like genotype P[6] strains in Taiwanese children. *J. Med. Microbiol.* **2012**, *61*, 990–997. [CrossRef]
38. Lorenzetti, E.; Da Silva Medeiros, T.N.; Alfieri, A.F.; Alfieri, A.A. Genetic heterogeneity of wild-type G4P[6] porcine rotavirus strains detected in a diarrhoea outbreak in a regularly vaccinated pig herd. *Vet. Microbiol.* **2011**, *154*, 191–196. [CrossRef]
39. Martella, V.; Ciarlet, M.; Bányai, K.; Lorusso, E.; Cavalli, A.; Corrente, M.; Elia, G.; Arista, S.; Camero, M.; Desario, C.; et al. Identification of a novel VP4 genotype carried by a serotype G5 porcine rotavirus strain. *Virology* **2006**, *346*, 301–311. [CrossRef]
40. Nyaga, M.M.; Tan, Y.; Seheri, M.L.; Halpin, R.A.; Akopov, A.; Stucker, K.M.; Fedorova, N.B.; Shrivastava, S.; Duncan Steele, A.; Mwenda, J.M.; et al. Whole-genome sequencing and analyses identify high genetic heterogeneity, diversity and endemicity of rotavirus genotype P[6] strains circulating in Africa. *Infect. Genet. Evol.* **2018**, *63*, 79–88. [CrossRef]

41. Li, D.D.; Duan, Z.J.; Zhang, Q.; Liu, N.; Xie, Z.P.; Jiang, B.; Steele, D.; Jiang, X.; Wang, Z.S.; Fang, Z.Y. Molecular characterisation of unusual human G5P[6] rotaviruses identified in China. *J. Clin. Virol.* **2008**, *42*, 141–148. [CrossRef]
42. Ahmed, K.; Dang, D.A.; Nakagomi, O. Rotavirus G5P[6] in child with diarrhoea, Vietnam. *Emerg. Infect. Dis.* **2007**, *13*, 1232–1235. [CrossRef]
43. Chieochansin, T.; Vutithanachot, V.; Phumpholsup, T.; Posuwan, N.; Theamboonlers, A.; Poovorawan, Y. The prevalence and genotype diversity of Human Rotavirus A circulating in Thailand, 2011–2014. *Infect. Genet. Evol.* **2016**, *37*, 129–136. [CrossRef]
44. Duan, Z.J.; Li, D.D.; Zhang, Q.; Liu, N.; Huang, C.P.; Jiang, X.; Jiang, B.; Glass, R.; Steele, D.; Tang, J.Y.; et al. Novel human rotavirus of genotype G5P[6] identified in a stool specimen from a Chinese girl with diarrhoea. *J. Clin. Microbiol.* **2007**, *45*, 1614–1617. [CrossRef] [PubMed]
45. Komoto, S.; Maeno, Y.; Tomita, M.; Matsuoka, T.; Ohfu, M.; Yodoshi, T.; Akeda, H.; Taniguchi, K. Whole genomic analysis of a porcine-like human G5P[6] rotavirus strain isolated from a child with diarrhoea and encephalopathy in Japan. *J. Gen. Virol.* **2013**, *94*, 1568–1575. [CrossRef] [PubMed]
46. Mladenova, Z.; Papp, H.; Lengyel, G.; Kisfali, P.; Steyer, A.; Steyer, A.F.; Esona, M.D.; Iturriza-Gómara, M.; Bányai, K. Detection of rare reassortant G5P[6] rotavirus, Bulgaria. *Infect. Genet. Evol.* **2012**, *12*, 1676–1684. [CrossRef] [PubMed]
47. Chilengi, R.; Rudd, C.; Bolton, C.; Guffey, B.; Masumbu, P.K.; Stringer, J. Successes, challenges and lessons learned in accelerating introduction of rotavirus immunisation in Zambia. *World J. Vaccines* **2015**, *5*, 43–53. [CrossRef]
48. Zambia Ministry of Health. The 2012 Annual Health Statistical Bulletin. 2014. Available online: https://www.moh.gov.zm/docs/reports/2012_Annual_Health_Statistical_Bulletin_Version_1.pdf (accessed on 18 March 2020).
49. Mpabalwani, M.; Oshitani, H.; Kasolo, F.; Mizuta, K.; Luo, N.; Matsubayashi, N.; Bhat, G.; Suzuki, H.; Numazaki, Y. Rotavirus gastro-enteritis in hospitalised children with acute diarrhoea in Zambia. *Ann. Trop. Paediatr.* **1995**, *15*, 39–43. [CrossRef]
50. Mpabalwani, E.M.; Simwaka, C.J.; Mwenda, J.M.; Mubanga, C.P.; Monze, M.; Matapo, B.; Parashar, U.D.; Tate, J.E. Impact of rotavirus vaccination on diarrhoeal Hospitalisations in children aged <5 Years in Lusaka, Zambia. *Clin. Infect. Dis.* **2016**, *62*, S183–S187. [CrossRef]
51. Mpabalwani, E.M.; Simwaka, J.C.; Mwenda, J.M.; Matapo, B.; Parashar, U.D.; Tate, J.E. Sustained impact of rotavirus vaccine on rotavirus hospitalisations in Lusaka, Zambia, 2009–2016. *Vaccine* **2018**, *36*, 7165–7169. [CrossRef]
52. WHO Vaccine-Preventable Diseases: Monitoring System. 2020 Global Summary. Available online: https://apps.who.int/immunization_monitoring/globalsummary/countries?countrycriteria%5Bcountry%5D%5B%5D=ZMB (accessed on 7 August 2020).
53. Mwenda, J.M.; Tate, J.E.; Parashar, U.D.; Mihigo, R.; Agócs, M.; Serhan, F.; Nshimirimana, D. African Rotavirus Surveillance Network: A brief overview. *Pediatr. Infect. Dis. J.* **2014**, *33*, S6–S8. [CrossRef]
54. Mwenda, J.M.; Burke, R.M.; Shaba, K.; Mihigo, R.; Tevi-Benissan, M.C.; Mumba, M.; Biey, J.N.; Cheikh, D.; Poy, A.; Zawaira, F.R.; et al. Implementation of rotavirus surveillance and vaccine introduction—World Health Organization African region, 2007–2016. *Morb. Mortal. Wkly. Rep.* **2017**, *66*, 1192–1196. [CrossRef]
55. Mwenda, J.M.; Ntoto, K.M.; Abebe, A.; Enweronu-Laryea, C.; Amina, I.; Mchomvu, J.; Kisakye, A.; Mpabalwani, E.M.; Pazvakavambwa, I.; Armah, G.E.; et al. Burden and epidemiology of rotavirus diarrhoea in selected African countries: Preliminary results from the African Rotavirus Surveillance Network. *J. Infect. Dis.* **2010**, *202*, S5–S11. [CrossRef] [PubMed]
56. Dong, H.J.; Qian, Y.; Huang, T.; Zhu, R.N.; Zhao, L.Q.; Zhang, Y.; Li, R.C.; Li, Y.P. Identification of circulating porcine-human reassortant G4P[6] rotavirus from children with acute diarrhoea in China by whole genome analyses. *Infect. Genet. Evol.* **2013**, *20*, 155–162. [CrossRef] [PubMed]
57. Yahiro, T.; Takaki, M.; Chandrasena, T.G.A.; Rajindrajith, S.; Iha, H.; Ahmed, K. Human-porcine reassortant rotavirus generated by multiple reassortment events in a Sri Lankan child with diarrhoea. *Infect. Genet. Evol.* **2018**, *65*, 170–186. [CrossRef] [PubMed]
58. Zhou, X.; Wang, Y.H.; Ghosh, S.; Tang, W.F.; Pang, B.B.; Liu, M.Q.; Peng, J.S.; Zhou, D.J.; Kobayashi, N. Genomic characterisation of G3P[6], G4P[6] and G4P[8] human rotaviruses from Wuhan, China: Evidence for interspecies transmission and reassortment events. *Infect. Genet. Evol.* **2015**, *33*, 55–71. [CrossRef] [PubMed]

59. Heylen, E.; Likele, B.B.; Zeller, M.; Stevens, S.; De Coster, S.; Conceição-Neto, N.; Van Geet, C.; Jacobs, J.; Ngbonda, D.; Van Ranst, M.; et al. Rotavirus surveillance in Kisangani, the Democratic Republic of the Congo, reveals a high number of unusual genotypes and gene segments of animal origin in non-vaccinated symptomatic children. *PLoS ONE* **2014**, *9*, e100953. [CrossRef] [PubMed]
60. Kaneko, M.; Do, L.P.; Doan, Y.H.; Nakagomi, T.; Gauchan, P.; Agbemabiese, C.A.; Dang, A.D.; Nakagomi, O. Porcine-like G3P[6] and G4P[6] rotavirus A strains detected from children with diarrhoea in Vietnam. *Arch. Virol.* **2018**, *163*, 2261–2263. [CrossRef] [PubMed]
61. Phan, M.V.; Anh, P.H.; Cuong, N.V.; Munnink, B.B.; Hoek, L.; My, P.T.; Tri, T.N.; Bryant, J.E.; Baker, S.; Thwaites, G.; et al. Unbiased whole-genome deep sequencing of human and porcine stool samples reveals circulation of multiple groups of rotaviruses and a putative zoonotic infection. *Virus Evol.* **2016**, *2*, 1–15. [CrossRef]
62. Wang, Y.H.; Kobayashi, N.; Zhou, D.J.; Yang, Z.Q.; Zhou, X.; Peng, J.S.; Zhu, Z.R.; Zhao, D.F.; Liu, M.Q.; Gong, J. Molecular epidemiologic analysis of group A rotaviruses in adults and children with diarrhoea in Wuhan city, China, 2000–2006. *Arch. Virol.* **2007**, *152*, 669–685. [CrossRef]
63. da Silva, M.F.; Tort, L.F.; Goméz, M.M.; Assis, R.M.; Volotão, E.d.M.; de Mendonça, M.C.; Bello, G.; Leite, J.P. VP7 Gene of human rotavirus A genotype G5: Phylogenetic analysis reveals the existence of three different lineages worldwide. *J. Med. Virol.* **2011**, *83*, 357–366. [CrossRef]
64. Green, K.Y.; Hoshino, Y.; Ikegami, N. Sequence analysis of the gene encoding the serotype-specific glycoprotein (VP7) of two new human rotavirus serotypes. *Virology* **1989**, *168*, 429–433. [CrossRef]
65. Martella, V.; Bányai, K.; Ciarlet, M.; Iturriza-Gómara, M.; Lorusso, E.; De Grazia, S.; Arista, S.; Decaro, N.; Elia, G.; Cavalli, A.; et al. Relationships among porcine and human P[6] rotaviruses: Evidence that the different human P[6] lineages have originated from multiple interspecies transmission events. *Virology* **2006**, *344*, 509–519. [CrossRef] [PubMed]
66. Burke, B.; Bridger, J.C.; Desselberger, U. Temporal correlation between a single amino acid change in the VP4 of a porcine rotavirus and a marked change in pathogenicity. *Virology* **1994**, *202*, 754–759. [CrossRef] [PubMed]
67. Mackow, E.R.; Shaw, R.D.; Matsui, S.M.; Vo, P.T.; Dang, M.N.; Greenberg, H.B. The rhesus rotavirus gene encoding protein VP3: Location of amino acids involved in homologous and heterologous rotavirus neutralization and identification of a putative fusion region. *Proc. Natl. Acad. Sci. USA* **1988**, *85*, 645–649. [CrossRef] [PubMed]
68. Arias, C.F.; Romero, P.; Alvarez, V.; López, S. Trypsin activation pathway of rotavirus infectivity. *J. Virol.* **1996**, *70*, 5832–5839. [CrossRef] [PubMed]
69. Steyer, A.; Poljšak-Prijatelj, M.; Barlič-Maganja, D.; Marin, J. Human, porcine and bovine rotaviruses in Slovenia: Evidence of interspecies transmission and genome reassortment. *J. Gen. Virol.* **2008**, *89*, 1690–1698. [CrossRef]
70. Zeller, M.; Heylen, E.; De Coster, S.; Van Ranst, M.; Matthijnssens, J. Full genome characterisation of a porcine-like human G9P[6] rotavirus strain isolated from an infant in Belgium. *Infect. Genet. Evol.* **2012**, *12*, 1492–1500. [CrossRef]
71. Zhang, S.; McDonald, P.W.; Thompson, T.A.; Dennis, A.F.; Akopov, A.; Kirkness, E.F.; Patton, J.T.; McDonald, S.M. Analysis of human rotaviruses from a single location over an 18-Year time span suggests that protein co-adaption influences gene constellations. *J. Virol.* **2014**, *88*, 9842–9863. [CrossRef]
72. Ciarlet, M.; Ludert, J.E.; Liprandi, F. Comparative amino acid sequence analysis of the major outer capsid protein (VP7) of porcine rotaviruses with G3 and G5 serotype specificities isolated in Venezuela and Argentina. *Arch. Virol.* **1995**, *140*, 437–451. [CrossRef]
73. Dyall-Smith, M.L.; Lazdins, I.; Tregear, G.W.; Holmes, I.H. Location of the major antigenic sites involved in rotavirus serotype-specific neutralisation. *Proc. Natl. Acad. Sci. USA* **1986**, *83*, 3465–3468. [CrossRef]
74. Kobayashi, N.; Taniguchi, K.; Urasawa, S. Analysis of the newly identified neutralisation epitopes on VP7 of human rotavirus serotype 1. *J. Gen. Virol.* **1991**, *72*, 117–124. [CrossRef]
75. Green, K.Y.; Sears, J.F.; Taniguchi, K.; Midthun, K.; Hoshino, Y.; Gorziglia, M.; Nishikawa, K.; Urasawa, S.; Kapikian, A.Z.; Chanock, R.M. Prediction of human rotavirus serotype by nucleotide sequence analysis of the VP7 protein gene. *J. Virol.* **1988**, *62*, 1819–1823. [CrossRef] [PubMed]

76. Gorziglia, M.; Larralde, G.; Kapikian, A.Z.; Chanock, R.M. Antigenic relationships among human rotaviruses as determined by outer capsid protein VP4. *Proc. Natl. Acad. Sci. USA* **1990**, *87*, 7155–7159. [CrossRef] [PubMed]
77. Bányai, K.; Martella, V.; Jakab, F.; Melegh, B.; Szűcs, G. Sequencing and phylogenetic analysis of human genotype P[6] rotavirus strains detected in Hungary provides evidence for genetic heterogeneity within the P[6] VP4 gene. *J. Clin. Microbiol.* **2004**, *42*, 4338–4343. [CrossRef]
78. Potgieter, A.C.; Page, N.A.; Liebenberg, J.; Wright, I.M.; Landt, O.; van Dijk, A.A. Improved strategies for sequence-independent amplification and sequencing of viral double-stranded RNA genomes. *J. Gen. Virol.* **2009**, *90*, 1423–1432. [CrossRef]
79. Kearse, M.; Moir, R.; Wilson, A.; Stones-Havas, S.; Cheung, M.; Sturrock, S.; Buxton, S.; Cooper, A.; Markowitz, S.; Duran, C.; et al. Geneious Basic: An integrated and extendable desktop software platform for the organization and analysis of sequence data. *Bioinformatics* **2012**, *28*, 1647–1649. [CrossRef] [PubMed]
80. Edgar, R.C. MUSCLE: A multiple sequence alignment method with reduced time and space complexity. *BMC Bioinform.* **2004**, *5*, 1–19. [CrossRef]
81. Katoh, K.; Standley, D.M. MAFFT multiple sequence alignment software version 7: Improvements in performance and usability. *Mol. Biol. Evol.* **2013**, *30*, 772–780. [CrossRef]
82. Tamura, K.; Stecher, G.; Peterson, D.; Filipski, A.; Kumar, S. MEGA 6: Molecular evolutionary genetics analysis version 6.0. *Mol. Biol. Evol.* **2013**, *30*, 2725–2729. [CrossRef]
83. Guindon, S.; Gascuel, O. A simple, fast, and accurate algorithm to estimate large phylogenies by maximum likelihood. *Syst. Biol.* **2003**, *52*, 696–704. [CrossRef]
84. Felsenstein, J. Confidence Limits on Phylogenies: An approach using the bootstrap. *Evolution* **1985**, *39*, 783–791. [CrossRef]
85. Frazer, K.A.; Pachter, L.; Poliakov, A.; Rubin, E.M.; Dubchak, I. VISTA: Computational tools for comparative genomics. *Nucleic Acids Res.* **2004**, *32*, 273–279. [CrossRef] [PubMed]

# Multiple Introductions and Predominance of Rotavirus Group A Genotype G3P[8] in Kilifi, Coastal Kenya, 4 Years after Nationwide Vaccine Introduction

Mike J. Mwanga [1], Jennifer R. Verani [2,3], Richard Omore [4], Jacqueline E. Tate [3], Umesh D. Parashar [3], Nickson Murunga [1], Elijah Gicheru [1], Robert F. Breiman [5], D. James Nokes [1,6] and Charles N. Agoti [1,7,*]

1. Kenya Medical Research Institute (KEMRI)-Wellcome Trust Research Programme, off Hospital Road, Kilifi 80108, Kenya; mikemwanga6@gmail.com (M.J.M.); nmurunga@kemri-wellcome.org (N.M.); egicheru@kemri-wellcome.org (E.G.); jnokes@kemri-wellcome.org (D.J.N.)
2. Centers for Disease Control and Prevention (CDC), KEMRI Complex, off Mbagathi Way, Village Market, Nairobi 00621, Kenya; qzr7@cdc.gov
3. Centers for Disease Control and Prevention (CDC), Atlanta, GA 30333, USA; jqt8@cdc.gov (J.E.T.); uap2@cdc.gov (U.D.P.)
4. KEMRI, Center for Global Health Research (KEMRI-CGHR), Kisumu 00202, Kenya; omorerichard@gmail.com
5. Hubert Department of Global Health, Rollins School of Public Health, Emory University, Atlanta, GA 30322, USA; rfbreiman@emory.edu
6. School of Life Sciences and Zeeman Institute (SBIDER), The University of Warwick, Coventry CV4 7AL, UK
7. School of Health and Human Sciences, Pwani University, Kilifi 80108, Kenya
* Correspondence: cnyaigoti@kemri-wellcome.org

**Abstract:** Globally, rotavirus group A (RVA) remains a major cause of severe childhood diarrhea, despite the use of vaccines in more than 100 countries. RVA sequencing for local outbreaks facilitates investigation into strain composition, origins, spread, and vaccine failure. In 2018, we collected 248 stool samples from children aged less than 13 years admitted with diarrheal illness to Kilifi County Hospital, coastal Kenya. Antigen screening detected RVA in 55 samples (22.2%). Of these, VP7 (G) and VP4 (P) segments were successfully sequenced in 48 (87.3%) and phylogenetic analysis based on the VP7 sequences identified seven genetic clusters with six different GP combinations: G3P[8], G1P[8], G2P[4], G2P[8], G9P[8] and G12P[8]. The G3P[8] strains predominated the season ($n = 37$, 67.2%) and comprised three distinct G3 genetic clusters that fell within Lineage I and IX (the latter also known as equine-like G3 Lineage). Both the two G3 lineages have been recently detected in several countries. Our study is the first to document African children infected with G3 Lineage IX. These data highlight the global nature of RVA transmission and the importance of increasing global rotavirus vaccine coverage.

**Keywords:** gastroenteritis; rotavirus; G3[P8]; phylogenetics; equine-like

## 1. Introduction

Following progressive introduction of rotavirus vaccines into national immunization programs (NIP) of more than 100 countries since 2006, a significant decline of rotavirus group A (RVA) disease burden has occurred [1,2]. However, despite these successes, RVA remains a leading cause of diarrhea morbidity and mortality [3,4], resulting in an estimated 128,500 deaths annually among under-5-year-olds, a majority occurring in low-income settings [5]. Consistently, licensed oral RVA vaccines have underperformed in low-income settings compared with high-income settings [6,7]. After monovalent Rotarix® vaccine was introduced into Kenya's NIP in July 2014, with doses given at 6 and 10 weeks of life, a multi-site case-control study found an overall 2-dose vaccine effectiveness of only 64% (95% confidence interval (CI): 35–80%) in under-5-year-olds [8]. In England, the same vaccine showed effectiveness of 77% (95% CI: 66–85%) [9].

In humans, RVA immunity is partly conferred by neutralizing antibodies directed against the VP4 (protease-sensitive) and VP7 (glycoprotein) viral capsid surface proteins that define P and G types, respectively [10]. These two viral proteins are highly diverse, with up to 36 different G and 51 different P types recorded to-date [11], some of which predominantly infect non-human animal species [12]. Among other factors, the higher number of co-circulating GP genotypes in low-income settings has been proposed to be a potential contributor to rotavirus vaccine underperformance [6].

Currently, there are four licensed and WHO pre-qualified RVA vaccines; all live attenuated and administered orally, but with different strain compositions. These are monovalent Rotarix® (G1P[8]), pentavalent RotaTeq® (5 reassortant viruses; G1, G2, G3, G4 and G6 genotypes in combination with P[8]), monovalent ROTAVAC® (G9P[11]) and pentavalent ROTASIIL® (5 reassortant viruses; G1, G2, G3, G4 and G9). All four vaccines were shown to be largely cross-protective against heterotypic strains in both clinical trials and following vaccine implementation in several settings [6,13]. Paradoxically, post-vaccine rollout, outbreaks caused by strains heterotypic to the vaccine in use have been sometimes reported in countries, occurring in patterns seeming to be influenced by the vaccine regimen in use [14–16].

Recent genotyping studies of RVA have found increased proportions of G2P[4], G3P[8] and G12P[8] genotypes in rotavirus vaccinating countries [14,16–18]. These genotypes appeared to play only a minor role in the pre-vaccine era; thus, their increasing prevalence is consistent with increased capacity in escaping vaccine immunity [12,19]. Furthermore, there have been several reports of human infection with equine-like G3 viruses suggestive of greater human vulnerability to antigenically novel RVA strains [20–29]. At the Kenya Medical Research Institute (KEMRI)—Wellcome Trust Research Programme (KWTRP), we have maintained a RVA surveillance at Kilifi County Hospital (KCH), located in rural coastal Kenya since 2009 [30]. The aim of the current analysis was to determine the genetic relatedness of the strains that were in circulation in the 2018 RVA season in Kilifi, their origins, global phylogenetic context, and role in the local sub-optimal vaccine performance.

## 2. Results

### 2.1. Study Population Characteristics

Between January and December 2018, 384 children aged less than 13 years were admitted to KCH with diarrhea as one of their illness symptoms. Of these, 208 (54.2%) were Kilifi Health and Demographic surveillance system (KHDSS) area residents (Figure S1). A stool sample was obtained from 248 (64.6%). The main reasons for non-sampling were death ($n = 13$), discharge or transfer before sample collection ($n = 22$), consent refusal ($n = 52$), or other ($n = 16$). Among study eligible children ($n = 384$), the distribution of the sampled and not sampled children differed significantly across age strata ($p = 0.002$) and discharge outcome ($p < 0.001$), Table 1. The distribution of the sampled and not sampled children were similar across sexes and by rotavirus vaccine eligibility status. The majority of the eligible participants were aged less than 2 years (68.2%) and were age eligible to have received one or two doses of rotavirus vaccine (83.6%). By EIA testing, RVA was detected in 55 children (22.2%), Figure 1a, 32 (58.1%) of which were KHDSS area residents. Fifty-one (92.7%) of the RVA positive children were age eligible to have received two doses of the RVA vaccine. Of these, the vaccination status was known for 36 (70.6%), of which 29 (80.6%) were confirmed to have received two doses of Rotarix® vaccine while the remainder (19.4%) received one dose, Table 1.

**Table 1.** A comparison of demographic characteristics of children with diarrhea admitted to Kilifi County Hospital (KCH) that were sampled versus those who were not sampled in 2018 and those that were RVA positive versus those that were RVA negative.

| Characteristic | All (%) | Sampled (%) | Unsampled (%) | p Value $ | RVA + ve (%) | RVA − ve (%) | p Value * |
|---|---|---|---|---|---|---|---|
| Number of patients | 384 | 248 (64.6) | 136 (35.4) | | 55 (22.2) | 193 (77.8) | |
| Sex | | | | 0.728 | | | 0.008 |
| Male | 210 (54.7) | 134 (54.0) | 76 (55.9) | | 21 (38.2) | 113 (58.6) | |
| Female | 174 (45.3) | 114 (46.0) | 60 (44.1) | | 34 (61.8) | 80 (41.5) | |
| Age | | | | | | | |
| Mean (SD) ¶ | 27.4 (29.9) | 26.4 (31.8) | 29.3 (26.1) | 0.352 | 19.6 (15.0) | 28.3 (35.0) | 0.073 |
| Median (IQR) δ | 16.8 (9.8–29.3) | 15.1 (9.4–24.1) | 19.9 (12.0–39.0) | 0.025 | 15.4 (9.9–20.8) | 15.1 (8.9–24.9) | 1.000 |
| Age group | | | | 0.002 | | | 0.254 |
| 0–11 months | 126 (32.8) | 92 (37.1) | 34 (25.0) | | 19 (34.6) | 73 (37.8) | |
| 12–23 months | 136 (35.4) | 92 (37.1) | 44 (32.4) | | 25 (45.5) | 67 (34.7) | |
| 24–59 months | 73 (19.0) | 34 (13.7) | 39 (28.7) | | 8 (14.6) | 26 (14.0) | |
| >60 months | 49 (12.8) | 30 (12.1) | 19 (14.0) | | 3 (5.5) | 27 (14.0) | |
| RVA vaccine eligibility | | | | 0.327 | | | 0.063 |
| Age eligible 2 dose | 317 (82.6) | 204 (82.3) | 113 (83.1) | | 51 (92.7) | 153 (79.3) | |
| Age eligible 1 dose | 4 (1.0) | 4 (1.6) | 0 (0.0) | | 0 (0.0) | 4 (2.1) | |
| Age ineligible | 63 (16.4) | 40 (16.1) | 23 (16.9) | | 4 (7.3) | 36 (18.7) | |
| Vaccination status (n = 321) | | | | 0.273 | | | 0.209 |
| Two dose eligible & received 2 doses | 165 (51.4) | 111 (53.4) | 54 (47.8) | | 29 (56.9) | 82 (52.2) | |
| Two dose eligible & received 1 dose | 24 (7.5) | 17 (8.2) | 7 (6.2) | | 7 (13.7) | 10 (6.2) | |
| One or 2 dose eligible but received none | 6 (1.8) | 2 (1.0) | 4 (3.5) | | 0 (0.0) | 2 (1.3) | |
| One or 2 dose eligible but status unknown | 126 (39.3) | 78 (37.5) | 48 (42.5) | | 15 (29.4) | 63 (40.1) | |
| Outcome (n = 379) | | | | <0.001 | | | 0.194 |
| Died | 38 (10.0) | 13 (5.3) | 25 (18.9) | | | 12 (6.3) | |
| Alive | 341 (90.0) | 234 (94.7) | 133 (81.1) | | | 180 (93.8) | |

¶ SD stands for standard deviation; δ IQR stands for interquartile range; $ p value for comparison of sampled and not sampled groups; * p value for comparison of RVA positive and negative groups.

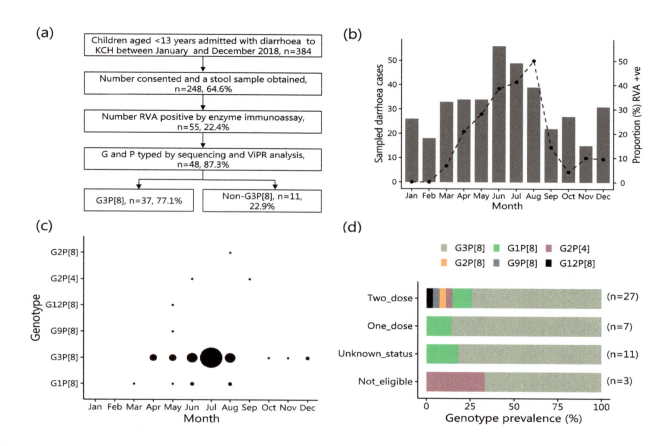

**Figure 1.** Summary of rotavirus group A (RVA) surveillance in Kilifi County Hospital (KCH) in 2018 and identified genotypes. Panel (**a**) sample flowgram from patient recruitment to VP4 and VP7 genotyping results for the RVA positives. Panel (**b**) monthly cases of diarrhea in children aged less than 13 years recorded at KCH in 2018 (grey bars) compared with monthly proportions of RVA positive samples (black dashed line on the secondary axis). Panel (**c**) the number of RVA positive samples by month in 2018 and by the GP genotype. The black circle size is proportional to the number of samples (the smallest indicates one sample and the largest is 13 samples). Panel (**d**) genotypes identified in children according to rotavirus vaccination status.

## 2.2. Characteristics of the RVA Infections and the Infected Children

RVA prevalence was higher in female compared to male children admitted with diarrhea (29.8% vs. 15.7%, $p = 0.008$), Table 1. RVA was detected in all months of 2018 except January and February Figure 1b. Diarrhea cases peaked in June while RVA prevalence peaked in August (50% of all collected samples were RVA positive). Sequencing and GP typing was successful for 48 (87.3%) of the 55 RVA-positive samples. Five G types (G1, G2, G3, G9 and G12) and two P types (P[4] and P[8]) were identified in the successfully sequenced samples. From these, six GP combinations were identified, namely: G3P[8] ($n = 37$, 77.1%), G1P[8] ($n = 6$, 12.5%), G2P[4] ($n = 2$, 4.2%), G2P[8] ($n = 1$, 2.1%), G9P[8] ($n = 1$, 2.1%) and G12P[8] ($n = 1$, 2.1%). The G3P[8] and G1P[8] strains were the only genotypes detected for > 2 months while the other four genotypes were detected sporadically (1–2 months), Figure 1c. The distribution of the infecting genotype (summarized as G3P[8] versus non-G3P[8]) did not diff significantly by sex, patient age, vaccination status or discharge outcome, Table 2 and Figure 1d.

**Table 2.** Characteristics of children whom were infected with rotavirus G3P[8] versus those whom were infected with non-G3P[8].

| Characteristic | Genotyped RVA (%) | G3P[8] (%) | Non-G3P[8] (%) | p Value |
|---|---|---|---|---|
| Number of patients | 48 | 37 (77.1) | 11 (22.9) | |
| Sex | | | | 0.248 |
| Male | 19 (39.6) | 13 (35.1) | 6 (55.6) | |
| Female | 29 (60.4) | 24 (64.9) | 5 (45.5) | |
| Age | | | | |
| Mean (SD #) | 19.3 (14.8) | 19.2 (13.3) | 19.5 (18.6) | 0.946 |
| Median (IQR δ) | 15.7 (9.9–20.4) | 15.9 (9.8–20.4) | 15.4 (7.8–23.1) | 1.000 |
| Age group | | | | 0.770 |
| 0–11 months | 17 (35.4) | 13 (35.1) | 4 (36.4) | |
| 12–23 months | 22 (45.8) | 17 (46.0) | 5 (45.6) | |
| 24–59 months | 7 (14.6) | 6 (16.2) | 1 (9.1) | |
| >60 months | 2 (4.2) | 1 (2.7) | 1 (9.1) | |
| RVA vaccine eligibility | | | | 0.658 |
| Age eligible 2 dose | 45 (93.8) | 35 (94.6) | 10 (90.9) | |
| Age eligible 1 dose | 0 (0.0) | 0 (0.0) | 0 (0.0) | |
| Age ineligible | 3 (6.3) | 2 (5.4) | 1 (9.1) | |
| RVA vaccination status among eligible (n = 45) | | | | 0.751 |
| Two dose eligible & received two doses | 27 (60.0) | 20 (57.1) | 7 (70.0) | |
| Two dose eligible & received one dose | 7 (15.6) | 6 (17.1) | 1 (10.0) | |
| One or 2 dose eligible but received none | 0 (0.0) | 0 (0.0) | 0 (0.0) | |
| One or 2 dose eligible but status unknown | 11 (24.4) | 9 (25.7) | 2 (20.0) | |
| Outcome | | | | 0.064 |
| Died | 1 (2.1) | 0 (0.0) | 1 (9.1) | |
| Alive | 47 (97.2) | 37 (100.0) | 10 (90.9) | |

# SD stands for standard deviation, δ IQR stands for interquartile range.

## 2.3. Genetic Diversity in the Sequenced Viruses

For the VP4 segment, a 579 nt long region (~25%) was recovered for 47 viruses (88.5%) while for the VP7 segment, a 644 nt long region (~65%) was recovered for 48 viruses (87.3%). One virus (KEN/KLF0879/2018), genotyped G9P[8], yielded a significantly shorter VP4 fragment relative to the other viruses (<500 nt) due to low quality sequencing data and was excluded from subsequent analyses. Consistent with the greater number of assigned G types ($n = 5$) compared to P types ($n = 2$) types, the range of pairwise nt differences was much greater in the VP7 (up to 203 nt differences) compared to VP4 segment (up to 87 nt differences), Figure 2a,b, respectively. A multi-modal distribution of nt differences was observed for both VP4 and VP7 segments. A total of 328 (~51%) and 141 (~24%) SNP positions were identified in the sequenced VP7 and VP4 fragments, respectively. Of the 48 sequenced samples, 22 (45.8%) yielded unique VP7 sequences while 17 (36.2%) gave unique VP4 sequences.

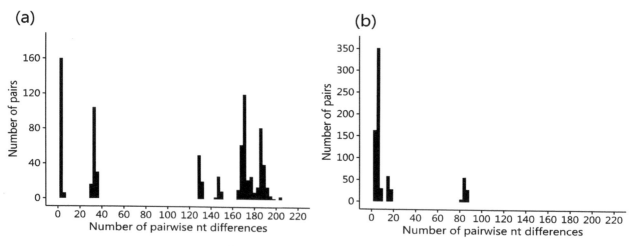

**Figure 2.** Genetic diversity in the sequenced RVA positives from Kilifi County Hospital (KCH). Panel (**a**) shows the distribution of pairwise nt differences in the sequenced portion of VP7 (644 nt long) of 48 RVA positives. Panel (**b**) shows the distribution of pairwise nt differences in the sequenced portion of VP4 (579 nt long) of 47 RVA positives.

## 2.4. Molecular Genetic Clusters

Using the range of pairwise nt differences observed in first modal distribution for the VP7 (0 to 20 nt differences, i.e., >97% nt similarity) to define a molecular genetic cluster, seven G clusters were assigned (named Clu_1-7). Members of a cluster were universally of same G type. All G type sequences identified to be of the same type formed a single cluster except G3P[8] that occurred in three clusters, named Clu_3/G3P[8], Clu_4/G3P[8] and Clu_5/G3P[8]. The temporal pattern of the assigned clusters is shown in Figure 3a. Most of the high incidence months (April to August) had multiple genetic clusters co-circulating, except for July, which had a single G3P[8] cluster. The reconstructed phylogenetic relationship between strains of the different G and P types sequenced is shown in Figure 3b,c. The VP7 phylogeny showed segregation of the seven clusters we identified from the pairwise nt difference analysis. The VP4 phylogeny showed less clear-cut phylogenetic clustering with respect to the assigned genetic clusters. The two phylogenies were not entirely congruent, a feature suggestive of reassortment in the local strains. The minimum spanning networks reconstructed for both the VP7 and VP4 sequences are shown in Figure 3d,e. Viruses in the same genetic cluster consistently had four or less nt differences to the closest next virus within the same genetic cluster.

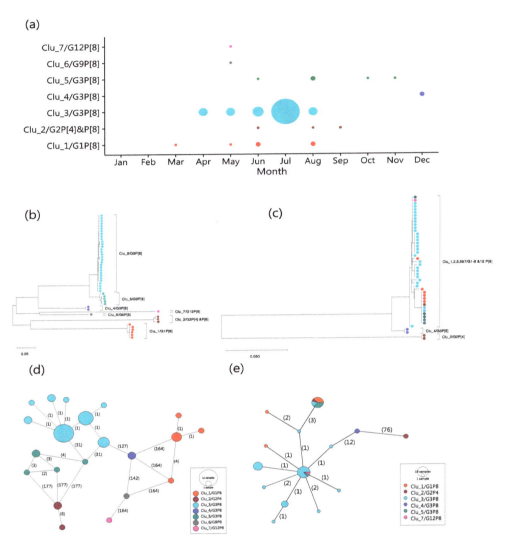

**Figure 3.** Temporal and genetic relatedness of the sequenced Kilifi rotaviruses. Panel (**a**) number of RVA positive samples by molecular genetic cluster and month. The circle sizes are proportional to the number of samples (the smallest indicates one sample and the largest is 13 samples). Panel (**b**) shows a Maximum Likelihood (ML) tree of the Kilifi 48 VP7 sequences. Panel (**c**) shows an ML tree of the Kilifi 47 VP4 sequences. Panel (**d**) shows the reconstructed POPART minimum spanning network from the 48 VP7 sequences. The vertexes represent the sequenced VP7 haplotypes. The size of the vertex is proportional to the number of haplotypes (identical sequences) and is colored by the assigned molecular genetic cluster. The numbers shown on the edges represent the number of nucleotide changes from one vertex (haplotype) to the next. Panel (**e**) same as panel (**d**) above but for the Kilifi 47 VP4 sequences.

## 2.5. Spatial Distribution of the Kilifi G3 Genetic Clusters

A few viruses in different VP7-based genetic clusters had identical VP4 sequences and we explored if these were spatially clustered. Twenty-eight of the 48 genotyped samples were from KHDSS area residents. The geographical distribution of all diarrhea admissions and the RVA positives by genetic cluster is shown in Figure S1. Cases of the predominant Clu_3/G3P[8] strains came from only a few locations although it appeared that road access (especially the Malindi-Mombasa highway) may have played a role in influencing which patients were turning up at KCH due to easier access.

## 2.6. Global Genetic Context of the Kilifi 2018 G3 Strains

A total of 338 G3 sequences from 26 countries fully met the criteria for inclusion as comparison data, including 39 previously collected in Kenya. The phylogeny derived from the combined Kilifi and global G3 viruses is shown in Figure 4a while Figure 4b shows the phylogenetic relatedness of all previous G3 sequences of RVA sampled in Kenya (5 locations including Kilifi).

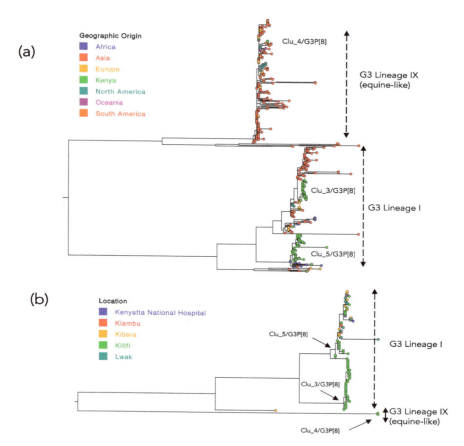

**Figure 4.** Global phylogeny derived from nucleotide sequences of G3 strains sampled between 2012–2018. (**a**) The phylogenetic tree reconstructed from 375 VP7 sequences of G3 type (338 collated from GenBank sampled across 26 countries including 39 from Kenya, and 37 G3 viruses sequenced in the current study) to determine the lineage and global context of the Kilifi sequences. The countries included were Australia, Belarus, Brazil, China, Dominican Republic, Ethiopia, Hungary, India, Indonesia, Italy, Japan, Kenya, South Korea, Kuwait, Nigeria, Pakistan, Peru, Russia, Spain, Taiwan, Thailand, USA, Uganda and Vietnam. The taxa for Kenya G3 sequences are provided by filled circles colored green and with the assigned Kilifi clusters names indicated next to the branches containing these sequences. Panel (**b**) a phylogeny of all Kenya G3 sequences ($n = 76$). The different colors of the filled circle symbols indicate the Kenya taxa distinguished by their location of sampling. The names assigned to the Kilifi clusters are indicated next to the nodes leading to their branches as similarly shown in panel (**a**).

A majority of the global viruses fell within two of nine previously identified G3 lineages [25]; Lineage I and equine-like G3 lineage (named Lineage IX). The Kilifi G3 sequences had representation in both these two lineages: Lineage I ($n = 35$, 94.6%) and equine-like G3 Lineage ($n = 2$, 5.6%). Viruses of the genetic cluster Clu_4/G3P[8] clustered with the equine-like G3 Lineage while the Kilifi G3 Lineage I viruses separated into two groups that corresponded to the Clu_3/G3P[8] cluster ($n = 30$) and the Clu_5/G3P[8] cluster ($n = 5$). The distribution of the pairwise nt differences in the compiled global G3 sequences dataset, like for the Kilifi G3 viruses, showed a multi-modal distribution (figure not shown). The first major trough was observed at 27 nt differences.

On applying the threshold used to identify the local molecular genetic clusters (>97% genetic similarity) on the global G3 dataset, 18 clusters were identified (Table S1). Of these, eight were singletons, six comprised of between 2 and 3 members and the remaining four clusters had 10, 47, 116 and 181 members. All the Kilifi G3 viruses fell in the three clusters that had the highest membership overall, Table S1. For each of the three Kilifi G3 genetic clusters we explored their closest genetic relative in the global dataset by network reconstructions (Figure 5). For the Kilifi Clu_3/G3P[8] the closest similar sequences were from India (G3P[8] collected in 2016) and Singapore (G3P[8] collected in 2016) that had 2 nucleotide differences Figure 5a. For the Kilifi Clu_4/G3P[8] (the equine-like G3 Lineage) the closest relative was from Taiwan (G3P[8] collected in 2016) with zero nucleotide difference in the sequenced region Figure 5b. For the Kilifi Clu_5/G3P[8] the closest relatives were from Kenya (G3P[6] collected in 2014) and Uganda (G3P[6] collected in 2013) that had zero and 2 nucleotide difference, respectively, Figure 5c. Overall, within these three major global G3 genetic clusters, clustering by country was common.

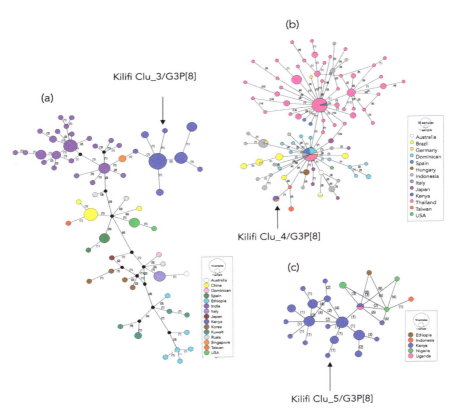

**Figure 5.** Haplotype network showing relationships of the identified global G3 lineages that included Kilifi viruses. Panel (**a**) shows the network for Lineage I cluster viruses that included the Kilifi Clu_3/G3P[8] strains. The vertices represent the VP7 haplotypes. The size of the vertex is proportional to the number of haplotypes (identical sequences) and is colored by the country of sampling. The numbers shown on the edges represent the number of nucleotide changes from one vertex (haplotype) to the next. Panel (**b**) and (**c**) have the same description as panel (**a**) above but represent Lineage IX (equine-like G3) cluster that included Kilifi Clu_4 G3P[8] and the Lineage I cluster that included Kilifi Clu_5 G3P[8] sequences, respectively.

## 3. Discussion

Four years after Kenya introduced Rotarix® vaccine into its NIP, multiple RVA GP genotypes circulated during the 2018 season in Kilifi, Kenya, with the G3P[8] genotype predominating at 67.2%. At this study site, the preceding two years (2016 and 2017) were dominated by the G2P[4] and G1P[8] genotypes, respectively, with only six cases of G3P[8] detected from September 2009 to December

2017 [30] and an additional three partially genotyped G3P[x] detected in 2013 [31]. The G3P[8] strains are partially heterotypic to the monovalent Rotarix® vaccine, which is comprised of an attenuated G1P[8] strain. During 2018, this local G3P[8] predominance is consistent with the previously documented season-to-season spatial-temporal fluctuations in the prevalence of RVA genotypes [12], hypothesized to be driven by the prevailing population-level immunity derived from natural infections and the use of vaccines [14].

Vaccination records were available for 70.6% of the children with an RVA positive test. Of these, 92.7% were age eligible to have received the two doses of Rotarix® vaccine and, in that subgroup, the vast majority (80.6%) had indeed received the full 2-dose series. However, overall, the vaccination status of these children did not appear to predict either their RVA diagnosis result or the infecting GP genotype. These findings, albeit from a single season and site, suggest that for these children who acquired an RVA infection despite one or two-dose vaccination, host factors rather than viral characteristics or vaccine composition may explain the vaccine failures. A follow-up study is planned.

At least seven distinct genetic clusters constituted the 2018 coastal Kenya RVA season. The VP7 sequences showed greater genetic diversity and provided a better phylogenetic resolution compared to the VP4 sequences. Each of the identified G types corresponded to a single genetic cluster except G3 viruses that segregated into three genetically distinct clusters. Strikingly, some samples with different G types yielded identical VP4 sequences, indicating that some of the children may have been infected by reassortant viruses or harbored mixed infections [25]. Our analyses improve understanding on the recent composition and transmission patterns of local RVA seasons, providing insight into the design of final stretch RVA control strategies following vaccine introduction.

Several recent studies have reported the increased proportion of G3P[8] strains, e.g., in Australia [14], Japan [32], Thailand [28], Indonesia [29], Pakistan [33], Dominican Republic [25], Brazil [34], Spain [20], Mozambique [24], Malawi [35] and Botswana [36]. The global G3 sequences available from GenBank showed extensive genetic diversity. The significance of this diversity in relation to human immune recognition should be investigated. Notably, recent years have also observed the emergence and global spread of a new G3 lineage named equine-like G3, of putative equine origin, assigned G3 Lineage IX [25]. Strains of G3 Lineage IX were first detected in 2013 in Japan and have since been widely detected in several other countries (Australia [21], Taiwan (unpublished data in GenBank), Indonesia [29], Thailand [28], USA [26], Dominican Republic [25], Brazil [34], Italy [23], Germany [27], Hungary [22] and Spain [20]). Our study is the first to document African children infection with the G3 Lineage IX. Continued surveillance to monitor whether this particular strain becomes endemic in Kenya and the wider Africa continent in the face of increased RVA vaccine coverage is important to optimize RVA vaccine-mediated control. Notably, recent studies in Botswana [36], Mozambique [24], Malawi [35] and Ethiopia [37] reported increased prevalence of G3 type viruses but sequencing data from these studies are not yet available.

Based on sequence data deposited in GenBank, the predominant Kilifi G3 cluster (Clu_3/G3P[8]) was the second most common genetic cluster globally. The closest sequences were from Singapore and India, both countries that did not yet have RVA vaccine in their NIP in 2018. The second most prevalent Kilifi G3 genetic cluster was Clu_5/G3P[8]. Notably, this cluster has not been detected frequently around the globe and the closest genetic links were Kenyan strains collected in Kiambu County (Central province) in July and August 2014 [38], Kilifi in 2017, and strains from Ethiopia (collection date: April 2016 [39]) and Uganda (collection date: January 2013 [40]), neighboring countries which included RVA vaccines in their NIP in 2013 and 2018, respectively. Although the Kilifi Clu_4/G3P[8] (equine-like G3 Lineage) was the least prevalent locally, it was the most prevalent globally. The closest relatives to the Kenyan strains were from Taiwan, a country yet to introduce RVA vaccination.

This study had some limitations. First, the sequence data from the cohort represents a single site and one season. Second, we only sequenced portions of the VP4 and VP7 segments. Whereas these data were adequate to assign genotypes, lineages and estimate the number of genetic clusters, whole genome sequences provide a better resolution in examining reassortment events, evolution in internal genes and studying genetic clusters [18,25,41]. Third, to determine the origin and pathways of spread of the imported genetic clusters, background sequence data from more countries and including populations neighboring coastal Kenya would have been ideal. Unfortunately, sequence data in public sequence databases to facilitate such phylogeographic analysis are currently limited. Fourth, the absence of significant epidemiological data for some variables e.g., vaccine status for ~30% of the RVA positive children and geographic origin for children from outside the KHDSS area limited our analyses.

In conclusion, the finding that >20% of diarrheal stools from children admitted to KCH with diarrhea in 2018 were RVA positive highlights that RVA is still a significant contributor to severe childhood diarrhea in coastal Kenya, despite the introduction of Rotarix® into Kenya's NIP in 2014. The cross-continent detection of the emerging equine-like G3 viruses and other typical human G3 strains demonstrates the global nature of RVA transmission. Strikingly, strains found circulating in the Kilifi population were most closely related to strains circulating in countries that were yet to introduce RVA vaccines into their NIP. This observation reminds of the global connectedness regarding pathogen movement and emphasizes the importance of vaccinating all eligible populations across the world, as failure to do so builds a reservoir for strains that continue to seed transmission in vaccinated populations. Identifying factors responsible for RVA vaccine underperformance in low-income settings is a priority research area that may support efforts to further reduce RVA burden. Our study did not ascertain that viral genetic diversity is a contributor to the vaccine underperformance in this setting. Studies investigating the relationship between RVA vaccine immunogenicity and infant characteristics, such as malnutrition, age at first RVA dose, concomitant receipt of oral polio vaccine (OPV), enteric co-infections and enteric dysbiosis may provide better insight into RVA vaccine performance characteristics.

## 4. Materials and Methods

### 4.1. Study Population and Location

KCH is the main referral hospital in Kilifi County (population size ~1.5 million people). The major economic activities in the county are subsistence farming, fishing and tourism [42]. An area around KCH (~900 km$^2$ with a population of ~300,000 people) is monitored by the KWTRP and is known as the KHDSS area [42], Figure S1. A high proportion of the patients seeking care at the KCH are KHDSS area residents [42]. Vaccination data of admitted children were collected using an electronic registry [8,43,44].

In the current analysis, stool samples were collected from eligible and consented pediatric patients admitted to KCH between January and December 2018 (the surveillance period), as part of the ongoing rotavirus surveillance program [8,31,43]. All children aged <13 years old admitted with diarrhea (defined as passing three or more watery stools in the last 24-h) were eligible for inclusion [8,31,43]. Following a review of demographic and clinical data collected by a clinical staff, parents or caregivers of eligible children were approached for consent, and a single stool sample was collected. The samples were immediately transferred into a cool box with ice blocks before transportation to the KWTRP for RVA testing and long-term storage at −80 °C.

### 4.2. Specimen Laboratory Processing

RVA in the stool samples was detected using ProSpecT™ enzyme immunoassay (EIA) kit (Oxoid, Basingstoke, UK) following the manufacturer's instructions. RVA positive samples were amplified in the VP4 and VP7 segments using One-step Reverse Transcriptase PCR Kit (Qiagen, Valencia, CA, USA) using previously published primers [45,46]. Successful amplification of the target regions was confirmed by the presence of expected bands (VP4: 660 bp and VP7: 881 bp) following gel electrophoresis of the PCR products. Products from successful PCRs were purified using GFX DNA purification kit (GFX-Amersham, Amersham, UK) and sequenced bi-directionally (both in forward and reverse directions) using Big Dye Terminator 3.1 (Applied Biosystems, Foster City, CA, USA) chemistry. The primers used during PCR amplification were used for sequencing on an ABI Prism 3130xl Genetic Analyzer (Applied Biosystems, Foster City, CA, USA).

### 4.3. Genotyping and Phylogenetic Analysis

The sequence reads were assembled using Sequencher v5.4.6 (Gene Codes Corp Inc., Ann Arbor, MI, USA). Nucleotide (nt) sequence alignments were prepared using MAFFT v7.222 and visualized using Aliview v1.8. G and P genotypes were determined using Virus Pathogen Resource (ViPR) online classification tool [47]. The best nt substitution model for the alignments were determined IQ-Tree v1.6.6 [48]. Phylogenetic trees were reconstructed using the maximum likelihood (ML) method in RaxML v8.2.12 [49] and MEGA v7 [50]. Support for the tree branching patterns was evaluated by 1000 bootstrap iterations.

### 4.4. Genetic Clusters

Molecular genetic clusters were defined from the distribution of pairwise nt differences of VP7 segment sequences. Pairwise nt differences were determined using pairsnp (https://github.com/gtonkinhill/pairsnp/). Viruses within the same molecular genetic clusters were those which pairwise nt differences occurred within the first modal distribution. Using this threshold, clusters were identified using the USEARCH algorithm [51]. Single nucleotide polymorphic (SNP) positions in alignments were assessed using parseSNP [52]. The minimum spanning networks between the RVA positive patients were reconstructed using POPART v1.70 program [53].

### 4.5. Comparison Dataset

The phylogenetic context of the locally predominant genotype in global RVA populations was investigated by co-analysis with similar G type strains sequence data deposited in GenBank. The search in GenBank was conducted in October 2020. The criteria for comparison data inclusion were (i) detection in a human stool/rectal swab specimen, (ii) sequence fully overlapping with the VP7 region sequenced for the Kilifi viruses, (iii) information on country and date of sampling available and (iv) sample collected in 2012–2018. G3 sequences collected previously from around Kenya including Kilifi were included in the analysis.

### 4.6. Statistical Analysis

Numerical data were analyzed in STATA v15.1. Continuous variables were summarized using various measures of dispersion. Differences between groups were assessed using a t-test or Wilcoxon rank-sum test. Binary data were summarized using proportions and comparison between groups made using either $\chi^2$ or Fisher's exact test (depending on group sample size). The 95% CI were presented for proportions and standard deviation for means. A $p$-value of <0.05 was considered significant.

### 4.7. Data Availability

Partial sequences for the VP7 and VP4 segments reported in this work have been deposited to GenBank database under the sequence accession numbers MN194408-MN194485 for VP7 and MN194325-MN194364 for VP4.

### 4.8. Ethical Statement

Before sample collection informed written consent was obtained from the child's parent or guardian. The Scientific Ethics Review Unit (SERU) board that sits at KEMRI, Nairobi, approved the study protocols (SERU#3049).

**Author Contributions:** Conceptualization, C.N.A., D.J.N., M.J.M. and R.F.B.; methodology, D.J.N., C.N.A. and M.J.M.; software, M.J.M. and C.N.A.; validation, C.N.A., E.G. and M.J.M.; formal analysis, C.N.A. and M.J.M.; investigation, C.N.A., M.J.M. and D.J.N. and E.G., resources, R.F.B., J.E.T., U.D.P. and D.J.N.; data curation, N.M., M.J.M. and C.N.A.; writing—original draft preparation, M.J.M. and C.N.A.; writing—review and editing, R.O., J.R.V., R.F.B., J.E.T., U.D.P. and D.J.N.; visualization, C.N.A. and M.J.M.; supervision, D.J.N. and C.N.A.; project administration, E.G., R.O., M.J.M., N.M. and D.J.N.; funding acquisition, D.J.N., R.O., J.R.V., J.E.T., U.D.P., R.F.B. All authors have read and agreed to the published version of the manuscript.

**Acknowledgments:** We thank the participants who provided samples for analysis, and the Clinical and Laboratory staff at Virus Epidemiology and Control group, KEMRI Wellcome Trust Research Programme for collection and processing the samples. This work is published with permission from Director KEMRI.

## References

1. Burnett, E.; Jonesteller, C.L.; Tate, J.E.; Yen, C.; Parashar, U.D. Global Impact of Rotavirus Vaccination on Childhood Hospitalizations and Mortality From Diarrhea. *J. Infect. Dis.* **2017**, *215*, 1666–1672. [CrossRef] [PubMed]
2. Steele, A.D.; Groome, M.J. Measuring Rotavirus Vaccine Impact in Sub-Saharan Africa. *Clin. Infect. Dis.* **2020**, *70*, 2314–2316. [CrossRef] [PubMed]
3. Operario, D.J.; Platts-Mills, J.A.; Nadan, S.; Page, N.; Seheri, M.; Mphahlele, J.; Praharaj, I.; Kang, G.; Araujo, I.T.; Leite, J.P.G.; et al. Etiology of Severe Acute Watery Diarrhea in Children in the Global Rotavirus Surveillance Network Using Quantitative Polymerase Chain Reaction. *J. Infect. Dis.* **2017**, *216*, 220–227. [CrossRef] [PubMed]
4. Iturriza-Gómara, M.; Jere, K.C.; Hungerford, D.; Bar-Zeev, N.; Shioda, K.; Kanjerwa, O.; Houpt, E.R.; Operario, D.J.; Wachepa, R.; Pollock, L.; et al. Etiology of Diarrhea Among Hospitalized Children in Blantyre, Malawi, Following Rotavirus Vaccine Introduction: A Case-Control Study. *J. Infect. Dis.* **2019**, *220*, 213–218. [CrossRef] [PubMed]
5. Troeger, C.; Khalil, I.A.; Rao, P.C.; Cao, S.; Blacker, B.F.; Ahmed, T.; Armah, G.; Bines, J.E.; Brewer, T.G.; Colombara, D.V.; et al. Rotavirus Vaccination and the Global Burden of Rotavirus Diarrhea Among Children Younger Than 5 Years. *JAMA Pediatr.* **2018**, *172*, 958–965. [CrossRef]
6. Steele, D.; Victor, J.; Carey, M.; Tate, J.; Atherly, D.; Pecenka, C.; Diaz, Z.; Parashar, U.; Kirkwood, C. Experiences with rotavirus vaccines: Can we improve rotavirus vaccine impact in developing countries? *Hum. Vaccines Immunother.* **2019**, *15*, 1215–1227. [CrossRef]
7. Willame, C.; Noordegraaf-Schouten, M.V.; Gvozdenović, E.; Kochems, K.; Oordt-Speets, A.; Praet, N.; Van Hoorn, R.; Rosillon, D. Effectiveness of the Oral Human Attenuated Rotavirus Vaccine: A Systematic Review and Meta-analysis—2006–2016. *Open Forum Infect. Dis.* **2018**, *5*, ofy292. [CrossRef]
8. Khagayi, S.; Omore, R.; Otieno, G.P.; Ogwel, B.; Ochieng, J.B.; Juma, J.; Apondi, E.; Bigogo, G.; Onyango, C.; Ngama, M.; et al. Effectiveness of Monovalent Rotavirus Vaccine Against Hospitalization With Acute Rotavirus Gastroenteritis in Kenyan Children. *Clin. Infect. Dis.* **2019**, *70*, 2298–2305. [CrossRef]
9. Walker, J.L.; Andrews, N.J.; Atchison, C.J.; Collins, S.; Allen, D.J.; Ramsay, M.E.; Ladhani, S.N.; Thomas, S.L. Effectiveness of oral rotavirus vaccination in England against rotavirus-confirmed and all-cause acute gastroenteritis. *Vaccine X* **2019**, *1*, 100005. [CrossRef]
10. Nair, N.; Feng, N.; Blum, L.K.; Sanyal, M.; Ding, S.; Jiang, B.; Sen, A.; Morton, J.M.; He, X.-S.; Robinson, W.H.; et al. VP4- and VP7-specific antibodies mediate heterotypic immunity to rotavirus in humans. *Sci. Transl. Med.* **2017**, *9*, eaam5434. [CrossRef]
11. RCWG. Rotavirus Classification Working Group: Newly Assigned Genotypes. Available online: https://rega.kuleuven.be/cev/viralmetagenomics/virus-classification/rcwg (accessed on 7 January 2020).
12. Sadiq, A.; Bostan, N.; Yinda, K.C.; Naseem, S.; Sattar, S. Rotavirus: Genetics, pathogenesis and vaccine advances. *Rev. Med. Virol.* **2018**, *28*, e2003. [CrossRef] [PubMed]
13. Leshem, E.; Lopman, B.; Glass, R.; Gentsch, J.; Bányai, K.; Parashar, U.; Patel, M. Distribution of rotavirus strains and strain-specific effectiveness of the rotavirus vaccine after its introduction: A systematic review and meta-analysis. *Lancet Infect. Dis.* **2014**, *14*, 847–856. [CrossRef]
14. Roczo-Farkas, S.; Kirkwood, C.D.; Cowley, D.; Barnes, G.L.; Bishop, R.F.; Bogdanovic-Sakran, N.; Boniface, K.; Donato, C.M.; Bines, J.E. The Impact of Rotavirus Vaccines on Genotype Diversity: A Comprehensive Analysis of 2 Decades of Australian Surveillance Data. *J. Infect. Dis.* **2018**, *218*, 546–554. [CrossRef] [PubMed]

15. Burke, R.M.; Tate, J.E.; Barin, N.; Bock, C.; Bowen, M.D.; Chang, D.; Gautam, R.; Han, G.; Holguin, J.; Huynh, T.; et al. Three Rotavirus Outbreaks in the Postvaccine Era—California, 2017. *MMWR Morb. Mortal. Wkly. Rep.* **2018**, *67*, 470–472. [CrossRef] [PubMed]
16. Pitzer, V.E.; Bilcke, J.; Heylen, E.; Crawford, F.W.; Callens, M.; De Smet, F.; Van Ranst, M.; Zeller, M.; Matthijnssens, J. Did Large-Scale Vaccination Drive Changes in the Circulating Rotavirus Population in Belgium? *Sci. Rep.* **2015**, *5*, 18585. [CrossRef] [PubMed]
17. Ianiro, G.; Micolano, R.; Di Bartolo, I.; Scavia, G.; Monini, M.; RotaNet-Italy Study Group. Group A rotavirus surveillance before vaccine introduction in Italy, September 2014 to August 2017. *Eurosurveillance* **2019**, *24*, 1800418. [CrossRef]
18. Ogden, K.M.; Tan, Y.; Akopov, A.; Stewart, L.S.; McHenry, R.; Fonnesbeck, C.J.; Piya, B.; Carter, M.H.; Fedorova, N.B.; Halpin, R.A.; et al. Multiple Introductions and Antigenic Mismatch with Vaccines May Contribute to Increased Predominance of G12P[8] Rotaviruses in the United States. *J. Virol.* **2018**, *93*, e01476-18. [CrossRef]
19. Santos, N.; Hoshino, Y. Global distribution of rotavirus serotypes/genotypes and its implication for the development and implementation of an effective rotavirus vaccine. *Rev. Med. Virol.* **2005**, *15*, 29–56. [CrossRef]
20. Arana, A.; Montes, M.; Jere, K.C.; Alkorta, M.; Iturriza-Gómara, M.; Cilla, G. Emergence and spread of G3P[8] rotaviruses possessing an equine-like VP7 and a DS-1-like genetic backbone in the Basque Country (North of Spain), 2015. *Infect. Genet. Evol.* **2016**, *44*, 137–144. [CrossRef]
21. Cowley, D.; Donato, C.M.; Roczo-Farkas, S.; Kirkwood, C.D. Emergence of a novel equine-like G3P[8] inter-genogroup reassortant rotavirus strain associated with gastroenteritis in Australian children. *J. Gen. Virol.* **2016**, *97*, 403–410. [CrossRef]
22. Dóró, R.; Marton, S.; Bartókné, A.H.; Lengyel, G.; Agócs, Z.; Jakab, F.; Bányai, K. Equine-like G3 rotavirus in Hungary, 2015—Is it a novel intergenogroup reassortant pandemic strain? *Acta Microbiol. Immunol. Hung.* **2016**, *63*, 243–255. [CrossRef] [PubMed]
23. Esposito, S.; Camilloni, B.; Bianchini, S.; Ianiro, G.; Polinori, I.; Farinelli, E.; Monini, M.; Principi, N. First detection of a reassortant G3P[8] rotavirus A strain in Italy: A case report in an 8-year-old child. *Virol. J.* **2019**, *16*, 64. [CrossRef] [PubMed]
24. João, E.D.; Munlela, B.; Chissaque, A.; Chilaúle, J.; Langa, J.; Augusto, O.; Boene, S.S.; Anapakala, E.; Sambo, J.; Guimarães, E.; et al. Molecular Epidemiology of Rotavirus A Strains Pre- and Post-Vaccine (Rotarix®) Introduction in Mozambique, 2012–2019: Emergence of Genotypes G3P[4] and G3P[8]. *Pathogens* **2020**, *9*, 671. [CrossRef] [PubMed]
25. Katz, E.M.; Esona, M.D.; Betrapally, N.; Leon, L.A.D.L.C.D.; Neira, Y.R.; Rey, G.J.; Bowen, M.D. Whole-gene analysis of inter-genogroup reassortant rotaviruses from the Dominican Republic: Emergence of equine-like G3 strains and evidence of their reassortment with locally-circulating strains. *Virology* **2019**, *534*, 114–131. [CrossRef]
26. Perkins, C.; Mijatovic-Rustempasic, S.; Ward, M.L.; Cortese, M.M.; Bowen, M.D. Genomic Characterization of the First Equine-Like G3P[8] Rotavirus Strain Detected in the United States. *Genome Announc.* **2017**, *5*, e01341-17. [CrossRef]
27. Pietsch, C.; Liebert, U. Molecular characterization of different equine-like G3 rotavirus strains from Germany. *Infect. Genet. Evol.* **2018**, *57*, 46–50. [CrossRef]
28. Tacharoenmuang, R.; Komoto, S.; Guntapong, R.; Upachai, S.; Singchai, P.; Ide, T.; Fukuda, S.; Ruchusatsawast, K.; Sriwantana, B.; Tatsumi, M.; et al. High prevalence of equine-like G3P[8] rotavirus in children and adults with acute gastroenteritis in Thailand. *J. Med. Virol.* **2020**, *92*, 174–186. [CrossRef]
29. Utsumi, T.; Wahyuni, R.M.; Doan, Y.H.; Dinana, Z.; Soegijanto, S.; Fujii, Y.; Juniastuti; Yamani, L.N.; Matsui, C.; Deng, L.; et al. Equine-like G3 rotavirus strains as predominant strains among children in Indonesia in 2015-2016. *Infect. Genet. Evol.* **2018**, *61*, 224–228. [CrossRef]
30. Mwanga, M.J.; Owor, B.E.; Ochieng, J.B.; Ngama, M.H.; Ogwel, B.; Onyango, C.; Juma, J.; Njeru, R.; Gicheru, E.; Otieno, G.P.; et al. Rotavirus group A genotype circulation patterns across Kenya before and after nationwide vaccine introduction, 2010–2018. *BMC Infect. Dis.* **2020**, *20*, 504. [CrossRef]
31. Owor, B.E.; Mwanga, M.J.; Njeru, R.; Mugo, R.; Ngama, M.; Otieno, G.P.; Nokes, D.J.; Agoti, C.N. Molecular

characterization of rotavirus group A strains circulating prior to vaccine introduction in rural coastal Kenya, 2002–2013. *Wellcome Open Res.* **2018**, *3*, 150. [CrossRef]

32. Thongprachum, A.; Chan-It, W.; Khamrin, P.; Okitsu, S.; Nishimura, S.; Kikuta, H.; Yamamoto, A.; Sugita, K.; Baba, T.; Mizuguchi, M.; et al. Reemergence of new variant G3 rotavirus in Japanese pediatric patients, 2009–2011. *Infect. Genet. Evol.* **2013**, *13*, 168–174. [CrossRef] [PubMed]

33. Umair, M.; Abbasi, B.H.; Sharif, S.; Alam, M.M.; Rana, M.S.; Mujtaba, G.; Arshad, Y.; Fatmi, M.Q.; Zaidi, S.Z. High prevalence of G3 rotavirus in hospitalized children in Rawalpindi, Pakistan during 2014. *PLoS ONE* **2018**, *13*, e0195947. [CrossRef] [PubMed]

34. Guerra, S.F.S.; Soares, L.S.; Lobo, P.S.; Júnior, E.T.P.; Júnior, E.C.S.; Bezerra, D.A.M.; Vaz, L.R.; Linhares, A.C.; Mascarenhas, J.D.P. Detection of a novel equine-like G3 rotavirus associated with acute gastroenteritis in Brazil. *J. Gen. Virol.* **2016**, *97*, 3131–3138. [CrossRef] [PubMed]

35. Mhango, C.; Mandolo, J.J.; Chinyama, E.; Wachepa, R.; Kanjerwa, O.; Malamba-Banda, C.; Matambo, P.B.; Barnes, K.G.; Chaguza, C.; Shawa, I.T.; et al. Rotavirus Genotypes in Hospitalized Children with Acute Gastroenteritis Before and After Rotavirus Vaccine Introduction in Blantyre, Malawi, 1997–2019. *J. Infect. Dis.* **2020**. [CrossRef]

36. Mokomane, M.; Esona, M.; Bowen, M.D.; Tate, J.; Steenhoff, A.; Lechiile, K.; Gaseitsiwe, S.; Seheri, L.; Magagula, N.; Weldegebriel, G.; et al. Diversity of Rotavirus Strains Circulating in Botswana before and after introduction of the Monovalent Rotavirus Vaccine. *Vaccine* **2019**, *37*, 6324–6328. [CrossRef]

37. Abebe, A.; Getahun, M.; Mapaseka, S.L.; Beyene, B.; Assefa, E.; Teshome, B.; Tefera, M.; Kebede, F.; Habtamu, A.; Haile-Mariam, T.; et al. Impact of rotavirus vaccine introduction and genotypic characteristics of rotavirus strains in children less than 5 years of age with gastroenteritis in Ethiopia: 2011–2016. *Vaccine* **2018**, *36*, 7043–7047. [CrossRef]

38. Wandera, E.A.; Komoto, S.; Mohammad, S.; Ide, T.; Bundi, M.; Nyangao, J.; Kathiiko, C.; Odoyo, E.; Galata, A.; Miring'U, G.; et al. Genomic characterization of uncommon human G3P[6] rotavirus strains that have emerged in Kenya after rotavirus vaccine introduction, and pre-vaccine human G8P[4] rotavirus strains. *Infect. Genet. Evol.* **2019**, *68*, 231–248. [CrossRef]

39. Gelaw, A.; Pietsch, C.; Liebert, U.G. Molecular epidemiology of rotaviruses in Northwest Ethiopia after national vaccine introduction. *Infect. Genet. Evol.* **2018**, *65*, 300–307. [CrossRef]

40. Bwogi, J.; Jere, K.C.; Karamagi, C.; Byarugaba, D.K.; Namuwulya, P.; Baliraine, F.N.; Desselberger, U.; Iturriza-Gomara, M. Whole genome analysis of selected human and animal rotaviruses identified in Uganda from 2012 to 2014 reveals complex genome reassortment events between human, bovine, caprine and porcine strains. *PLoS ONE* **2017**, *12*, e0178855. [CrossRef]

41. Jere, K.C.; Chaguza, C.; Bar-Zeev, N.; Lowe, J.; Peno, C.; Kumwenda, B.; Nakagomi, O.; Tate, J.E.; Parashar, U.D.; Heyderman, R.S.; et al. Emergence of Double- and Triple-Gene Reassortant G1P[8] Rotaviruses Possessing a DS-1-Like Backbone after Rotavirus Vaccine Introduction in Malawi. *J. Virol.* **2017**, *92*, 92. [CrossRef]

42. Scott, J.A.G.; Bauni, E.; Moisi, J.C.; Ojal, J.; Gatakaa, H.; Nyundo, C.; Molyneux, C.S.; Kombe, F.; Tsofa, B.; Marsh, K.; et al. Profile: The Kilifi Health and Demographic Surveillance System (KHDSS). *Int. J. Epidemiol.* **2012**, *41*, 650–657. [CrossRef] [PubMed]

43. Otieno, G.P.; Bottomley, C.; Khagayi, S.; Adetifa, I.; Ngama, M.; Omore, R.; Ogwel, B.; Owor, B.E.; Bigogo, C.; Ochieng, J.B.; et al. Impact of the Introduction of Rotavirus Vaccine on Hospital Admissions for Diarrhea Among Children in Kenya: A Controlled Interrupted Time-Series Analysis. *Clin. Infect. Dis.* **2019**, *70*, 2306–2313. [CrossRef] [PubMed]

44. Adetifa, I.M.; Bwanaali, T.; Wafula, J.; Mutuku, A.; Karia, B.; Makumi, A.; Mwatsuma, P.; Bauni, E.; Hammitt, L.L.; Nokes, D.J.; et al. Cohort Profile: The Kilifi Vaccine Monitoring Study. *Int. J. Epidemiol.* **2016**, *46*, 792–792h. [CrossRef]

45. Gómara, M.I.; Cubitt, D.; Desselberger, U.; Gray, J. Amino Acid Substitution within the VP7 Protein of G2 Rotavirus Strains Associated with Failure To Serotype. *J. Clin. Microbiol.* **2001**, *39*, 3796–3798. [CrossRef] [PubMed]

46. Simmonds, M.K.; Armah, G.; Asmah, R.; Banerjee, I.; Damanka, S.; Esona, M.; Gentsch, J.R.; Gray, J.J.; Kirkwood, C.; Page, N.; et al. New oligonucleotide primers for P-typing of rotavirus strains: Strategies for typing previously untypeable strains. *J. Clin. Virol.* **2008**, *42*, 368–373. [CrossRef]

47. Pickett, B.E.; Greer, D.; Zhang, Y.; Stewart, L.; Zhou, L.; Sun, G.; Gu, Z.; Kumar, S.; Zaremba, S.; Larsen, C.N.; et al. Virus Pathogen Database and Analysis Resource (ViPR): A Comprehensive Bioinformatics Database and Analysis Resource for the Coronavirus Research Community. *Viruses* **2012**, *4*, 3209–3226. [CrossRef] [PubMed]
48. Nguyen, L.-T.; Schmidt, H.A.; Von Haeseler, A.; Minh, B.Q. IQ-TREE: A Fast and Effective Stochastic Algorithm for Estimating Maximum-Likelihood Phylogenies. *Mol. Biol. Evol.* **2015**, *32*, 268–274. [CrossRef]
49. Stamatakis, A. Using RAxML to Infer Phylogenies. *Curr. Protoc. Bioinform.* **2015**, *51*, 6–14. [CrossRef]
50. Kumar, S.; Stecher, G.; Tamura, K. MEGA7: Molecular Evolutionary Genetics Analysis Version 7.0 for Bigger Datasets. *Mol. Biol. Evol.* **2016**, *33*, 1870–1874. [CrossRef]
51. Edgar, R.C. Search and clustering orders of magnitude faster than BLAST. *Bioinformatics* **2010**, *26*, 2460–2461. [CrossRef]
52. Taylor, N.E.; Greene, E.A. PARSESNP: A tool for the analysis of nucleotide polymorphisms. *Nucleic Acids Res.* **2003**, *31*, 3808–3811. [CrossRef] [PubMed]
53. Leigh, J.W.; Bryant, D. POPART: Full-feature software for haplotype network construction. *Methods Ecol. Evol.* **2015**, *6*, 1110–1116. [CrossRef]

# Permissions

All chapters in this book were first published by MDPI; hereby published with permission under the Creative Commons Attribution License or equivalent. Every chapter published in this book has been scrutinized by our experts. Their significance has been extensively debated. The topics covered herein carry significant findings which will fuel the growth of the discipline. They may even be implemented as practical applications or may be referred to as a beginning point for another development.

The contributors of this book come from diverse backgrounds, making this book a truly international effort. This book will bring forth new frontiers with its revolutionizing research information and detailed analysis of the nascent developments around the world.

We would like to thank all the contributing authors for lending their expertise to make the book truly unique. They have played a crucial role in the development of this book. Without their invaluable contributions this book wouldn't have been possible. They have made vital efforts to compile up to date information on the varied aspects of this subject to make this book a valuable addition to the collection of many professionals and students.

This book was conceptualized with the vision of imparting up-to-date information and advanced data in this field. To ensure the same, a matchless editorial board was set up. Every individual on the board went through rigorous rounds of assessment to prove their worth. After which they invested a large part of their time researching and compiling the most relevant data for our readers.

The editorial board has been involved in producing this book since its inception. They have spent rigorous hours researching and exploring the diverse topics which have resulted in the successful publishing of this book. They have passed on their knowledge of decades through this book. To expedite this challenging task, the publisher supported the team at every step. A small team of assistant editors was also appointed to further simplify the editing procedure and attain best results for the readers.

Apart from the editorial board, the designing team has also invested a significant amount of their time in understanding the subject and creating the most relevant covers. They scrutinized every image to scout for the most suitable representation of the subject and create an appropriate cover for the book.

The publishing team has been an ardent support to the editorial, designing and production team. Their endless efforts to recruit the best for this project, has resulted in the accomplishment of this book. They are a veteran in the field of academics and their pool of knowledge is as vast as their experience in printing. Their expertise and guidance has proved useful at every step. Their uncompromising quality standards have made this book an exceptional effort. Their encouragement from time to time has been an inspiration for everyone.

The publisher and the editorial board hope that this book will prove to be a valuable piece of knowledge for researchers, students, practitioners and scholars across the globe.

# List of Contributors

**Francesco Napolitano, Abdoulkader Ali Adou, Alessandra Vastola and Italo Francesco Angelillo**
Department of Experimental Medicine, University of Campania "Luigi Vanvitelli", Via L. Armanni, 5 80138 Naples, Italy

**Joshua Oluoch Amimo**
Department of Animal Production, Faculty of Veterinary Medicine, University of Nairobi, Nairobi 00625, Kenya
Biosciences of East and Central Africa-International Livestock Research Institute, (BecA-ILRI) Hub, Nairobi 00100, Kenya

**Eunice Magoma Machuka and Edward Okoth**
Biosciences of East and Central Africa-International Livestock Research Institute, (BecA-ILRI) Hub, Nairobi 00100, Kenya

**Ulrich Desselberger**
Department of Medicine, University of Cambridge, Addenbrooke's Hospital, Cambridge CB2 0QQ, UK

**Konstantin P. Alekseev, Anton G. Yuzhakov and Taras I. Aliper**
N. F. Gamaleya National Research Center for Epidemiology and Microbiology, Gamaleya Str. 18, Moscow 123098, Russia
Federal State Budget Scientific Institution "Federal Scientific Centre VIEV", Moscow 109428, Russia

**Aleksey A. Penin**
A. N. Belozersky Institute of Physico-Chemical Biology, Lomonosov Moscow State University, Moscow 119991, Russia
Institute for Information Transmission Problems of the Russian Academy of Sciences, Moscow 127051, Russia
Laboratory of Extreme Biology, Institute of Fundamental Biology and Medicine, Kazan Federal University, Kazan 420021, Russia
Department of Genetics, Faculty of Biology, Lomonosov Moscow State University, Moscow 119991, Russia

**Alexey N. Mukhin and Tatyana V. Grebennikova**
N. F. Gamaleya National Research Center for Epidemiology and Microbiology, Gamaleya Str. 18, Moscow 123098, Russia

**Kizkhalum M. Khametova, Anna S. Moskvina, Maria I. Musienko, Alexandr M. Mishin, Alexandr P. Kotelnikov and Oleg A. Verkhovsky**
Independent Non-Profit Organization "Diagnostic and Prevention Research Institute for Human and Animal Diseases", Moscow 123098, Russia

**Sergey A. Raev**
Federal State Budget Scientific Institution "Federal Scientific Centre VIEV", Moscow 109428, Russia
Independent Non-Profit Organization "Diagnostic and Prevention Research Institute for Human and Animal Diseases", Moscow 123098, Russia

**Eugeny A. Nepoklonov**
The Ministry of Agriculture of the Russian Federation, Orlikov Pereulok 1/11, Moscow 107139, Russia

**Diana M. Herrera-Ibata and Douglas G. Marthaler**
Veterinary Diagnostic Laboratory, College of Veterinary Medicine, Kansas State University, 1800 Denison Ave, Manhattan, KS 66502, USA

**Frances K. Shepherd**
Department of Veterinary and Biomedical Sciences, College of Veterinary Medicine, University of Minnesota, St. Paul, MN 55108, USA

**Joseph J. Malakalinga**
Food and Microbiology Laboratory, Tanzania Bureau of Standards, Ubungo Area, Morogoro Road/Sam Nujoma Road, Dar es Salaam, Tanzania
Southern African Centre for Infectious Disease Surveillance (SACIDS), Africa Centre of Excellence for Infectious Diseases of Humans and Animals in Eastern and Southern Africa (ACE), Sokoine University of Agriculture (SUA), Chuo Kikuu, SUA, Morogoro, Tanzania

**Gerald Misinzo**
Southern African Centre for Infectious Disease Surveillance (SACIDS), Africa Centre of Excellence for Infectious Diseases of Humans and Animals in Eastern and Southern Africa (ACE), Sokoine University of Agriculture (SUA), Chuo Kikuu, SUA, Morogoro, Tanzania

## List of Contributors

**George M. Msalya**
Department of Animal, Aquaculture and Range Sciences, College of Agriculture, Sokoine University of Agriculture, Morogoro, Tanzania

**Rudovick R. Kazwala**
Department of Veterinary Medicine and Public Health, College of Veterinary Medicine and Biomedical Sciences, Sokoine University of Agriculture, Morogoro, Tanzania

**Raúl Pérez-Ortín, Susana Vila-Vicent, Noelia Carmona-Vicente, Cristina Santiso-Bellón, Jesús Rodríguez-Díaz and Javier Buesa**
Department of Microbiology, School of Medicine, University of Valencia and Clinical Microbiology Service, Hospital Clínico Universitario de Valencia, Instituto de Investigación INCLIVA, 46010 Valencia, Spain

**Arnold W. Lambisia**
Kenya Medical Research Institute (KEMRI)-Wellcome Trust Research Programme, Centre for Geographic Medicine Research-Coast, Kilifi 230-80108, Kenya
Department of Biochemistry, Jomo Kenyatta University of Agriculture and Technology, Juja 62000-00200, Kenya

**Sylvia Onchaga and Clement S. Lewa**
Kenya Medical Research Institute (KEMRI)-Wellcome Trust Research Programme, Centre for Geographic Medicine Research-Coast, Kilifi 230-80108, Kenya

**Nickson Murunga**
Kenya Medical Research Institute (KEMRI)-Wellcome Trust Research Programme, Centre for Geographic Medicine Research-Coast, Kilifi 230-80108, Kenya

**Steven Ger Nyanjom**
Department of Biochemistry, Jomo Kenyatta University of Agriculture and Technology, Juja 62000-00200, Kenya

**Charles N. Agoti**
Kenya Medical Research Institute (KEMRI)-Wellcome Trust Research Programme, Centre for Geographic Medicine Research-Coast, Kilifi 230-80108, Kenya
School of Health and Human Sciences, Pwani University, Kilifi 195-80108, Kenya

**Matías Castells**
Laboratorio de Virología Molecular, CENUR Litoral Norte, Centro Universitario de Salto, Universidad de la República, Rivera 1350, Salto 50000, Uruguay
Instituto Nacional de Investigación Agropecuaria (INIA), Plataforma de Investigación en Salud Animal, Estación Experimental la Estanzuela, Ruta 50 km 11, Colonia 70000, Uruguay

**Rubén Darío Caffarena**
Instituto Nacional de Investigación Agropecuaria (INIA), Plataforma de Investigación en Salud Animal, Estación Experimental la Estanzuela, Ruta 50 km 11, Colonia 70000, Uruguay
Facultad de Veterinaria, Universidad de la República, Alberto Lasplaces 1620, Montevideo 11600, Uruguay

**María Laura Casaux, Carlos Schild, Franklin Riet-Correa and Federico Giannitti**
Instituto Nacional de Investigación Agropecuaria (INIA), Plataforma de Investigación en Salud Animal, Estación Experimental la Estanzuela, Ruta 50 km 11, Colonia 70000, Uruguay

**Samuel Miño and Viviana Parreño**
Sección de Virus Gastroentéricos, Instituto de Virología, CICVyA, INTA Castelar, Buenos Aires 1686, Argentina

**Felipe Castells**
Doctor en Veterinaria en Ejercicio Libre, Asociado al Laboratorio de Virología Molecular, CENUR Litoral Norte, Centro Universitario de Salto, Universidad de la República, Rivera 1350, Salto 50000, Uruguay

**Daniel Castells**
Centro de Investigación y Experimentación Dr. Alejandro Gallinal, Secretariado Uruguayo de la Lana, Ruta 7 km 140, Cerro Colorado, Florida 94000, Uruguay

**Matías Victoria and Rodney Colina**
Laboratorio de Virología Molecular, CENUR Litoral Norte, Centro Universitario de Salto, Universidad de la República, Rivera 1350, Salto 50000, Uruguay

**Júlia Sambo and Esperança Guimarães**
Instituto Nacional de Saúde (INS), Maputo 1008, Mozambique
Instituto de Higiene e Medicina Tropical, Universidade Nova de Lisboa, 1349-008 Lisbon, Portugal

**Simone S. Boene**
Instituto Nacional de Saúde (INS), Maputo 1008, Mozambique
Centro de Biotecnologia, Universidade Eduardo Mondlane, Maputo 3453, Mozambique

**Jorfélia Chilaúle, Elda Anapakala and Diocreciano Bero**
Instituto Nacional de Saúde (INS), Maputo 1008, Mozambique

**Orvalho Augusto**
Faculdade de Medicina, Universidade Eduardo Mondlane, Maputo, Mozambique
Harris Hydraulics Laboratory, Department of Global Health, University of Washington, Seattle, WA 98195-7965, USA

**Jason M. Mwenda**
African Rotavirus Surveillance Network, Immunization, Vaccines and Development Program, WHO Regional Office for Africa, Brazzaville, Congo
World Health Organization, Regional Office for Africa, Brazzaville, Congo

**Isabel Maurício**
Instituto de Higiene e Medicina Tropical, Universidade Nova de Lisboa, 1349-008 Lisbon, Portugal
Global Health and Tropical Medicine, Instituto de Higiene e Medicina Tropical, Universidade Nova de Lisboa, 1349-008 Lisbon, Portugal

**Hester G. O'Neill**
Department of Microbial, Biochemical and Food Biotechnology, University of the Free State, Bloemfontein 9301, South Africa

**Nilsa de Deus**
Instituto Nacional de Saúde (INS), Maputo 1008, Mozambique
Departamento de Ciências Biológicas, Universidade Eduardo Mondlane, Maputo 3453, Mozambique

**Meylin Bautista Gutierrez, Alexandre Madi Fialho, Adriana Gonçalves Maranhão, Fábio Correia Malta, Juliana da Silva Ribeiro de Andrade, Rosane Maria Santos de Assis, Sérgio da Silva e Mouta, Marize Pereira Miagostovich, José Paulo Gagliardi Leite and Tulio Machado Fumian**
Laboratory of Comparative and Environmental Virology, Oswaldo Cruz Institute, Oswaldo Cruz Foundation, Avenida Brasil 4365, Rio de Janeiro 21040-900, Brazil

**Peter N. Mwangi, Milton T. Mogotsi, Sebotsana P. Rasebotsa and Martin M. Nyaga**
Next Generation Sequencing Unit, Division of Virology, Faculty of Health Sciences, University of the Free State, Bloemfontein 9300, South Africa

**Mapaseka L. Seheri**
Diarrhoeal Pathogens Research Unit, Sefako Makgatho Health Sciences University, Medunsa 0204, Pretoria, South Africa

**Valantine N. Ndze**
Faculty of Health Sciences, University of Buea, Buea, Cameroon

**Francis E. Dennis**
Noguchi Memorial Institute for Medical Research, University of Ghana, LG581, Legon, Ghana

**Khuzwayo C. Jere**
Centre for Global Vaccine Research, Institute of Infection and Global Health, University of Liverpool, Ronald Ross Building, 8 West Derby Street, Liverpool L69 7BE, UK
Malawi-Liverpool-Wellcome Trust Clinical Research Programme, College of Medicine, University of Malawi, Blantyre 312225, Malawi

**Benilde Munlela**
Instituto Nacional de Saúde (INS), Distrito de Marracuene, Maputo 3943, Mozambique
Centro de Biotecnologia, Universidade Eduardo Mondlane, Maputo 3453, Mozambique

**Eva D. João, Assucênio Chissaque, Adilson F. L. Bauhofer and Marta Cassocera**
Instituto Nacional de Saúde (INS), Distrito de Marracuene, Maputo 3943, Mozambique
Instituto de Higiene e Medicina Tropical (IHMT), Universidade Nova de Lisboa, UNL, Rua da Junqueira 100, 1349-008 Lisbon, Portugal

**Celeste M. Donato**
Enteric Diseases Group, Murdoch Children's Research Institute, 50 Flemington Road, Parkville, Melbourne 3052, Australia
Department of Paediatrics, the University of Melbourne, Parkville 3010, Australia
Biomedicine Discovery Institute and Department of Microbiology, Monash University, Clayton 3800, Australia

**Amy Strydom**
Department of Microbial, Biochemical and Food Biotechnology, University of the Free State, 205 Nelson Mandela Avenue, Bloemfontein 9301, South Africa

**Jerónimo Langa and Jorfélia J. Chilaúle**
Instituto Nacional de Saúde (INS), Distrito de Marracuene, Maputo 3943, Mozambique

**Idalécia Cossa-Moiane**
Instituto Nacional de Saúde (INS), Distrito de Marracuene, Maputo 3943, Mozambique
Institute of Tropical Medicine (ITM), Kronenburgstraat 43, 2000 Antwerp, Belgium

**Bianca F. Middleton**
Global and Tropical Health, Menzies School of Health Research, Charles Darwin University, Darwin 0810, Australia
Division of Women, Children and Youth, Royal Darwin Hospital, Darwin 0810, Australia

# List of Contributors

**Margie Danchin**
Department of Paediatrics, University of Melbourne, Melbourne 3052, Australia
Murdoch Children's Research Institute, Melbourne 3052, Australia
Department of General Medicine, Royal Children's Hospital, Melbourne 3052, Australia

**Helen Quinn**
The National Centre for Immunisation Research and Surveillance (NCIRS), The Children's Hospital at Westmead, Sydney 2145, Australia
Faculty of Medicine and Health, Westmead Clinical School, The University of Sydney, Westmead 2145, Australia

**Anna P. Ralph**
Global and Tropical Health, Menzies School of Health Research, Charles Darwin University, Darwin 0810, Australia
Division of Medicine, Royal Darwin Hospital, Darwin 0810, Australia

**Nevada Pingault**
Department of Health Western Australia, Communicable Disease Control Directorate, Perth 6004, Australia

**Mark Jones and Marie Estcourt**
Health and Clinical Analytics, School of Public Health, The University of Sydney, Sydney 2006, Australia

**Tom Snelling**
Global and Tropical Health, Menzies School of Health Research, Charles Darwin University, Darwin 0810, Australia
Wesfarmers Centre for Vaccine and Infectious Diseases, Telethon Kids Institute, Perth 6009, Australia
School of Public Health, Curtin University, Perth 6102, Australia

**Zoe Yandle, Suzie Coughlan, Jonathan Dean, Gráinne Tuite, Anne Conroy and Cillian F. De Gascun**
UCD National Virus Reference Laboratory, University College Dublin, Dublin 4, Ireland

**Wairimu M. Maringa**
Next Generation Sequencing Unit, Division of Virology, Faculty of Health Sciences, University of the Free State, Bloemfontein 9300, South Africa

**Julia Simwaka**
Virology Laboratory, Department of Pathology & Microbiology, University Teaching Hospital, Adult and Emergency Hospital, Lusaka 10101, Zambia

**Evans M. Mpabalwani**
Department of Paediatrics & Child Health, School of Medicine, University of Zambia, Ridgeway, Lusaka RW50000, Zambia

**Ina Peenze and Mathew D. Esona**
Diarrhoeal Pathogens Research Unit, Faculty of Health Sciences, Sefako Makgatho Health Sciences University, Medunsa, Pretoria 0204, South Africa

**M. Jeffrey Mphahlele**
Diarrhoeal Pathogens Research Unit, Faculty of Health Sciences, Sefako Makgatho Health Sciences University, Medunsa, Pretoria 0204, South Africa
South African Medical Research Council, 1 Soutpansberg Road, Pretoria 0001, South Africa

**Mike J. Mwanga and Elijah Gicheru**
Kenya Medical Research Institute (KEMRI)-Wellcome Trust Research Programme, off Hospital Road, Kilifi 80108, Kenya

**Jennifer R. Verani**
Centers for Disease Control and Prevention (CDC), KEMRI Complex, off Mbagathi Way, Village Market, Nairobi 00621, Kenya
Centers for Disease Control and Prevention (CDC), Atlanta, GA 30333, USA

**Richard Omore**
KEMRI, Center for Global Health Research (KEMRI-CGHR), Kisumu 00202, Kenya

**Jacqueline E. Tate and Umesh D. Parashar**
Centers for Disease Control and Prevention (CDC), Atlanta, GA 30333, USA

**Robert F. Breiman**
Hubert Department of Global Health, Rollins School of Public Health, Emory University, Atlanta, GA 30322, USA

**D. James Nokes**
Kenya Medical Research Institute (KEMRI)-Wellcome Trust Research Programme, off Hospital Road, Kilifi 80108, Kenya
School of Life Sciences and Zeeman Institute (SBIDER), The University of Warwick, Coventry CV4 7AL, UK

# Index

## A
Acute Gastroenteritis, 9, 17, 28, 39, 56, 77, 95, 110-112, 115, 124-125, 127, 142, 155, 158, 171, 173, 179, 184, 186, 189, 221-223
Adenovirus, 15, 57, 66-76, 79, 122, 173, 175, 180-182
Agarose Gel Electrophoresis, 14, 107
Amino Acid, 30, 35-36, 42, 55, 123, 126, 129, 131-132, 134, 136-137, 139, 142, 145, 151-153, 156, 191, 195, 200-201, 203, 207, 223
Antigenic Drift, 42, 180
Astrovirus, 66-76, 79, 81, 94, 173, 175, 180-182, 187
Avitaminoses, 17, 20

## B
Bayesian Analysis, 143-144, 154
Binary Classification, 113, 127, 144, 189

## C
Capsid Protein, 31, 207-208
Concomitant Infections, 56, 62
Confidence Intervals, 3, 58, 92, 108, 168, 183

## D
Detection Rates, 31, 115-116, 120-121, 180
Diarrheal Disease, 12, 27, 122, 140, 144
Dna Sequencing, 114

## E
Enteric Disease, 30-31, 37
Enteric Nervous System, 19, 24
Enteric Pathogens, 12, 21, 27, 75, 93
Environmental Enteropathy, 20, 22-23, 25, 28, 169
Enzyme Immunoassay, 43, 47, 201, 219
Enzyme-linked Immunosorbent Assay, 57, 106
Evolutionary Analysis, 143, 147, 156, 158

## F
Fecal Samples, 12-14, 16, 31, 38, 43, 90, 116, 155

## G
Gastrointestinal Disease, 30, 56, 229
Gene Segments, 30-31, 37, 81, 90, 98, 127, 135, 141, 143-144, 189-193, 200-201, 207
General Practitioners, 1, 179, 183
Genetic Diversity, 13, 30, 37, 40-42, 47, 49-50, 52, 54, 80-81, 94, 96, 154, 200, 214, 218-219
Genome Constellation, 126, 128, 135, 144-145
Genome Copies, 80-82, 92, 114, 117
Genotype Diversity, 19, 51, 109, 111, 123, 172-174, 177, 179, 181, 184, 205-206, 221

Genotypes Circulation, 118, 121
Group C Rotavirus, 12, 15
Gut Microbiota, 21, 26-27

## H
Heterotypic Strains, 104, 162, 180, 210
Histo-blood Group Antigens, 22, 56-57, 59, 61, 63-64

## I
Illness Symptoms, 76, 210
Immune Responses, 19-22, 24, 26, 28
Immune System, 20-22, 25, 28
Interspecies Transmission, 42, 49, 54, 80-81, 89-90, 92-93, 98, 109, 123, 188-189, 200-201, 204-207

## L
Lactobacillus Rhamnosus, 21, 27
Lewis Antigens, 56-57, 61-62
Lewis B Positive, 56, 59-60, 62
Lewis Gene, 57

## M
Malnutrition, 17, 20-22, 25, 56, 219
Molecular Epidemiology, 19, 78, 94, 97, 110, 112-113, 125, 158, 173, 222-223
Monoclonal Antibodies, 24, 42, 57, 131, 134

## N
Neonatal Calf Diarrhea, 80-82
Next Generation Sequencing, 31, 126, 138, 155, 188, 190
Non-structural Proteins, 17, 41, 113, 127, 144
Norovirus, 64-79, 125, 173, 175-176, 180-183, 185, 187
Novel Genotypes, 50, 95, 110, 112, 180, 186
Nucleic Acid, 14, 37, 75, 111, 114, 159
Nucleotide Sequence, 42, 113, 135, 144, 146, 156, 207

## O
Odds Ratios, 3, 58, 92, 108
Open Reading Frames, 128, 145

## P
Pediatrician, 6-8
Phosphate-buffered Saline, 14, 57, 91, 137, 202
Phylogenetic Analysis, 15, 30, 39-40, 42, 54, 83, 89, 92, 95, 110, 114, 117-118, 121, 128, 131, 134, 136, 139-140, 143, 154, 156, 158, 160, 191, 195, 198-200, 203, 207-209, 220

Point Mutations, 42, 49, 51, 98
Polymerase Chain Reaction, 12, 47, 67, 91, 94, 111, 123-124, 159, 187, 221
Probe Binding Sites, 73, 75-76

## R
Reassortant Strains, 49-50, 118, 121, 136, 154, 198
Reoviridae, 31, 41, 81, 113, 127, 144, 189
Reverse Primer, 73, 91, 228
Rna Polymerase, 17, 127
Rotarix Vaccine, 41-43, 46-47, 49-50, 62, 64, 165, 170, 173, 180
Rotavirus Gastroenteritis, 1-3, 5-8, 23-25, 54, 56, 63, 78, 110, 123, 140, 168-171, 180, 184-186, 221
Rotavirus Infection, 1-9, 19, 24, 26-27, 29, 41, 43, 46-47, 49, 53-54, 56-57, 60-64, 78, 98, 105-106, 109-110, 124, 144, 155, 157, 161-164, 169-170, 173, 179-181, 183, 185, 200
Rotavirus Strain, 24, 42, 46-47, 49-52, 54, 56, 64, 93, 95, 98, 104, 109-111, 122-125, 140-142, 157, 168, 172, 187-188, 204-207, 222
Rotavirus Vaccine, 1-3, 5-6, 9-10, 17, 20, 23-29, 41-43, 50-54, 57, 63-64, 66-68, 70, 72, 75-78, 98, 104, 106, 108-111, 122-126, 140-141, 158-159, 161-162, 165-166, 168-172, 174, 179, 181, 184-186, 190, 200, 206, 209-210, 221-223

## S
Sapovirus, 66-76, 78-79, 173, 175, 180-182, 185, 187
Secretor Phenotype, 57, 61-62
Secretor Status, 29, 56, 58, 60-61, 63-65, 225-226, 228-233
Strain Diversity, 46-47, 49-51, 56, 97, 104-106, 109, 122, 140

## V
Vaccination Status, 8-9, 154-155, 170, 175, 210-213, 218
Vaccine Development, 41, 180
Vaccine Efficacy, 17, 20, 22, 25, 28, 42, 57, 162, 172, 181
Vaccine Strain, 41-42, 46, 49, 141, 146, 150-152, 156
Vetbiochim, 31, 38
Viral Load, 80-82, 88, 92, 112, 115-117, 120
Viral Proteins, 41, 98, 144, 189, 210
Vitamin A Supplementation, 20-21, 26

## W
Whole-genome Sequencing, 42, 50, 126, 138, 205

## Z
Zinc Deficiency, 17, 20, 25

Printed in the USA
CPSIA information can be obtained
at www.ICGtesting.com
LVHW050715061023
760082LV00014B/259